THE
BREASTFEEDING
ATLAS

Fifth Edition

Barbara Wilson-Clay, BSEd

Kay Hoover, M Ed, IBC

418 color photographs and explanatory text

The Breastfeeding Atlas
Fifth edition

Barbara Wilson-Clay, BSEd, IBCLC, FILCA
Kathleen L. Hoover, M Ed, IBCLC, FILCA

LactNews Press
12710 Burson Drive
Manchaca, Texas 78652, USA

Edited by Anna Swisher, MA, IBCLC
Cover design by Paulomi Shah
Back cover photo of Barbara Wilson-Clay by Christina Lord

www.BreastfeedingMaterials.com

Library of Congress Control Number: 2013915429

ISBN 0-9672758-7-3

Previous Editions copyrighted 1999, 2002, 2005, 2008

Printed in the United States of America

TABLE OF CONTENTS

We dedicate this edition to Chris Mulford, RN, BSN, IBCLC

Preface to the Fifth Edition

The Breastfeeding Atlas is meant to be a practical book, containing photos, observations, and case studies from our own experience, backed up by evidence from the research literature. For the Preface to this edition, we have invited colleagues from around the world to share a piece of advice or a clinical tip that they personally value. Below, we present their Pearls for Practice:

Avoid drawing any conclusions until you have seen the baby and done a full evaluation. It is so easy to tell the mother what you think is going on and then realize it is something completely different after you get more information. If the dad or partner is in the room, be sure to include them with eye contact during the consultation. Many want to be involved and sometimes feel left out.

> Judy Eastburn, BS, IBCLC, RLC
> USA

Mums often ask "One breast or two?" We need to learn more about the baby before immediately answering this question. What is the frequency of feeding? What are the lengths of feeds? How many wet and dirty diapers (nappies) is the baby producing? What about spitting up (possets)? This information will help us guide the mother. Some babies do better using one breast at a feed; others need both breasts, swapping frequently during feeds. It's all about looking at the baby and the mother in front of you and not relying on an automatic or scripted response.

> Sue Cox, AM, BM, FILCA
> Tasmania

We try to avoid using antibiotics as a first choice of treatment for cracked nipples because of rising antibiotic resistance in many common bacteria. I have had good experience using topical antisepetics on nipples that become cracked in the hospital. Antiseptics can prevent infection and help cure existing infections. In Poland, we use octenidine hydrochloride. Octenidine is a germicidal agent with wide antibacterial, antiviral, and anticandidal spectrum, and also prevents bacteria from producing biofilms. I advise the mother to use the antiseptic spray on her nipple 3 to 4 times a day after feeding. The taste is bitter, so the mother must rinse her nipple before the next feeding. I suggest using the antiseptic until the wound begins to heal. When the wound doesn't improve, I take a culture (smear) and at that point would precribe an antibiotic according to the results.

> Monika Zukowska-Rubik, Pediatrician, IBCLC
> Poland

Maximize the milk intake for the high-risk baby who stays on the mother/baby unit. If the baby is being monitored for blood sugar levels (late preterm, SGA, diabetic mom), keep the baby skin-to-skin as much as possible. Have mom hand express at least 4 times the first day. Jane Morton's research on the importance of hand expression in the first few days to increase maternal milk production verifies what I have long suspected: even the best breast pump can't entirely duplicate the effect of the mom's hands. I think with more proactive lactation support for at-risk dyads in the first 24 to 48 hours we could prevent some of the hypoglycemia, jaundice, and weight loss that so often occurs in these types of babies.

> Rebecca Mannel, BS, IBCLC, FILCA
> USA

When assessing a breastfeed, to avoid giving the mother the impression of judging her, ask her if the LC may observe how her BABY is breastfeeding (not how the MOTHER is breast-feeding). This tip is originally from UNICEF/WHO (2009) Baby-Friendly Hospital 20 hour course, and it's a great suggestion. Also, sometimes older babies unintentionally bite their mothers' nipple just before falling asleep. One La Leche League Leader suggests the following from her own experience. Before baby bites, carefully watch and listen to the baby's breathing in out. When the baby is breathing out, place a finger near the areola and quickly push the breast against the baby's mouth. The baby will release the breast without waking.

> Hiroko Hongo MSW, MHSc, IBCLC
> Japan

Many people don't know that exclusively breastfeeding mothers get more sleep and have more energy than moms who are mixed or formula feeding. If a mother is depressed, be sure to support her breastfeeding because research shows that breastfeeding protects maternal mood because it lowers stress. For survivors of abuse, let them know that breastfeeding can lessen the impact of previous sexual assault on mothers' mood and sleep.

> Kathleen Kendall-Tackett, PhD, IBCLC, FAPA
> USA

Begin the consultation with the baby and mother skin-to-skin. This will tell you a lot about the relationship. Ask the mother if she would like you to use her cellphone to take a picture of her breastfeeding.

> Nikki Lee, RN, BSN, MS, IBCLC, CCE, CIMI, ANLC, CKC
> USA

Almost all the mothers I consult with need "mothering" first. Many of them do not have a mother present in their lives. Their mother may be deceased or live in another state or country. The new mother needs to have her own emotional "tank" filled before she can truly mother her own baby. She may need help developing basic strategies for when to eat and sleep, and encouragement to follow her own instincts.

> Deborah Erhrhardt, BA, IBCLC
> USA

Thanks to all who submitted ideas to this section. We encourage everyone to document their cases, publish their observations, and share their tips so that others may benefit from their clinical experiences. As we hope The Breastfeeding Atlas proves, pictures amplify the learning process. We advise LCs everywhere to pick up a camera and expand the library of breastfeeding images.

Barbara Wilson-Clay
Kay Hoover
2013

Introduction

Breastfeeding is a robust, biologically stable activity so central to our evolutionary identity that it names the class of animals to which we belong. Healthy, term, human babies, placed on their mothers' abdomens after birth, share with other mammals the instinctive ability to crawl to the nipple and begin breastfeeding (Righard 1990, Colson 2008). The completion of this journey and a satisfactory first breastfeed might rightly be called the natural culmination of a normal birth. The very survival of our species attests to the fact that for millennia, under all sorts of conditions, many of us, gently assisted by our mothers, successfully made that journey.

Uncertainties and even dangers have always surrounded the birth process, and some mothers and babies are more vulnerable than others. Studies show that approximately one-third of women experience difficulties initiating breastfeeding, or have babies who exhibit "suboptimal" breastfeeding behaviors in the first week after birth (Dewey 2003). Feeding difficulties increase the risk of untimely weaning or early introduction of breast milk substitutes. Even if no clinical feeding problems exist, many infants and mothers experience disruptive hospital policies that interfere with normal establishment of breastfeeding (AAP 2012). The personal and societal costs of suboptimal breastfeeding are significant.

Common sense must prevail in breastfeeding assessment. The inability to feed is quickly recognized as a symptom of illness or dysfunction when it affects an older child, an elderly person, or even a household pet. However, the poorly breastfeeding infant frequently waits many days before being assisted. This contributes to increased family stress and risk of complications for the infant.

When women encounter breastfeeding difficulties, many state that they do not feel they received adequate support (McLeod 2002). Brenner (2011) reports that most mothers in the US want to breastfeed and are trying to do so, but they face multiple barriers to maintaining breastfeeding.

This phenomenon is not unique to the US. Despite intensive counseling at birth and during the immediate postpartum period in a baby-friendly hospital in Bangalore, India, complementary feeding was introduced as early as one month among 44 percent of infants, and only 14.2 percent were exclusively breastfeeding at 6 months (Samuel 2011). The reason for the introduction of early complementary feeding in this study was primarily a crying infant and the parent's perception that the infant was hungry. Home and community-oriented approaches to address barriers, provide information, and improve breastfeeding duration rates must augment improvements in hospital care and should be instituted in all countries.

In spite of health and economic advantages of breastfeeding, breastfeeding mothers report experiencing societal bias and receive many mixed messages about their feeding choice (Smith 2011). Lactation-related care is unavailable in many communities. Medical care providers in busy practices often lack the time to provide comprehensive lactation support, and may inadvertently send out signals to mothers that their questions and concerns are burdensome and time-consuming. And yet, research affirms that breastfeeding duration can best be increased through "specific advice" (Labarere 2005). Therefore, health workers must be trained both to respect normal breastfeeding and to recognize deviations from the norm in order to help mothers solve problems in a timely manner.

Breastfeeding support requires patience, empathy, and good counseling skills. Additionally, a greater emphasis on evidence-based care requires that health care providers understand that stressful pregnancies or complicated deliveries often negatively affect the course of early lactation (Chen 1998, Hall 2002). Care providers must develop the ability to distinguish between dyads with uncomplicated situations who primarily require encouragement, and those who need special assistance. For dyads with complications, the support they receive must be timely and their care must often be extended beyond the immediate hospital stay with provisions for continued follow-up in the community.

Early hospital discharge often results in the breastfeeding mother and baby being sent home before the onset of copious milk production and before feeding is well-established. Many infants are discharged with weight loss of 7 percent or greater; a factor that contributes to lethargic feeding (AAP 2012). While the first pediatric evaluation may occur in a timely manner, it may be several weeks before the baby is weighed again. During this time, well-meaning individuals may try to reassure the new mother, telling her to ignore her accurate perceptions of poor feeding (Ramsay 1996). At the next check-up, these mothers are often dismayed to discover that their infant has not gained weight adequately and that their milk supply has been affected.

While rare, some breastfeeding babies suffer harm during these intervals (Rand 2001). This has led to the reporting of sensational stories that have chosen to focus on the risks of breastfeeding (Helliker 1994) rather than on a failure of the health care system to provide adequate follow-up care (Davis 2013). The American Academy of Pediatrics (AAP) recommends that all breastfeeding infants be medically evaluated at 3 to 5 days (48 to 72 hours after discharge), so that mothers and babies who are at risk for feeding problems can be identified and helped. A visit at 2 to 3 weeks of age should be routinely scheduled to monitor weight gain and provide additional support and encouragement to the mother during this critical period (AAP 2012).

International Board Certified Lactation Consultants (IBCLCs) are increasingly involved on maternal child health care teams. They have special expertise in lactation management. IBCLCs are required to re-certify by examination at 10-year intervals in order to remain current with advances in lactation science. Lactation consultants (LCs) do not seek to replace medical advice or traditional sources of cultural support from family members and peers in the community. They seek to ensure that women have access to care designed to enable them to meet their breastfeeding goals. Women with complicated problems may need frequent follow-up until their situations stabilize, and they often form strong and sustaining relationships with their LCs.

A Cochrane Review reports that breastfeeding education has a significant positive effect on increasing initiation rates compared to routine care (Dyson 2005). Giving birth at a hospital that employs an IBCLC is associated with increased likelihood of breastfeeding at discharge for full term and for preterm babies (Castrucci 2006, 2007). Witt, et al. (2012) validate the importance of an early postpartum visit with an IBCLC, and documented significantly increased breastfeeding initiation and short- and long-term breastfeeding duration rates when routine lactation consultation was provided in a pediatric practice setting.

Because following the 10 Steps of the Baby-Friendly Hospital Initiative (BFHI) positively impacts breastfeeding rates, many countries have made support of the BFHI a priority (WHO 2012).

The Health and Economic Implications of Breastfeeding

Research documents that formula-fed infants in developed as well as developing countries have higher rates of morbidity and mortality from infectious diseases (Duijits 2010). Benefits of breastfeeding are not only observed for common illnesses of infancy, but for more serious illnesses such as pneumonia, severe lower respiratory tract infection, leukemia, and sudden infant death syndrome (SIDS). The benefits of breast milk feeding extend into childhood and even adulthood, impacting cardiovascular fitness and risk of obesity (Labayen 2012).

The positive impact of breastfeeding is increased with exclusivity. Six months of exclusive breastfeeding confers the most protection, with partial or mixed breastfeeding producing better health outcomes than formula feeding (Meyers 2009).

In stressed economies, breastfeeding offers substantial savings both to families and nations. Bartick (2010) analyzed current costs and compared them to projected costs if 80 and 90 percent of US families complied with current recommendations to exclusively breastfeed their babies for 6 months. With 90 percent compliance, the US would save $13 billion per year and prevent an estimated 911 infant deaths.

In spite of this information, many hospital practices remain stubbornly entrenched even though they have been demonstrated to undermine exclusive breastfeeding. For example, a survey of 3,209 US maternity sites conducted from 2006 to 2007 found that 91 percent of hospitals distributed formula sample packs in violation of the WHO Code and despite the recommendations of the 10 Steps of the BHFI and numerous governmental and health promotion organizations (Merewood 2010). Citing cost contraints, many hospitals have delayed changing maternity practices. However, DelliFraine (2011) provided an economic assessment of the costs of becoming a baby-friendly site and found that it is a relatively cost-neutral process for a typical acute care hospital. Changes in hospital accreditation requirements and pressure from consumer groups will hopefully spur improvements and increase the trend toward more compliance with currently accepted standards of care (Joint Commission 2010).

In 2011, the US Surgeon General issued a *Call to Action to Support Breastfeeding* (US Department of Health and Human Services 2011). Actions to improve breastfeeding and to eliminate barriers will be part of a national campaign in the United States to promote and monitor breastfeeding in a more consistent manner.

Globally, the cost of not breastfeeding includes more than the economic implications of increased morbidity and mortality. There are hidden economic realities that affect everyone, including the cost of purchasing formula and bottles, fuel costs to heat and clean bottles, and the environmental costs related to formula production, distribution, and container waste processing (International Women Count Network 2000). Lactation activists have found cost analysis data useful in legislative efforts being undertaken in various locales to argue for policy changes to remove breastfeeding barriers (Kramer 2001, Wilson-Clay 2005).

In 2001, the US Centers for Disease Control (CDC) began including breastfeeding-related questions in the National Immunization Survey (NIS). NIS breastfeeding information is now available in the form of a Breastfeeding Report Card for geographic areas within the US. The information in this report includes socio-demographic data useful to policy-makers seeking to identify areas where new programs might improve breastfeeding rates (CDC 2011).

Improvements in data collection have helped identify both the progress that has been made and the work that remains to be done. The incidence of any breastfeeding increased in the US from 68.3 percent in 1999 to 76.5 percent in 2013. However, US rates of exclusive breast-feeding at 3 months and 6 months have consistently failed to reach target goals, especially in certain geographical regions and among black and unmarried mothers. 2013 data report that only 37.7 percent of US infants were exclusively breastfed at 3 months, and only 16.4 percent at 6 months (CDC 2012). US Healthy People 2020 goals call for increasing breastfeeding initiation rates to 81.9 percent, with 60.6 percent continuation at 6 months, and 34.1 percent breastfeeding at one year. The 2020 target goals for exclusivity at 3 months call for 42.6 percent and 25.5 percent at 6 months (US DHHS 2010).

To address stalled progress in duration of exclusive breast-feeding, new goal areas have been added to the Healthy People 2020 objectives. These include increasing work-place support for lactating women, reducing the proportion of newborns who receive formula supplementation in the first 2 days from 24.2 percent to 14.2 percent, and increasing the proportion of births that occur in facilities that provide recommended care for lactating mothers from 2.9 percent to 8.1 percent. While this last goal seems quite modest, there is a hopeful trend in the US toward broader acceptance of the policies expressed in the WHO 10 Steps to promote baby-friendly hospitals.

What changes are needed? The US Preventative Services Task Force (2003) analyzed available data to evaluate interventions demonstrated to be effective in preventing early introduction of complementary feeds or weaning. The task force affirmed the importance of early maternal contact with newborns (skin-to-skin care), rooming-in, and the avoidance of formula supplementation without medical necessity.

It is important to note that low rates of duration for exclusive breastfeeding are not unique to the US. A Cochrane Review described breastfeeding rates in many countries as "resistant to change" (Britton 2007). Both social and physiological factors appear to influence breastfeeding outcomes. Early use of

formula and premature weaning continue to undermine duration goals worldwide.

Cultural issues strongly influence infant feeding decisions. An Australian study found that 5 percent of women discontinue breastfeeding prior to hospital discharge because of pre-pregnancy feeding decisions, based on whether their own mother breastfed and on the perception that the baby's father prefers formula feeding (Scott 2001). North American and Australian studies identify embarrassment and concerns about breastfeeding in public as major barriers (Sheeshka 2001).

Moral norms were identified as the most predictive variable influencing the intention to breastfeed in socioeconomically deprived pregnant teenagers in the UK (Dyson 2010). In this population, breastfeeding was viewed as a morally inappropriate behavior, and associated with "sexuality of the breast" and embarrassment. The authors conclude that "Existing breastfeeding promotion activities are likely to continue to fail...in the absence of effective strategies to change the underlying negative moral norms toward breast-feeding." Such studies are important because breastfeeding advocates are typically so passionate in support of the activity that it can be difficult to perceive that others may view breastfeeding through an entirely different framework.

Qualitative studies report that many mothers continue to report dissatisfaction with their experiences of breastfeeding. Women in these studies tend to rate social support as being more important than health service support, but this may result from their impression of health service support as being unavailable, too time consuming, or as providing unhelpful and conflicting advice (McInnes 2008). Additionally, infant feeding disorders appear to be less well tolerated by emotionally fragile mothers and those who lack social support (Abadie 2001). These mothers are at increased risk for early weaning.

The opinions and practices of health care providers also influence women's breastfeeding decisions (Lu 2001, Taveras 2004). Studies indicate that families face frustration caused by inconsistent or non-supportive information from caregivers (Freed 1993, Taveras 2004). However, clinicians complain of limited time to provide this care for breastfeeding problems. The need for preventative care suggests that additional resources and assistance should be added to traditional sources of support, at least until the culture of breastfeeding revives.

Without this support, many new mothers wean in the first week postpartum (Hall 2002). Many others wean between 1 and 4 weeks (Lewallen 2006). They quit because of difficulties in getting the baby to latch, sore nipples, and concerns about low milk production. They wean because they are returning to school or work and have not received information or the institutional support that enables them to continue breastfeeding. Lack of familial and cultural support are critical factors in the weaning decision.

The Breastfeeding Atlas

Many books describe normal breastfeeding. The goal of this book is to use photos, case studies and evidence-based management strategies to improve the assessment skills of those charged with supporting mothers and babies. Breastfeeding is an activity with various phases. A hospital-based LC may only see mothers in the earliest stages of lactation. The LC working in a human donor milk bank may never be called upon to help a mother latch her baby to the breast. And yet it is critical for all LCs in any practice setting to acquire the skills to assist a mother who develops a problem during any stage of lactation.

In addition to assisting in the development of professional assessment skills, many users of *The Breastfeeding Atlas* have discovered that sharing a photo with a breastfeeding mother enhances the counseling experience. Mothers often describe feeling reassured to discover their problem is not unique. In this way, photos provide an opportunity to establish rapport, educate, and empower mothers.

A Note from the Authors About Clinical Photography

How do clinicians approach a woman about taking photographs or videos? Sometimes a woman's situation is so distressing that it is best to forego a request to take a picture. In some cases, the woman's cultural background and issues related to modesty preclude such a request. However, many women are extremely generous when informed that a photo of their problem might be useful in helping other women in the future, and in educating HCPs who assist with breastfeeding. Both authors are sensitive to privacy issues and aware of concerns about the exploitation of clients. In some cases, if a photo or video was taken during a consultation, we waived or reduced the consultation fee. Some mothers received a model fee. All individuals whose photos are included in *The Breastfeeding Atlas* signed a consent form.

Clinical photographers must have a Consent To Photograph form that clarifies issues of use. In most cases, close-up views are selected to eliminate identifying features. In accordance with the ethical requirement to protect the confidentiality and privacy of the client, names are not used. Consent forms make clear that the photos and videos will be used only for educational purposes and to promote breastfeeding. A sample photo consent form developed by Kay

Hoover can be viewed at www.BreastfeedingMaterials.com. ILCA has a standard consent to photograph release form that is available on the ILCA website: www.ILCA.org.

Photographs, Intellectual Property, and Copyright Law

The IBLCE Code of Professional Conduct for IBCLCs requires that they "Respect intellectual property rights" (IBLCE 2011). Photographs, like written work, belong to their creators. Clinical photographs are challenging to acquire, in part because the opportunity to obtain a specific image depends upon chance. Copying, reproducing, and distributing photos or videos without permission violates copyright law and the IBLCE Code of Conduct. Please obtain prior written permission from the authors about the use of any of the photos from *The Breastfeeding Atlas*.

Abadie V, Andre A, Zaouche A, et al. Early feeding resistance: a possible consequence of neonatal oro-oesophageal dyskinesia. *Acta Paediatrica* 2001; 90(7):738-45.

American Academy of Pediatrics (AAP) Section on Breastfeeding. Breastfeeding and the use of human milk. *Pediatrics* 2012; 129(3):e827-841.

Bartick M, Reinhold A. The burden of suboptimal breastfeeding in the United States: a pediatric cost analysis. *Pediatrics* 2010; 125(5):e1048-e1056.

Brenner MG, Buescher ES. Breastfeeding: a clinical imperative. *J Womens Health* 2011; 20(12):1767-1763.

Britton C, McCormick FM, Renfrew MJ, et al. Support for breastfeeding mothers. *Cochrane Database of Systematic Reviews* 2007; Issue 1.

Castrucci BC, Hoover KL, Lim S, et al. A comparison of breatfeeding rates in an urban birth cohort among women delivering infants at hospitals that employ and do not employ lactation consultants. *Journal of Public Health Management Practice* 2006; 12(6):578-585.

Castrucci BC, Hoover KL, Lim S, et al. Availability of lactation counseling services influences breastfeeding among infants admitted to neonatal intensive care units. *American Journal of Health Promotion* 2007; 21(5):410-415.

Centers for Disease Control (CDC). Breastfeeding Report Card-United States, 2012. Division of Nutrition, Physical Activity, and Obesity, National Center for Chronic Disease Prevention and Health Promotion, Centers for Disease Control and Prevention, Atlanta, GA, US. Accessed July 2013.

Chen D, Nommsen-Rivers L, Dewey K, et al. Stress during labor and delivery and early lactation performance. *American Journal of Clinical Nutrition* 1998; 68(2):335-344.

Colson SD, Meek JH, Hawdon JM. Optimal positions for the release of primitive neonatal reflexes stimulating breastfeeding. *Early Human Development* 2008; 84(7):441-449.

Davis LS, Is the medical community failing breastfeeding moms? *Time*, Jan 2, 2012.

DelliFraine J, Langabeer J 2nd, Williams JF, et al. A cost analysis of Baby-Friendly Hospitals. *Pediatrics* 2011; 127(4):e989-e994.

Dewey K, Nommsen-Rivers L, Heinig M, et al. Risk factors for suboptimal infant breastfeeding behavior, delayed onset of lactation, and excess neonatal weight loss. *Pediatrics* 2003; 112(3):607-619.

Duijts L, Jaddoe VW, Hofman A, et al. Prolonged and exclusive breastfeeding reduces the risk of infectious diseases in infancy. *Pediatrics* 2010; 126(1):e19-e25.

Dyson L, Green JM, Rendfrew MJ, et al. Factors influencing the infant feeding decision for socioeconomically deprived pregnant teenagers: the moral dimension. *Birth* 2010; 37(2):141-149.

Dyson L, McCormick F, Renfrew MJ. Interventions for promoting the initiation of breastfeeding. *The Cochrane Database of Systematic Reviews* 2005; Issue 3.

Freed G. Breast-feeding: time to teach what we preach. *Journal of the American Medical Association* 1993; 269(2):243-44.

Hall R, Mercer A, Teasley S, et al. A breast-feeding assessment score to evaluate the risk for cessation of breast-feeding by 7 to 10 days of age. *Journal of Pediatrics* 2002; 141(5):659-64.

Helliker K. Dying for milk. *Wall Street Journal* (1994, July 22), A1, A4.

International Board of Lactation Consultant Examiners (IBLCE). The Code of Professional Conduct for International Board Certified Lactation Consultants. Falls Church, VA: IBLCE, 2011. www.iblce.org. Accessed March, 2012.

International Women Count Network and World Alliance for Breastfeeding Action, Women & Work Task Force. *The Milk of Human Kindness.* London and Philadelphia: Crossroads Books, 2000.

Kramer M, Chalmers B, Hodneff E, et al. Promotion of breastfeeding intervention trial (PROBIT): a randomized trial in the Republic of Belarus. *Journal of the American Medical Association* 2001; 285(4):413-420.

Labarere J, Gelbert-Baudino N, Ayral A-S, et al. Efficacy of breastfeeding support provided by trained clinicians during an early, routine, preventive visit: a prospective, randomized, open trial of 226 mother-infant pairs. *Pediatrics* 2005; 115(2):139-146.

Labayen I, Ruiz JR, Ortega FB, et al. Exclusive breastfeeding duration and cardiorespiratory fitness in children and adolescents. *American Journal of Clinical Nutrition* 2012; 95(2):498-505.

Lewallen L. A review of instruments used to predict early breastfeeding attrition. *Journal of Perinatal Education* 2006; 15(1):26-41.

Lu M, Lange L, Flusser W, et al. Provider encouragement of breastfeeding: evidence from a national survey. *Obstetrics and Gynecology* 2001; 79(2):290-295.

McInnes RJ, Chambers JA. Supporting breastfeeding mothers: qualitative synthesis. *Journal of Advanced Nursing* 2008; 62(4):407-427.

McLeod D, Pullon S, Cookson T. Factors influencing continuation of breastfeeding in a cohort of women. *Journal of Human Lactation* 2002; 18(4):335-343.

Merewood A, Grossman X, Cook J, et al. US hospitals violate WHO policy on the distribution of formula sample packs: results of a national survey. *Journal of Human Lactation* 2010; 26(4):363-367.

Meyers D. Breastfeeding and health outcomes. *Breastfeeding Medicine* 2009; 4(S1):S-13-S-15.

Ramsey M, Gisel E. Neonatal sucking and maternal feeding practices. *Developmental Medicine and Child Neurology* 1996; 38(1):34-47.

Rand S, Kolberg A. Neonatal hypernatremic dehydration secondary to lactation failure. *Journal of the American Board of Family Practice* 2001; 14(2):155-158.

Righard L, Alade M. Effect of delivery room routines on success of first breast-feed. *Lancet* 1990; 336(8723):1105-1107.

Samuel TM, Thomas T, Bhat S, et al. Are infants born in baby-friendly hospitals being exclusively breastfed until 6 months of age? *European Journal of Clinical Nutrition* 2012; 66:459-465.

Scott J, Landers M, Hughes R, Binns C. Psychosocial factors associated with abandonment of breastfeeding prior to hospital discharge. *Journal of Human Lactation* 2001; 17(1):24-30.

Sheeshka J, Potter B, Valaitis R, et al. Women's experiences breastfeeding in public places. *Journal of Human Lactation* 2001; 17(1):31-38.

Smith JL, Hawkinson K, Paull K. Spoiled milk: an experimental examination of bias against mothers who breastfeed. *Personality & Social Psychology Bulletin* 2011; 37(7):867-878.

Taveras E, Ruovei L, Grummer-Strawn L, et al. Opinions and practices of clinicians associated with continuation of exclusive breastfeeding. *Pediatrics* 2004; 113(4):e283-290.

The Joint Commission 2010. www.jointcommission.org. Accessed March 2012.

US Department of Health and Human Services, Healthy People 2020.

US Department of Health and Human Services, *The Surgeon Generals's Call to Action to Support Breastfeeding*, Washington, DC. Office of the Surgeon General; 2011.

US Preventative Services Task Force. Behavioral interventions to promote breastfeeding: recommendations and rationale. *Annals of Family Medicine* 2003; 1(2):79-80.

Wilson-Clay B, Rourke J, Bolduc M, et al. Learning to lobby for pro-breastfeeding legislation. *Journal of Human Lactation* 2005; 2(2):191-200.

Witt AM, Smith S, Mason MJ, et al. Integrating routine lactation consultant support into a pediatric practice. Breastfeeding Medicine 2012; 7(1):38-42.

World Health Organization (WHO) *Percentage of BFHI Services in 28 Countries.* Compiled from Country Reports for the 2012 WHO Meeting for Country BFHI Coordinators.

Infant State and Infant Assessment

Learning to "read" the baby is one of the great challenges each new parent faces. It is a skill feeding specialists also require. This chapter reviews issues related to infant assessment, including the concept of infant state, which provides a useful system to help classify infant behavior and interpret infant body language. Also reviewed are infant tone, movement, color, unusual body posture, and physical anomalies that may affect breastfeeding.

Careful assessment helps explain why a baby has difficulty breastfeeding. The explanation may not matter to the health care provider, but it matters to the mother, who may otherwise blame herself for failing one of the earliest tasks of motherhood (Redshaw 2012).

It is critical to educate parents about any underlying medical conditions that interfere with breastfeeding. Information empowers parents and enhances their willingness and ability to follow care plans. Explain that breastfeeding may not improve until the infant is treated, recovers, or matures. If the milk supply is protected, breastfeeding can usually, at some point, be safely and successfully initiated. Families in such situations need information about the value of receiving human milk feedings, even if the child cannot directly breastfeed.

Lactation Acuity

The concept of *patient acuity* refers to matching the severity of an illness to the intensity of the care required to treat it. In health care, acuity is an important determinant of patient safety and outcomes. It also assists in determining staffing needs so that optimal care can be provided. Mannel (2011) developed an evidence-based definition of *lactation acuity* to help identify mother-baby couplets at risk for premature weaning. Higher acuity breastfeeding patients require higher skill and knowledge levels from the people providing their care.

Developed at Oklahoma University Medical Center and implemented in several US hospitals in 2010, 3 levels of lactation acuity were described. Acuity level 1 patients require basic education and routine management. They can be cared for by nursing staff who have basic breastfeeding knowledge and competency.

Acuity level 2 patients have more complicated maternal and infant characteristics. These may include cesarean section delivery, delayed initiation of breastfeeding, newborn birth trauma, or suboptimal milk transfer leading to the medical decision to supplement. These hospital patients should be cared for by an IBCLC, sometimes referred to in the US as a Registered Lactation Consultant (RLC). Patients should be referred to an IBCLC in the community for early follow-up after discharge.

Acuity level 3 patients require in-depth care by an IBCLC and will require ongoing care. Their characteristics may include pathological engorgement, maternal mastitis, breast abscess, induced lactation, maternal breast complications (including breast surgeries and anomalies), and maternal illness or other surgery. Infant characteristics include NICU admission, late preterm birth, small for gestational age, multiple births, hyperbilirubinemia, hypoglycemia, congenital defects, oral/motor dysfunction (tight frenulum, hyper or hypotonia), and excess infant weight loss (>7 percent before discharge.)

It should be noted that some instances of early excessive infant weight loss may be associated with the administration of intravenous fluids (IV fluids) to women during labor. *Diuresis* (increased urination) of extra fluids by the infant appears to occur only during the first 24 hours (Noel-Weiss 2011). This phenomenon has prompted some people to recommend delaying the first weight until Day 2. If an infant is still losing on Day 2, diuresis-related weight loss should no longer be suspected, and feeding should be evaluated carefully. Supplementation decisions should always be made on a case-by-case basis. Excess weight loss in the first 24 hours might require only watchful waiting if the baby is of normal weight and the mother had a large volume of IV fluids during labor. Excess weight loss in a low birth weight baby might prompt a decision to immediately supplement with hand expressed colostrum.

When high acuity problems occur, lactation management typically consists of 3 key actions summarized as follows: Feed the baby. Protect the milk supply. Preserve breast focus. The infant's caloric intake must be protected with appropriate supplementation, ideally with mother's own milk. Simultaneously, the milk supply must be protected to prevent involution and down-regulation. Accurate information about breast milk expression (pumping and hand expression) must be provided. The goal is to enable successful breastfeeding once problems resolve. Transitioning the mother and baby away from dependence on the first 2 interventions will be easier if "breast focus" has been preserved. Practices such as skin-to-skin holding help both mother and baby remain oriented to breastfeeding. Nipple shields and supplemental feeding devices can also assist in protecting breast focus.

Lactation interventions are time-consuming and occur when women are recovering from childbirth and engaged in the adjustment to motherhood. A woman's ability to follow a lactation care plan may be subverted unless she is also provided with counseling support and receives help from her family.

The Stable Baby

Identifying the level of lactation acuity begins with accurrate assessment of the infant. Als (1986) describes *state stability* as the manifestation of appropriate sleep patterns, rhythmical, robust crying, and the ability to self-quiet. Color, tone, and respiration appear normal and behavioral cues do not reveal stress or pain (Herr 2006). Stable babies are consolable and responsive. These infants can latch onto the breast with minimal assistance.

The Stressed Baby

Infants who are stressed also behave in characteristic ways. Their behaviors include: whimpering, strained fussing, gaze aversion, or staring. Parents describe irritability, crying, inconsolability, worried alertness, and restlessness. Motor activity (the way the baby moves) can reveal stress (Als 1982). Stress cues may manifest as *hypotonia* (the baby appears flaccid or limp) or *hypertonia* (the baby appears rigid or stiff). Stressed babies flail their arms and legs. They stiffen, splay their fingers, startle frequently, arch, grimace, and twitch. The mildly stressed infant may begin to yawn, sneeze, or hiccup. The severely stressed baby may vomit, gasp, cry, gag, show skin color changes, and, in extreme cases, experience seizures. Because it can be difficult to differentiate stress-related cues from certain neurological disorders, the persistence of significant stress cues should be reported to the baby's medical care providers.

Alertness as an Indicator of Infant State

Brazelton (1984) described state from the point of view of variations in levels of infant alertness. Feeding typically can take place in 4 of these states, but babies are difficult to breastfeed while in a deep sleep state or during intense crying. Rousing or calming must usually occur to help move the baby into a state more conducive to effective feeding. Individual babies may feed better in one state than another.

Infant States:

- deep sleep
- light sleep
- drowsy
- quiet alert
- active alert
- crying

Gestational age, maturity, neurological status, and health affect state stability and influence which level of alertness predominates in an individual infant. Preterm babies spend a great deal of time asleep. Conditions such as jaundice may make babies lethargic or irritable, affecting their availability to feed. Babies who are injured or ill may experience such discomfort that they become too distracted to feed effectively.

Whenever a baby is breastfeeding poorly, it is important to observe an entire feeding. The point at which a baby begins to act stressed during a feeding can provide clues that may indicate the cause of the stress. For example, a baby exiencing respiratory distress may stuggle with fatigue-related aspiration. To protect themselves from choking, they may discontinue feeding after only a few minutes of sucking and fail to consume sufficient milk.

The Sleepy Baby

Excessive infant sleepiness has various causes. Sleepiness may be associated with neuromaturation or growth restriction. Preterm and small-for-gestational-age (SGA) infants show less organized state behavior, act sleepy, and often give indistinct feeding cues (Buckley 2006, Lawrence 2011). Sometimes medications may cause sleepiness. For example, hydrocodone is a narcotic commonly used to manage postpartum pain. While moderate dosages appear acceptable during breastfeeding, several case reports describe excessive sedation of newborns exposed to this medication. Infants who display excessive lethergy should be referred for medical examination (Anderson 2007).

The baby who is sleepy at the beginning of a feed may simply need assistance moving into a more alert state. Some babies breastfeed better if blankets are unwrapped, since small reductions in ambient temperature can improve alertness (Elder 1970). However, parents should be taught to identify signs of thermal stress such as shivering and skin mottling. Preterm and SGA infants are at increased risk for cold stress and need to be kept warm (Narchi 2010, Raju 2006).

Some sleepy babies rouse when undressed and placed in a more upright position. Sometimes it helps to put them on a flat surface and gently roll them from side to side. Some parents rouse sleepy babies by speaking in animated tones or playing lively music. A lit room is more stimulating than a dark one; however harsh lighting may be stressful for some infants. Light stroking touches can be rousing, although the baby's response to light touch should be observed. Some infants, particularly those with sensory defensiveness disorders, cannot tolerate ticklish touch and become agitated and distracted by it. They respond more positively to firm touch.

Babies who fall asleep before completing a full feed may have stamina issues caused by neurological prematurity, injury, or illness. These infants may gain weight slowly. They also require medical evaluation. To compensate for the infant's inability to complete feedings, the mother must alter her approach to feedings. Pumping may be necessary to provide milk for supplementation and to stimulate the milk supply. If the mother is willing, many short feeds at breast can sometimes compensate for a baby's inability to sustain feedings of a normal length. Infant weight gain should be monitored.

The Hypersensitive Baby

Hypersensitive babies have difficulty making smooth transitions between states. Feeding may be facilitated by decreasing environmental stimuli. Dimming the lights and providing quiet often helps calm a baby who cannot tolerate distractions. Firm touch is preferable as light touch may provoke stress reactions. Irritable, disorganized babies may profit from rhythmic rocking. Such babies often breastfeed better when warm, drowsy, and relaxed. Avoid prolonged, tight, straight-leg swaddling in order to permit normal hip development and prevent developmental dysplasia of the hip (van Sleuwen 2007, Wang 2012).

Views of Infant State

The infant in **Fig. 1** is in a state of deep sleep. If feeding cannot be delayed until the infant wakes on his own, the mother may use gentle rousing techniques to induce him to breastfeed. This 7 day-old Hispanic infant demonstrates normal skin color, facial tone, and symmetry. Well defined facial features indicate normal facial muscle tone. The *philtrum* is the midline groove that extends from the top of the lip to the nose. Observe the well defined philtrum and shape of the baby's upper lip.

The shape of the philtrum and the shape of the upper lip are genetically determined, vary somewhat between different racial groups, and may be affected by various syndromes and by infant facial tone. A smooth philtrum and thin upper lip may indicate Fetal Alcohol Syndrome (FAS) (The FAS Diagnostic & Prevention Network 2012).

The infant pictured in **Fig. 1** demonstrates the ability to maintain lip closure while asleep, one indicator of normal facial tone. Full-term infants such as this boy typically are born with well developed fat pads in the cheeks. The fat pads give the cheeks their rounded appearance and stabilize sucking by preventing cheek collapse.

Contrast the appearance of the infant in **Fig 1** with that of the sleeping infant in **Fig. 2**. This infant is also in a deep sleep state. However, this infant is slightly jaundiced, which may be contributing to a more pronounced degree of lethargy. Note this infant's inability to maintain lip closure during sleep. This may indicate poor facial tone, or perhaps the infant has nasal congestion requiring mouth breathing. Both poor facial tone or blocked breathing may contribute to feeding difficulty.

The infant in **Fig. 3** is in a light sleep state. Her eyes are closed, but her hand-to-mouth behavior indicates she may be receptive to feeding.

The 6 week-old baby in **Fig. 4** is drowsy. He is enjoying non-nutritive sucking (NNS) while sucking his thumb. Comfort sucking is a self-soothing behavior for infants.

Contrast the facial expression of the infant pictured in **Fig. 4** with that of the obviously stressed baby in **Fig. 5**. This drowsy baby is also engaged in NNS. However, the baby's frown indicates an unpleasant reaction to the experience. It may be the taste or odor of soap on his dad's just-washed hand. Perhaps the size or depth of penetration of the father's thumb has triggered the infant's gag reflex. The frown and grimace are behavioral stress cues, and the parent correctly responded by removing his thumb.

The bright-eyed baby boy in **Fig. 6** is 4 days old and demonstrates state stability. His calm, focused facial expression is typical of an infant in the quiet alert state. Following an uncomplicated, unmedicated delivery, this baby went to the breast within moments of birth and fed vigorously. He recovered his birth weight by Day 3. Here he exhibits an early feeding cue, raising his hand to his mouth.

The infant in **Fig. 7** is 6 days old. Note his kicking feet and how he reaches for the crib toy. This infant is in an active alert state. His ability to lift his limbs, turn toward and interact with the graphic of a human face demonstrates normal muscle tone, good eye-hand coordination, and the capacity to enthusiastically engage with his environment (Klaus 2000).

Fig. 8 provides an example of an alert infant demonstrating motoric stress cues. His body language reveals tension and distress. This is revealed by the presence of facial grimacing, finger splaying, toe curling and rigidity of the limbs (Als 1986, Herr 2006). The shaved area on the head and the presence of monitoring wires suggest that this baby has undergone recent medical procedures, some of which may have been painful. Pain increases the risk of morbidity, disrupts parent-infant bonding and may interfere with breastfeeding. While this infant may lack stamina to sustain normal feeds, breastfeeding is an important way to help newborns manage pain (Gray 2002, Shah 2006). If not medically contraindicated, skin-to-skin holding helps reduce crying and facilitates parental attachment (Moore 2012).

Fig. 9 also illustrates a stressed infant. She is 3 weeks old and 3 oz (85 g) below birth weight. Infants who fail to thrive often present with anxious facial expressions and manifest a worried alert appearance. If failure to thrive (FTT) is severe, the infant may lack the energy to cry and will appear apathetic (Lawrence 2011).

Crying refers to a specific infant behaviorial state. It also refers to a significant stress cue. Crying can be a normal response to hunger, undressing, diaper changing, or to any form of handling that startles the baby. Inconsolable crying may be a sign that the baby is ill or in pain (Short 2004). It is relatively common for fussy infants without fever who are under 4 months of age to have urinary tract infections. Urine evaluation can rule out infection as a cause of excessive infant crying (Freedman 2009).

The infant in **Fig. 10** is crying. Note the elevated, retracted tongue tip. An elevated tongue-tip can block the nipple, make latching on difficult. Crying also interferes with safe swallowing, It is important to calm a crying baby before attempting to feed in order to prevent aspiration. Notice this infant's thin cheeks and the deep creases under the eyes. These features suggest a lack of development of the subcutaneous fat pads in the cheeks. The upper lip line lacks definition. This may indicate poor lip tone. Poor lip and cheek tone may interfere with the baby's ability to form a strong seal at breast.

The infant shown in **Fig. 10** may be preterm or have experienced intrauterine growth restriction (IUGR), resulting in low birth weight. Both prematurity and being born SGA may affect feeding ability (Lawrence 2011). Excessive crying in such infants may be a sign of hunger. Breastfeeding typically improves as infants mature and gain weight, size, and stamina. Temporary supplementation may be required, ideally with mother's own pumped milk or donor human milk from an approved source. If neither are available, formula may be used until the mother's milk supply can be established.

Fig. 11 illustrates a satiated baby who is spitting up milk. Observe the remains of a wet burp dribbling from the corner of her mouth. In contrast to the peaceful facial expression of this baby, a newborn whose vomiting interferes with growth typically appears distressed and thin. Such infants should be medically evaluated to rule out illness,

bowel blockage, swallowing disorders, or gastroesophageal reflux disease (GERD).

It is important to note that mothers with milk over supply may also report that their babies frequently spit up after feeding. Parents may describe both types of infants as exhibiting fussy or "colicky" behavior. Infant weight gain is the critical determinant and the distinguishing factor that guides the type of lactation management provided. If weight gain is normal and the infant is happy, the LC merely reassures. In the case of over supply, the LC helps the mother manage breast engorgement and gives advice on how to avoid overfeeding the infant (See Ch. 11). She may explore alternative feeding positions so the baby is not overwhelmed by rapid milk flow. Conversely, in the case of a poorly gaining baby, the milk supply and the baby's intake require support. If not already under medical care, the LC must refer the poorly gaining infant to the primary health care provider for evaluation.

Assessing the Skin

Visual evaluation of the newborn includes assessment of the skin. Parents and lactation consultants may sometimes encounter infants who have unusual rashes. The infant in **Fig. 12** has a newborn rash. Newborn rash moves around. It seems to fade and then darken within minutes.

The infant in **Fig. 13** however, was ill and required hospitalization. *Petechiae* (red rash) may be a sign of *neonatal sepsis* (Short 2004). In neonates, symptoms of sepsis (bloodstream infection) are often nonspecific. Only one or two subtle signs of illness may be present in a baby who otherwise appears to be well. Community-based LCs provide a safety net for infants who are discharged within 48 hours. Because neonates may develop sepsis prior to the first well-baby checkup, rashes, low body temperature, fever, or excessive lethargy should be reported immediately to the baby's health care provider to ensure medical evaluation.

Normal infant skin temperature should feel warm and dry to the touch. Newborns during the first 2 days who are not held in skin-to-skin contact with their mother may have difficulty maintaining thermal stability (Anderson 2003). On the other hand, many infants are overdressed and kept so warm that they are difficult to rouse. Being too warm increases the risk of Sudden Infant Death Syndrome (SIDS) (AAP 2011).

The infant in **Fig. 14** shows signs of cold stress. The marbled look of her skin is called *mottling*. Some parents may not be able to identify signs of cold stress. They need help identifying mottling, shivering, or bluish coloration of the skin as indicators that their baby is cold. Preterm infants and SGA infants are especially at risk for *hypothermia*, (severe cold stress) that occurs when the body loses heat so rapidly that it cannot maintain a normal core body temperature. Acute difficulty in maintaining proper body temperature can be as dangerous as fever and, like fever, is also a sign of infection. The healthy, full-term infant in **Fig. 14** had been undressed for weighing and got chilled. She rapidly recovered and the mottling disappeared when she was placed skin-to-skin with her mother and both were covered with blankets. Owing to the size of their heads in proportion to their bodies (as compared to an adult), babies lose a great deal of heat through their heads. Soft hats or caps protect against heat loss.

Babies with Birth Trauma

Birth trauma may complicate the baby's ability to breastfeed. Birth trauma that impacts feeding may be apparent upon examination or may be revealed by taking a history and discovering, for example, that the birth required forceps or vacuum extraction (Caughey 2005). Infants express their reaction to pain in their behavior and body language. They may become more lethargic or more irritable. Increased parental holding and breastfeeding have been demonstrated to help infants manage pain (Gray 2002, Carbajal 2003, Campbell-Yeo 2011). Parents should be encouraged to contact the baby's doctor to report any concerns.

A forceps delivery after a long labor has left the 3 day-old baby in **Fig. 15** bruised and distressed. Discharged from the hospital without having established breastfeeding, this infant was difficult to rouse, producing scant wet diapers, and no stooling. Positioning the baby at the breast was difficult. She cried when her head was turned or touched in certain ways. Spoon-feeding expressed colostrum to the baby provided caloric energy that helped her breastfeed for brief periods, although her sucking was not vigorous.

Breastfeeding while side-lying in bed proved to be the least stressful feeding position for the baby in **Fig. 15**. Side-lying (see Ch. 6) increased the baby's postural stability and took pressure off her head and neck. At follow-up on Day 5, the baby still demonstrated poor stamina. She fell asleep before taking in a normal amount of milk (as determined by pre- and post-feed intake weights on an electronic scale sensitive to 2 g). Her mother had previously been instructed to use a hospital-grade pump to bring in and protect her milk supply.

The mother was encouraged to continue pumping until the baby demonstrated the ability to take full feeds at breast. Small amounts of pumped milk continued to be used at the beginning of feedings to rouse the baby. The mother was taught to observe for signs of fatigue and instructed to offer the remainder of the pumped milk if the baby fell asleep too quickly at breast. By Day 12 the baby appeared to be recovering from the most severe effects of the birth trauma. At that point, pumping and supplemental feeding were discontinued and breastfeeding proceeded uneventfully.

The 1 week-old baby seen in **Fig. 16** experienced an extremely stressful birth. Observe the abrasion on his head that resulted from vacuum extraction. The baby cried during most of his waking moments. Note his arched back and his clenched arm. This infant refused to be held close to the breast in spite of repeated attempts. The mother believed that his breast-refusing behavior resulted from a helper in the hospital pushing on the baby's head to get him to latch. Upon discharge, his mother had been instructed to pump her milk and deliver it in a Special Needs Feeder ™ (formerly called a Haberman Feeder). Stressed infants often have difficulty coordinating safe swallowing when milk flow rates are too rapid. Parents can avoid the expense of special bottles by employing external pacing techniques when using regular bottles (see Ch. 14).

The community-based LC providing follow-up care for the infant pictured in **Fig. 16** suggested bottle-feeding the baby in a flexed position, with his hips up against his mother's abdomen. Hip flexion prevents arching and helped this mother stabilize the baby's head position for safer swallowing. Note that the mother has placed her supporting hand at the base of the baby's neck where it will not touch his wounded head. Over time, as the baby recovered from the birth trauma, the mother began to bottle-feed closer to her body, eventually bottle-feeding in a breastfeeding position (See **Fig. 336**). This strategy helped begin the transition of the baby to the breast. The baby continued to be partially bottle-fed with a standard bottle after his mother returned to work.

The 5 day-old infant seen in **Fig. 17** has bruises on the scalp resulting from internal fetal monitoring. The LC makes note of bruising during her assessments of the infant because it increases the risk of developing jaundice (ABM 2010).

This mother also was incorrectly taught to latch her baby by shoving the baby's head into her breast. The baby responded by crying and struggling during latch. To remedy this breast-refusing behavior, the mother was advised to increase skin-to-skin holding in a non-feeding context, and to give the baby more control over latching. If the baby appeared to need assistance, the mother was taught to bring the baby's shoulders closer without touching the head. Once the baby stopped associating latching with pain, breastfeeding improved.

Assessing the Head and Neck for Molding, Asymmetries, and Torticollis

Localized cranial molding is common in newborns. The rate of occurrence is 13 percent in singletons; 56 percent of twins exhibit some degree of cranial asymmetry. Risk factors for localized cranial molding include instrument-assisted vaginal delivery, prolonged labor, primiparity, infant birth position, and male gender (Peitsch 2002). Infants with abnormal head shape and cranial asymmetry (*plagiocephaly*) require careful evaluation if they experience breastfeeding difficulty. Unusual head shape has an association with an increased risk of torticollis (twisted neck) and range-of-motion limitations that may impact breastfeeding (Hummel 2005, Walls 2006). Affected infants may refuse one or both breasts. Parents often misinterpret the infant's signals of distress and pain to mean that the baby dislikes breastfeeding. Creative positioning helps some infants; others require more intensive interventions such as chiropractic, massage, or physical therapy. In some cases, alternative feeding must be employed until improvement occurs. The LC must counsel about protection of the milk supply whenever an infant refuses the breast.

Muscular spasms or rigidity in the neck and shoulders contribute to jaw clenching, and may influence the baby to prefer the breast he can turn toward most easily. Limitations in range-of-motion, muscle rigidity, and any pulling of the head to one side impair the baby's ability to latch. These problems also affect the baby's ability to seal the lips around the breast. Poor lip seal impacts the baby's ability to maintain suction. The baby may compensate by clenching with the jaws in order to hold onto the breast, causing the mother to have sore nipples. Mothers in such situations often say, "My baby has a strong suck," when, in fact, the suck is weak and the baby's compensations are uncomfortable.

The infant in **Fig. 18** spent the final weeks of gestation in a breech position and was delivered by cesarean section. Because he was wedged in one position, the baby's ear was flattened level with his skull. Over time the ear position will probably normalize and is not, in itself, dangerous. However, the flattened ear is a marker that alerts the LC to closely observe for other problems that may have developed owing to this baby's inability to move freely during fetal development. The baby may not be capable of full range-of-motion or may have developed torticollis (Hummel 2005). These issues may affect the ability to breastfeed normally. On a positive note, observe how

the infant in **Fig. 18** maintains a closed lip position during sleep. This suggests that this infant has normal lip tone. The LC evaluates both strengths and weaknesses in each infant assessment.

The 4 day-old infant in **Fig. 19** has marked cranial molding (a narrow head). The baby also experienced significant bruising during a long second stage of labor that lasted approximately 3 hours. These are infant risk factors for poor breastfeeding and the mother described the infant's early feeding behavior as "lethargic." Delayed lactogenesis II has been attributed to stressful labor with a long second stage (Chen 1998, Dewey 2003). During her home visit on Day 4, the LC observed flaccid breasts and noted additional maternal-related breastfeeding risk factors. The mother had breast surgery within the past year to remove an intraductal papilloma from her right breast. Consider the breast as the face of a clock. An incision scar was visible at the areolar edge extending laterally from 10 o'clock to 12 o'clock. The breast tissue under the scar was lumpy and tender to the touch, and the baby seemed to have greater difficulty breastfeeding on that side. Both of the mother's nipples were abraded.

The infant had lost 8 percent of birth weight and appeared jaundiced, but alert during the consultation. The mother reported an adequate number of wet, but few soiled diapers.

The LC showed the woman how to help the baby get a deeper latch, and the mother reported immediate improvement in her level of comfort during breastfeeding. A test weight indicated that the baby took 30 ml of milk from the left, but only 4 ml from the right, surgically affected, breast.

Because of the multiple infant and maternal risk factors in this case, the LC recommended "insurance pumping" and suggested that the parents offer pumped milk to the baby after feeds until the stool output increased. The mother was advised to rinse her nipples with warm water after feedings and to apply purified lanolin to help heal the nipples (Dennis 2012). Pumping and breastfeeding with an improved latch helped increase the milk in both breasts. The mother did not develop mastitis. Infant stooling rapidly increased. All interventions were withdrawn within 2 days. The baby regained her birth weight by Day 10 and was still breastfeeding at last contact at 18 months.

Fig. 20 shows a photo of 6 week-old twins. The twin on the right required surgery to correct prematurely fused cranial sutures to allow room for her brain to grow normally. This is an example of dangerous cranial malformation.

The head of the infant in **Fig. 21** was molded by low engagement in the mother's pelvis during the latter weeks of pregnancy. During the delivery, the baby sustained a cranial bruise called a *cephalohematoma* (a collection of effused blood that forms under the tissue that covers the skull). Such infants may require temporary supplementation with pumped milk if their feeding stamina is affected.

Breast Preference

Occasionally a baby will breastfeed on one breast while refusing the other. Various factors can contribute to unilateral breast refusal. The baby may have experienced birth trauma resulting in a painful muscle injury or torticollis (Hutchinson 2004). A broken clavicle creates similar discomfort. Sometimes the problem is related to maternal nipple anatomy; for example, one nipple may lack elasticity, leading the baby to prefer the one that is easier to grasp.

One of the authors (KH) worked with a mother whose baby would only breastfeed in the cradle position lying on his right side. At 5 months, he finally became willing to lie on his left side and accept both breasts in the cradle position. At 1 year of age he was diagnosed with sensory integration dysfunction. There are case reports of babies who rejected one breast because they are blind in one eye. They prefer to nurse on the breast that allows them to see their mothers while feeding (Harm 2001). Similarly, infants who are deaf in one ear may become upset when their hearing ear is blocked.

Infant Pain and Stress

Fig. 22 shows the heel of an infant born at 37 weeks gestation who is being monitored for hyperbilirubinemia. Heel sticks are the most common way to draw blood from newborns to perform newborn screening tests and to monitor jaundice levels. Frequent heel sticks or other unpleasant stimuli resulting from necessary medical care may cause some infants to develop patterns of sensory defensiveness that interfere with feeding. For instance, infants who have been vigorously suctioned or intubated may have injured vocal cords (indicated by raspy cries) and sore throats. They may react with stress when they experience oral penetration, whether from a long maternal nipple, bottle teat, finger, or pacifier. This may be revealed in aversive behavior, refusal to feed, or as an easily activated gag reflex.

The infant in **Fig. 23** has a painful lump on his spine resulting from a *lumbar puncture* (spinal tap). Lumbar punctures, circumcision and intramuscular injections are other examples of the types of painful experiences that may cause babies to "shut down" and become difficult to comfortably position or to rouse for feeding. While guidelines have been developed to help in the management of neonatal pain, pain management is hampered by a lack of awareness among some health care professionals. Many parents do not realize that newborns experience pain.

If a procedure is painful to adults, it should be considered painful to newborns. Because neural inhibitory mechanisms are lacking in preterm infants, they are especially at risk for increased sensitivity to pain compared to more mature infants, older children, and adults. Repeated noxious stimuli can lead to chronic neuropathic states, resulting in normally innocuous stimuli being perceived as painful. Consequently, it is important to minimize and manage neonatal pain in order to promote normal growth and development (Duhn 2004).

As in adults, adequate treatment of pain is associated with decreased clinical complications. Anand (2001) described 3 types of interventions:

- **Environmental:** reduce noise and light; group medical procedures to allow babies rest periods.
- **Behavioral:** breastfeed or use breastmilk or glucose and pacifiers during painful procedures.
- **Pharmacological:** use anesthetics or analgesics as ordered by the physician.

Jaundice

Neonatal jaundice is common, occuring to some degree in most newborns (ABM 2011). It typically resolves within the first weeks after birth unless calories are restricted. However, because of the risk of bilirubin toxicity, infants should be monitored to screen for those who might develop severe hyperbilirubinemia, bilirubin encephalopathy or kernicterus (ABM 2011). Risk factors for exaggerated neonatal jaundice include a positive Coombs' test, ABO incompatibility, prematurity, starvation (poor caloric intake), dehydration, and vacuum-assisted delivery (Bertini 2001). Cephalohematoma or significant bruising are also considered risk factors.

Lethargy and poor arousal are common in babies with hyperbilirubinemia. LCs may be called upon to support the mother whose infant needs increased milk intake to reduce bilirubin levels. It is beyond the scope of this book to undertake a thorough examination of all the issues related to jaundice; however, it must be emphasized that poor caloric intake contributes to and may result from jaundice. An aim of therapy with such babies is to increase stooling, since bowel movements are the major route of excretion of bilirubin. To increase stooling, calories must be increased. The infant should get 8 to 12 effective feedings during each 24 hours. The mother should pump to protect her milk supply, and supplement with her own milk, if needed.

Compare the skin color of the 4 day-old Caucasian baby in **Fig. 24** with his father's arm. This baby is jaundiced on the face, trunk, and palms. As bilirubin levels increase there is a *cranio-caudal* (head to foot) progression of discoloration of the skin.

The family of the infant shown in **Fig. 24** had been keeping their house dark to encourage the baby to sleep. Taking the baby from a dimly lit room into sunlight helped the parents identify that their baby's jaundice had worsened. The baby needed help rousing and needed more calories. Information motivated the parents to begin using temporary interventions to improve feeding.

Pressing a finger on the skin of a baby and observing the underlying color of the skin can identify the presence of jaundice (Short 2004). See **Figs. 24** and **25**. However, visual inspection of infants to gauge their bilirubin level is felt to be unreliable, particularly in non-Caucasian populations. Serum levels provide more accurate information. Safe levels of bilirubin depend on many factors including birth weight and gestational age. The smaller and less mature the infant, the greater the concern there is with jaundice, particularly if visible jaundice occurs in the first 24 hours of age. The AAP (2004) recommends that term infants with risk factors and those who are visibly jaundiced before 24 hours of age receive diagnostic testing regardless of feeding method.

Bilirubin levels are most likely to peak on day 3-5, after hospital discharge. These peaks sometime occur before the first scheduled pediatric follow-up visit. The community-based lactation consultant may be consulted about poor breastfeeding during this time period and may observe jaundice in an infant that requires immediate medical evaluation. In such cases, the LC advises the parents to seek care, and alerts the health care provider regarding the infant.

Fig. 26 pictures an infant wearing a fiberoptic device to lower the bilirubin concentration. Using this "bili blanket" permits the baby to be held and to breastfeed during treatment. It does not require that the baby's eyes be protected, and allows the baby to receive treatment at home.

In **Fig. 27** an infant with ABO incompatibility receives the more traditional form of phototherapy with special lights over the bed requiring eye patches. This treatment temporarily disrupts holding and may alter feeding frequency. Newer bili beds are being designed with lights under the baby, negating the need for blindfolds. Keeping the mother and jaundiced infant in close proximity during treatment may be one way to ensure frequent breastfeeding. Breastfeeding and breastmilk feeds are not contraindicated when a baby is jaundiced, although the baby may be difficult to rouse and may feed poorly. Feeding water is not recommended as a method to lower bilirubin (Lawrence 2011). The mothers's milk supply in such situations requires protection with pumping and hand expression. Parents require specific counseling and reassurance that newborn jaundice typically resolves without consequences with appropriate care (Kemper 1989).

Als H. A synactive model of neonatal behavioral organization: development in the premature infant and for support of infants and parents in the neonatal intensive care environment. *Physical and Occupational Therapy in Pediatrics* 1986; 6:3-53.

Als H. Toward a synactive theory of development: promise for the assessment and support of infant individuality. *Infant Mental Health Journal* 1982; 3(4):229-243.

Academy of Breastfeeding Medicine (ABM). ABM Protocol Committee. ABM Clinical Protocol #22: Guidelines for management of jaundice in the breastfeeding infant equal to or greater than 35 weeks' gestation. *Breastfeeding Medicine* 2010; 5(2):87-93.

American Academy of Pediatrics (AAP). Clinical Practice Guidelines Subcommittee on Hyperbilirubinemia. Management of hyperbilirubinemia in the newborn infant 35 or more weeks of gestation. *Pediatrics* 2004; 114(1):297-316.

American Academy of Pediatrics (AAP), Task Force on Sudden Infant Death Syndrome. SIDS and other sleep-related infant deaths: expansion of recommendations for a safe infant sleeping environment. *Pediatrics* 2011; 128; e1341.

Anand K. The International Evidence-Based Group for Neonatal Pain: Consensus Statement for the Prevention and Management of Pain in the Newborn. *Archives of Pediatric and Adolescent Medicine* 2001; 155(2):173-180.

Anderson PO, Sauberan JB, Lane JR, et al. Hydrocodone excretion into breast milk: the first two reported cases. *Breastfeeding Medicine* 2007; 2(1):10-14.

Bertini G, Dani C, Tronchin M, et al. Is breastfeeding really favoring early neonatal jaundice? *Pediatrics* 2001; 107(3):e41.

Brazelton T. *Neonatal Behavioral Assessment Scale.* Philadelphia, PA: J.B. Lippincott, 1984.

Buckley KM, Charles GE. Benefits and challenges of transitioning preterm infants to at-breast feedings. *International Breastfeeding Journal* 2006; 1:13.

Campbell-Yeo M, Fernandes A, Johnston C. Procedural pain management for neonates using nonpharmacological strategies: part 2: mother-driven interventions. *Advances in Neonatal Care* 2011; 11(5):312-318.

Carbajal R, Veerapen S, Couderc S, et al. Analgesic effect of breastfeeding in term neonates: randomized controlled trial. *British Medical Journal* 2003; 326(7379):13-15.

Caughey AB, Sandberg PL, Zlatnik MG, et al. Forceps compared with vacuum: rates of neonatal and maternal morbidity. *Obstetrics & Gynecology* 2005; 106(5 Pt 1):908-912.

Chen D, Nommsen-Rivers L, Dewey K. Stress during labor and delivery and early lactation performance. *American Journal of Clinical Nutrition* 1998; 68(2):335-344.

Dennis CL, Schottle N, Hodnett E, et al. An all-purpose nipple ointment versus lanolin in treating painful damaged nipples in breastfeeding women: a randomized, controlled trial. *Breastfeeding Medicine* 2012; 7(6):473-479.

Dewey K, Nommsen-Rivers L, Heinig MJ, et al. Risk factors for suboptimal infant breastfeeding behavior, delayed onset of lactation, and excess neonatal weight loss. *Pediatrics* 2003; 112(3):607-619.

Duhn L, Medves J. A systematic integrative review of infant pain assessment tools. *Advances in Neonatal Care* 2004; 4(3):126-140.

Elder M. The effects of temperature and position on the sucking pressure of newborn infants. *Child Development* 1970; 41(1):95-102.

Fetal Alcohol Syndrome Network. Website:www.depts.washington.edu/fasdpn/htmls/research/htm. Accessed May 2012.

Freedman SB, Al-Harthy N, Thull-Freedman J. The crying infant: diagnostic testing and frequency of serious underlying disease. *Pediatrics* 2009; 123(3): 841-848.

Gartner L. Jaundice and the Breastfed Baby, in J Riordan K Wambach. *Breastfeeding and Human Lactation* (4th edition). Sudbury. MA: Jones and Bartlett, 2010; pp. 365-378.

Gray L, Miller L, Philipp B, et al. Breastfeeding is analgesic in healthy newborns. *Pediatrics* 2002; 109(4):590-593.

Harm LS. In your words; not quite perfect. *American Baby* 2001; 63(2):58.

Herr K, Coyne P, Key T, et al. Pain assessment in the nonverbal patient: position statement with clinical practice recommendations. *Pain Management Nursing* 2006; 7(2):44-52.

Hummel P, Fortado D. Impacting infant head shapes. *Advances in Neonatoal Care* 2005; 5(6):329-340.

Hutchison BL, Hutchinson LA, Thompson JM, et al. Plagiocephaly and brachycephaly in the first two years of life: a prospective cohort study. *Pediatrics* 2004; 114(4):970-980.

Kemper K, Forsyth B, McCarthry P. Jaundice, terminating breastfeeding, and the vulnerable child. *Pediatrics* 1989; 84(5):773-778.

Klaus M, Klaus P. *Your Amazing Newborn*. Boston, MA: Da Capo Press, 2000.

Lawrence RA, Lawrence RM. *Breastfeeding: A Guide for the Medical Profession* (7th edition). Philadelphia, PA: Elsevier Mosby, 2011; pp. 343, 346-347, 492, 542-543.

Mannel R. Defining lactation acuity to improve patient safety and outcomes. *Journal of Human Lactation* 2011; 27(2):163-170.

Moore E, Anderson G, Bergman N, et al. Early skin-to-skin contact for mothers and their healthy newborn infants. *The Cochrane Database of Systematic Reviews* 2012 Issue 5. Article Number CD003519. www.thecochranelibrary.com. Accessed May 2012.

Narchi H, Skinner A, Williams B. Small for gestational age neonates -- are we missing some by only using standard population growth standards and does it matter? *Journal of Maternal, Fetal, and Neonatal Medicine* 2010; 23(1):48-54.

Noel-Weiss J, Woodend AK, Peterson W, et al. An observational study of associations among maternal fluids during parturition, neonatal output, and breastfed newborn weight loss. *International Breastfeeding Journal* 2011; 6:9.

Peitsch W, Keefer C, La Brie R, et al. Incidence of cranial asymmetry in newborns. *Pediatrics* 2002; 110(6):e72.

Raju TN, Higgins RD, Stark AR, et al. Optimizing care and outcome for late-preterm (near-term) infants: a summary of the workshop sponsored by the National Institute of Child Health and Human Development. *Pediatrics* 2006; 118(3):1207-1214.

Redshaw M, Henderson J. Learning the hard way: expectations and experiences of infant feeding support. *Birth* 2012; 39(1):21-29.

Shah PS, Aliwalas LL, Shah V. Breastfeeding or breast milk for procedural pain in neonates. *The Cochrane Database of Systematic Reviews* 2006; Issue 3. Article Number: CD004950. www.thecochranelibrary.com. Accessed May 2012.

Short M. Guide to a systematic physical assessment in the infant with supected infection and/or sepsis. *Advances in Neonatal Care* 2004; 4(3):141-153.

van Sleuwen B, Engleberts A, Boere-Boonekamp M, et al. Swaddling: a systematic review. *Pediatrics* 2007; 120(4):e1097.

Walls V, Glass R. Mandibular asymmetry and breastfeeding problems: experience from 11 cases. *Journal of Human Lactation* 2006; 22(3):328-334.

Wang E, Liu T, Li J, et al. Does swaddling influence developmental dysplasia of the hip? An experimental study of the traditional straight-leg swaddling model in neonatal rats. *Journal of Bone Joint Surgery American Volume* 2012, 94(12):1071-1077.

Infant Orofacial Assessment and Feeding Reflexes

It is important to assess infant facial structures, tone and feeding reflexes because deficits or anomalies may affect the ability to breastfeed. It is beyond the LC's scope of practice to diagnose or to remedy all such problems, but the LC must be able to identify and accurately report weaknesses that increase the risk of lactation failure (see Ch. 2). After obtaining permission from the patient or client, the LC shares these observations with the primary care provider. This satisfies the ethical requirement stated in the International Board of Lactation Consultant Examiners' Code of Professional Conduct that the IBCLC: "Report accurately and completely to other members of the health care team" (IBLCE 2011).

Speech-Language Pathologists (SLPs), Physical Therapists (PTs), and Occupational Therapists (OTs) are trained to assess neuromuscular performance and to treat deficits. Working within such referral networks, the LC broadens her own assessment skills and educates other health care professionals about the importance of human milk, especially for compromised infants.

Assessment of the Oral Structures

Oral structures change over time with maturation and growth. Changes in the first 4 to 6 months of life can be dramatic. Both structure and function can be affected by prematurity, injury, congenital malformation, neurological deficit, or illness. Each of these occurrences can negatively affect breastfeeding (Ogg 1975).

The Lips

The baby uses the lips to draw the breast into the mouth (Wolf 1992). The lips work with the tongue to form a seal around the breast (Genna 2013b). Lip seal facilitates the creation of negative pressure (suction) inside the mouth. Poor lip seal impairs the amount of suction the baby can create and maintain. Frequent loss of suction results in the baby losing the breast and requires the baby to constantly re-latch. This causes breastfeeding to become tiring and the baby may fall asleep before taking a full feeding. Residual milk must then be expressed to protect the milk supply from down regulation. Pumped milk should be fed to the baby to protect growth.

The lips normally are smoothly flanged around the breast. Weak lip seal and frequent release of the breast may indicate poor motoric and muscular control of the lips. Prematurity, excessive weight loss, neuromuscular deficits, or illness contribute to generalized weakness that may

be expressed as difficulty maintaining lip seal. However, it is important to assess breast support and positioning. Poor positioning and poor support of a heavy breast can also cause the infant to lose the breast.

Both decreased and excessive lip tone can be problematic. Assess the lips by observing the baby's ability to open, round (see **Fig. 39**), and shape the lips. The infant should be able to maintain a closed lip position awake and asleep, and to control saliva secretions. It is unusual for infants to drool until the onset of teething (Morris 1977). While it is normal for a teething baby to drool, excessive drooling in a young infant can indicate that the infant is having difficulty swallowing. Drooling is a warning sign that the infant may be easily overwhelmed by larger volumes of fluid and should prompt closer assessment for aspiration.

Gentle digital pressure against the lips should generate some resistance. In other words, the baby's lips should be responsive to touch. The LC should observe the baby's ability to seal on a finger, the breast, or a bottle teat. For some infants with weak facial tone, it will be easier and require less effort for them to seal on narrow objects. Some infants who appear to seal well on a finger or narrow bottle teat tire quickly when trying to sustain a seal on a wide-based object such as a breast.

Uniform lip seal should be visually assessed. Sometimes, what appears to be a problem at the lips is actually an issue involving the jaw or tongue that affects lip seal. For example, jaw asymmetry can make it impossible for an infant to seal the lips uniformly. Poor jaw grading (opening the mouth too wide) may break lip seal and result in loss of suction. The cupped sides of the infant's tongue on the breast help seal the corner of the lips during breastfeeding. If tongue mobility is restricted (as in tongue-tie) the sides of the tongue cannot cup and cannot assist in forming lip seal.

Clicking or Smacking Sounds and Milk Leaking

Weak lip seal may result in loss of the breast and loss of milk during feeding. It may be revealed by intermittent breaks in suction with resultant clicking or smacking sounds. Leaking or spilling milk during breast or bottle-feeding may be observed at the corners of the mouth or the mother may notice wet clothing. Milk leaking and noisy feeding may also indicate weakness of the muscles of the soft palate, a submucosal cleft palate, tongue-tie, or other oral anomaly.

Intermittent breaks in lip seal and smacking sounds do not always indicate weak lip tone or a structural anomaly. Breaking the seal may also be a strategy that a baby deliberately employs when trying to manage a milk flow rate that is too rapid. Thus, mothers with strong let-down reflexes may observe clicking or smacking sounds and milk leaking during breastfeeding. Their baby has learned to release the seal in order to slow down the milk flow rate.

When assessing infants who make smacking sounds or leak milk, it is important to look at the whole picture. If the infant is gaining weight robustly and the milk supply is ample, smacking sounds are probably not an indication of a problem. On the other hand, if an infant is gaining poorly, and has difficulty completing feeds, smacking sounds and milk leaking may reveal dysfunction.

Lip Retraction

Lip retraction is sometimes caused by a tight upper labial frenum (**Fig. 28**). Lip retraction is also a compensation a baby may employ to grip the breast when lip tone is weak (**Fig. 29**), or the baby is tongue-tied. Lip retraction may contribute to the formation of sucking blisters as pictured in **Fig. 30**. Often described as "normal," sucking blisters might better be characterized as "common." The creation of blisters or calluses on skin is a sign of friction trauma. The rough calluses formed on the lips can irritate the nipples, generally around the base. Mothers can use a finger to gently flange the lip. A light coat of purified lanolin applied to the baby's lips can soften sucking blisters.

Therapeutic Exercises to Strengthen Lip Tone

The brief use of firm pressure stimulus (tapping, stretching, stroking) of the *orbicularis oris* muscle around the lips prior to feeding, as in **Fig. 31**, may improve tone and help strengthen the baby's ability to form a competent lip seal (Alper 1996). Use of a finger, bottle teat, or a pacifier with a round-shaped nipple to play "tug of war" with the baby is an exercise that can assist in strengthening lip tone.

The Cheeks

Subcutaneous fat deposits in the cheeks provide structural support for oral and pharyngeal function. Cheek stability influences lip seal (Wolf 1992). Preterm or low birth weight infants often have immature development of subcutaneous fat pads in their cheeks. By placing a gloved finger inside and a thumb outside a baby's cheek (**Fig. 32**), the LC can assess the thickness of subcutaneous fat deposits. Thin cheeks contribute to difficulty creating sufficient suction. Collapsing cheeks create an appearance of "dimpling" (see **Fig. 125**). Observation of dimpling

during feeding suggests shallow latch, loss of suction, or lack of cheek stability.

Low tone (hypotonia) can contribute to poor cheek stability. The use of external counter-pressure can improve cheek stability by decreasing the intra-oral space (see **Fig. 351** and **Fig. 352**). Decreasing the space inside the mouth diminishes the effort the baby must exert to create the vacuum necessary to generate suction. As the baby gains weight, the fat deposits in the cheeks will increase, generally resulting in improved feeding stability.

Appearance: Form Influences Function

The LC is alert to abnormal infant appearance because it may reveal functional problems that affect feeding. Physiological function is supported by normal development. Abnormal development of the skull and facial skeleton may alter function of the brain, vision, airway, mastication, and speech (Beals 2004). Abnormal facial muscle development or inhibited movement during the fetal period may also lead to facial deformations that affect function (Hall 2010).

Dysphagia refers to disruption in the swallowing process. Infants with facial malformation are at higher risk for dysphagia and respiratory and nutritional complications (Baudon 2009). Dysphagia may have behaviorial consequences such as *neonatal feeding resistance* (Abadie 2001). This term describes an aversion that develops because the infant cannot safely coordinate breathing and swallowing and becomes afraid to eat. Some cases of breast refusal and non-organic failure to thrive have been attributed to aversive behavior caused by dysphagia.

The Jaws

The jaws provide stability for the movements of the tongue, lips, and cheeks (Wolf 1992). Normal jaw movements are rhythmic and graded. In other words, the jaw excursions are neither too wide nor too narrow during feeding. Opening and closing motions are smooth, and regular. Arrhythmic jaw movements and inconsistent degree of jaw excursions signify disorganization of sucking. Jaw asymmetry and abnormally wide jaw excursions break the seal at breast with resultant loss of suction. To compensate, the infant may clench the jaws to hold onto the breast, causing pain for the mother. Milk intake often suffers. This pattern is described as a dysfunctional suck (Palmer 1993a).

Just as some infants have difficulty staying latched because of jaw excursions that are too wide, some babies cannot open wide enough. Injury at the joint of the jaw (*temporomandibular joint* or TMJ) and hypertonic facial tone cause narrow jaw opening and shallow latch. Jaw closure occuring on the nipple shaft increases the risk of sore nipples.

Sometimes a narrow gape is not caused by a problem with the jaws, but reveals a weakness of the tongue or lips. The baby may compensate by using excessive jaw clenching as a strategy to hold the breast in the mouth. Providing breast support helps reduce the work of feeding for a baby struggling to hold onto the breast.

The position of the adult jaw is normally neutral, with lower and upper gums approximating. Infants have somewhat receding lower jaw structures because the lower jaw development is less than 40 percent complete at birth. Head circumference increases by an average of 5 cm during the first 5 months after birth, and the lower jaw begins to move anteriorly (forward) at a rapid pace (Ranly 1998).

The forward growth of the *mandible* (lower jaw) during the first 3 years of life changes the profile, typically correcting the somewhat receding chin normally observed in the infant. Some infants have significantly receding chins, true *retrognathia*. This characteristic can be familial or associated with specific chromosomal disorders. Receding chin may also result from intrauterine position that inhibits jaw development (for example, certain breech presentations).

Fig. 33 shows an infant with a receding chin. Note also the slight anomaly in the ear development.

Observe the marked jaw asymmetry of the 8 day-old infant pictured in **Figs. 34** and **35**. His position *in utero* negatively affected the development of the shape of his head and pushed his jaw to the side. The infant was unable to latch successfully to the breast. The LC and mother observed cheek dimpling as he fed. Nipple shields appear to reduce the work of feeding for some infants, but use of a shield failed to improve this baby's sucking ability. His mother pumped her milk for 4.5 months, but the baby never transitioned to the breast.

Receding chin, high-arched or cleft palates, and defects of the soft palate all pose structural challenges to breastfeeding that are difficult to overcome. Repositioning is one of the few interventions that might assist an infant with such problems.

In the case of the infant whose receding chin impairs breastfeeding, it may help to position the baby with his head tilted back, so that the lower jaw pushes into the breast. This may improve latch and may prevent painful jaw closure on the nipple shaft. (See Ch. 18 for more discussion related to receding chin.)

Asymmetries of the face may be associated with abnormal jaw development, asymmetrical muscle tone, injury, torticollis, or facial nerve paralysis associated with forceps delivery or conditions such as *neonatal asymmetric crying facies* (Smith 1981, Sapin 2005, Wall 2006). Neck position also influences jaw function. It is difficult to achieve full range of motion of the jaws with the chin tucked (hyperflexion of the head). Breastfeeding is facilitated when the mother provides appropriate postural support that flexes the baby at the hips and supports the head in a neutral or extended position.

The Tongue

If the full range of motion of the tongue is impaired, many oral functions may be negatively affected, including speech, dentition, and feeding. Appearance is also altered. The tongue must be able to lift, extend, lateralize and cup. During breastfeeding, the degree of tongue extension impacts nipple soreness. (An extended tongue pads the breast from compression by the lower gum.) A combination of suction and peristaltic tongue movements extract milk from the breast. Tongue lift is important because it determines the distance that the tongue will then drop in a piston-like manner, creating negative pressure (Geddes 2008). The tongue also must be mobile enough to form a central groove and generate a peristaltic wave that controls the direction of fluids during swallowing (Wolf 1992, Woolridge 2012, Burton 2013). As previously described, the curled sides of the tongue also assist in sealing the lips at the corners of the mouth (See **Fig. 381**).

The normal tongue is soft rather than rigid, and is capable of the elastic maneuvers described above. (See Ch. 17 for a full discussion of range-of-motion issues related to tongue function.) The tongue is normally thin and mobile rather than thick and bunched. The tip is rounded (Ogg 1975) rather than notched, square, or heart-shaped (Philipp 2012). Tongue tone should be excellent and may be assessed with gentle digital pressure on the mid-section of the tongue. The tongue should resist when pressed, pressing back up against the finger. When a gloved finger is inserted (pad side up) to assess sucking, the LC should observe that the tongue extends over the lower gum ridge, and sense the tongue cupping around the digit, moving rhythmically with pressure against the finger.

If the tongue cannot move properly, individuals cannot breathe, suck, or swallow efficiently. Conversely, problems with free range-of-motion of the body or issues related to swallowing and breathing may generate abnormal tongue movements.

Abnormal presentations of the tongue include ankyloglossia (tongue-tie), short, bunched, retracted, or flat tongue (one that cannot easily form a central groove). Tongue protrusion can result from low tone and chromosomal disorders such as Down Syndrome. One of the authors (BWC) has observed tongue asymmetry as the result of forceps injury that affected the nerves of the tongue.

Abnormally high muscle tone can cause tongue retraction. As the head pulls back and the baby arches from the effects of hypertonia, the tongue drops back. Flexion of the baby at the hips may help control such arching, but it is important to try to determine why the infant is arching. Some infants with airway obstructions such as *tracheomalacia* may arch their bodies to try to hold open a collapsing trachea. These infants may aspirate if forced to swallow large volumes of liquid. External pacing techniques help prevent aspiration (See Ch. 14).

Tongue-tip elevation can make insertion of the breast difficult (see **Fig. 44**). A nipple shield sometimes can be used to help a baby drop the tongue into a position that makes it easier to latch.

The Palates

The hard palate is a thin plate of bone located in the roof of the mouth. It provides stability to the structures of the mouth (Wolf 1992). The hard palate opposes the tongue, forming a surface that provides a back guard that grades tongue movement.

The soft palate is a muscular flap that lifts during swallowing to seal off the opening to the nasopharynx to prevent food from entering the nose. It drops when the posterior tongue rises to form a sealed oral cavity during sucking. "The coordination between the tongue and soft palate may reflect the process by which the tongue is timed to pump liquid by moving it into an enclosed space, compressing it, and allowing it to leave by a specific route through the pharynx" (Goldfield 2010). A sealed oral cavity facilitates creation of negative pressure and suction (Ramsay 2004b).

The angle of the slope of the palate should be smooth and moderate, and both palates should be intact, with no evidence of a cleft. The shape of the hard palate should accommodate the tongue (Bosma 1977). Familial narrow, arched, or grooved palates can occur. As was mentioned in the discussion about jaw formation, genetic, skeletal and muscular development both determine and affect function. Hard palate shape may sometimes be influenced

by intrauterine breech position that prevents the tongue from elevating to spread and shape the developing bony structures. In a similar way, tongue-tie may prevent the tongue from shaping the hard palate during fetal development.

BWC has observed that infants with tongue-tie often have high or bubble-shaped hard palates. Observe the bubble shape of the palate of the 2 week-old infant pictured in **Fig. 36**. He was born with a tongue-tie and was unable to breastfeed. His frenulum membrane was clipped on Day 5 and healed well. However, he still cannot lift his tongue above the midline. (Imagine the midline as an invisible line drawn from the corners of the lips when the mouth is open wide.) Lack of ability to lift the tongue to the upper gum ridge is an indication that the tongue is still abnormally adhered to the floor of the mouth. This characterizes a *Stage 4 tongue-tie* and requires more extensive surgery to remediate (Genna 2013a). For a full discussion of ankyloglossia, see Ch. 17.

Long periods of intubation can create grooves in the palate or contribute to narrow, arched palates (Wolf 1992). Babies with genetic syndromes such as Turner Syndrome often have grooved (channeled) hard palates (see **Figs. 364, 408-409**).

The soft palate is a muscle. Stamina influences muscle performance. Poor stamina may lead to fatigue aspiration when a weak baby begins to lose control of soft palate muscle function. Loss of ability to seal the rear of the oral cavity may not be evident at first. It becomes more noticeable as the feeding progresses and the baby tires. If aspiration occurs because of a cleft of the soft palate or because of a muscle stamina problem, the baby may sound congested or have stuffy breathing. Parents or health care providers may observe excess nasal debris from aspirated milk that has accumulated in the nose. More information about clefts of the palate can be found in Ch. 18.

The Nose

The nasal passages should be assessed (Alper 1996) when unusual breathing is noted. Congested breathing during and after feeds may be a sign of aspiration. Organisms prioritize breathing over eating, and some instances of early feed termination or outright breast rejection may be connected with inability to breathe adequately while feeding. On rare occasions, abnormally small nasal openings are observed. The 4 week-old infant in **Fig. 37** has abnormally small nares. His mother had been attempting to breastfeed him, but each time she held him firmly at her breast, he panicked and fought to push away so he could breathe through his mouth. The LC concluded that when his mouth was full, his nostrils were not sufficiently large to permit him to adequately breathe through his nose.

The LC observed similar behavior when this baby drank from a bottle. He appeared to hold his breath, gulping milk, and then pushed away and panted, struggling to catch his breath (see **Fig. 332**). Feedings were miserable for both mother and baby until the LC demonstrated external pacing techniques (see Ch. 14). Within 24 hours of instituting paced bottle-feeding, this baby calmed down for feedings. His mother reported that slowing down feedings produced "a totally different baby."

Neither the LC nor the pediatrician thought to refer this infant to a pediatric Ear Nose and Throat specialist (ENT) for evaluation of the narrow nasal passages. However, the mother later shared that the baby continued to have breathing issues and was assessed for sleep apnea and snoring at 9 months. The ENT remarked that it would have been possible to enlarge the small nasal passages with a dilation procedure at an earlier age when the cartilage was maleable.

As previously mentioned, nasal congestion in the absence of respiratory illness may be related to fluid aspiration during feedings. Debris may accumulate in the nose, causing congestion. If the parents report or the LC identifies audible nasal congestion, an alternative explanation may be that the baby is having difficulty managing a forceful milk ejection. The baby may also have a problem with coordinating sucking and swallowing with breathing.

In cases where obstructed nasal breathing is observed, the mother may be able to assist the baby by changing the nursing position or by softening the breast before the baby latches. Expressing a small amount of milk reduces the spray pressure of the first milk ejection (let-down reflex), making it easier for the baby to cope with the milk flow rate. Upright, reclined, and side-lying positions help some babies. The mother should experiment with alternative positions to see if any help the baby better manage the milk flow-rate from the breast.

Any time a mother notices that her baby is having difficulty with respiration, she should allow the baby to release the breast periodically in order to rest and to prevent apnea. If the mother is supplementing, she may find it necessary to assume more responsibility for the pace of feedings, pausing frequently to match the speed of delivery of milk to the baby's breathing. This helps the baby reorganize his breathing, assists the baby in learning how to self-pace, and helps protect the baby from developing behavioral aversions to feeding (see Ch. 14).

Respiratory distress in the infant always requires evaluation by a medical professional. Swallowing disorders and conditions such as gastroesophageal reflux disease (GERD) contribute to respiratory distress and often impact breastfeeding. Diagnostic tests are available to evaluate infants with breathing or swallowing disorders. As infants grow and mature, some conditions (such as GERD) may resolve. Other infants will require treatment with medication or occupational therapy.

Feeding Reflexes

Normal infants are born with reflexes that assist with feeding. These reflexes include:

- Rooting
- Swallowing
- Sucking
- Gagging
- Coughing

Prematurity, injury, illness, or congenital disorders may affect feeding reflexes. If a feeding reflex is depressed or hyperactive, a baby may have difficulty feeding normally. The LC's assessment should include observation of the presence or absence of functional feeding reflexes. The LC reports abnormal findings to the physician.

The Rooting Reflex

The rooting reflex helps the baby locate the nipple. Rooting behavior is present at birth and extinguishes between 2 to 4 months of age, although some experts feel it may persist longer in breastfed infants (Morris 1977). If the rooting reflex is absent or is diminished, it may signal poor tactile receptivity or poor neural integration. If the rooting reflex is hyperactive, the baby may be easily distracted and become frustrated while trying to latch.

The Swallowing Reflex

Swallowing develops early in fetal life (12-14 weeks gestation) with ingestion of amniotic fluid. The volume of the fluid, the delivery of fluid to the back of the tongue, and the reaction of chemical receptors in the larynx and pharynx trigger swallowing in the infant (Woolridge 1986, Wolf 1992).

Abnormalities of the tongue and palate interfere with safe swallowing and are risk factors for aspiration. Swallowing dysfunction is distressing. It feels like drowning, and can result in feeding aversion and breast refusal.

The Sucking Reflex

Sucking behavior has been observed *in utero* as early as 13 weeks gestation (Hafstrom 2000). By 28 weeks, disorganized and random mouthing patterns are observed. By 32 weeks, stronger sucking with a burst-pause pattern begins to occur. By 34-35 weeks gestational age, some preterm infants can sustain a stable sucking rhythm that allows them to feed effectively (Brake 1988). Feeds at this stage are generally brief and preterm infants fatigue quickly (Meier 2007).

A Premature Infant Oral Motor Intervention (PIOMI) was developed (Lessen 2011) to provide exercises to increase control of movements for the lips, cheeks, jaw and tongue of preterm infants. The invervention consists of internal and external stimulation according to a specific protocol with finger stroking. In a randomized, blinded clinical trial, beginning at 29 weeks gestational age, the infants who received the once-daily exercises tolerated them well, transitioned to total oral feedings 5 days sooner, and were discharged 2.6 days earlier than controls.

Sucking is stimulated by touch pressure on the lips and tongue (Wolf 1992), and by stroking of the posterior palate near the junction of the hard and soft palates (Woolridge 1986, Ramsay 2004b).

Sucking is categorized into two modes: nonnutritive (NNS) and nutritive (NS). NNS develops earlier and matures at about 37 weeks. NNS sucking patterns change with maturity. Both the number of sucks in each burst and suction pressure increase as the baby develops. Bursts of NNS are more rapid than NS, and appear to affect behavioral state. NNS has been observed to decrease stress in preterm infants. Preterm infants experience reduced length of hospitalization when given opportunities for NNS (Premji 2000, Pinelli 2005). Premji suggests that NNS may also play a role in stimulating fibers in the oral cavity that activate the vagal nerve, influencing the levels of gastrointestinal hormones that affect digestion.

NNS can occur as the baby sucks on a pacifier, a finger, or an emptied (just pumped) breast (Narayanan 1991). It is characterized by rapid, shallow sucking and a lack of swallowing. The rate of sucking is 6-8 sucks for each swallow.

Nutritive sucking occurs solely in the presence of fluid transfer and is more organized (Glass 1994). The sucking rate is slower than in NNS. Some breath holding (brief apnea) occurs during NS because of the pauses for swallowing. Breathing rate increases during the pauses between sucking bursts and may be observed as light panting (Geddes 2006).

The terms NS and NNS are often used incorrectly to describe effective versus ineffective suck. The LC must recognize that within a breastfeeding session, sucking rates are variable and the baby may alter back and forth between NNS and NS depending upon the milk flow rates before, during, and after each milk ejection.

Ultrasound is a noninvasive method of breast examination previously used primarily to detect breast abnormalities in nonlactating women. Milk ejection can be visualized by ultrasound techniques. Visualization verifies that milk flow rate is low before milk ejection occurs. Human mammary glands do not store milk in large ducts close to the nipple. In fact, milk appears to reflux or flow in reverse back up into the smaller ducts and ductules of the breast for storage between milk ejections. Therefore milk is not readily available unless released by the milk ejection (Ramsay 2004a).

Some clinicians have described the baby's rapid sucking pattern during the initial part of a breastfeed as "start-up" or "call-up" sucking. Rapid sucking appears to trigger the let-down or milk ejection reflex. Ramsay observed that a typical milk ejection lasted for approximately 1.5 minutes, during which time the baby's sucking rate was observed to change to the slower NS pattern. The higher milk flow rates during milk ejection necessitate a slowing of the sucking rate to accommodate the need of the infant to take a breath after several swallows.

The normal, term infant maintains coordinated, sustained nutritive sucking. The LC may describe this to parents by pointing out that infants generally feed in sucking bursts of 10-30 sucks before pausing briefly to rest (Bamford 1992, Palmer 1993a, Taki 2010). Then they launch into another vigorous burst of sucking. This sucking pattern is repeated several times, and correlates well with observations from Ramsay's (2004a) ultrasound studies that document multiple milk ejections during normal breastfeeding sessions.

Some parents verbalize concerns about infants "using the breast as a pacifier." While the majority of milk transfer occurs early in the feeding, milk intake continues to occur during the later part of a breastfeed, when the breast feels less full and the sucking rate slows. While the mother may not sense all the milk ejections (Ramsay 2004a), the baby is still obtaining milk, and the hind milk is higher in calories.

Research demonstrates that observation alone is not sufficient to assess milk intake in the at-risk infant. Whenever an infant experiences feeding difficulties or there is concern about intake, an accurate scale should be used for assessment (Meier 1994, Sachs 2002).

Abnormal Sucking

Abnormal sucking increases the risk of insufficient milk intake and poor growth. The LC must be able to distinguish between babies who are sucking effectively and those whose sucking rhythms and patterns reveal dysfunction (McBride 1987, Palmer 1993b). It should be noted, however, that ultrasound studies reveal differences in tongue movement between NS and NNS, suggesting that there is an altered sucking action when milk flow is absent (Sakalidis 2012). If abnormal sucking is suspected, the LC must first evaluate whether the milk supply is adequate to rule out altered sucking patterns as the result of low milk flow.

An absent or diminished suck might indicate:

- Central nervous system immaturity (CNS), prematurity
- CNS abnormality (various syndromes)
- Prenatal CNS insults such as exposure to drugs
- Asphyxia, trauma, stroke, sepsis
- Congenital problems (heart disease, hypothyroidism)

A weak suck might indicate:

- CNS abnormalities associated with hypotonia
- Myasthenia gravis or infant botulism
- Medullary lesions
- Abnormalities of the muscles

An uncoordinated suck, marked by mistiming of normal motions or by interference from hyperactive reflexes might indicate:

- History of asphyxia
- Perinatal cerebral insults
- CNS malformations

The variability of sucking patterns over the course of a normal feed should not be confused with the feeding behavior characteristic of a baby who is unable to suck effectively. The impaired infant typically goes to the breast with closed eyes and appears unable to sustain normal nutritive sucking episodes. Short, shallow, choppy jaw excursions, lack of swallowing, and flat behavioral affect are abnormal signs. Test weights are critical to verify the impression that the baby is not transferring milk normally.

Changes in feeding behavior can result from injury or reveal the onset of disease. One of the authors (KH) observed changes in her son's sucking ability at 9 months of age. His increasing low tone, weakened suck, and feed-ing difficulties eventually led to the diagnosis of a brain tumor (see **Fig. 356**).

The Gag Reflex

The gag reflex protects the baby's airway from large objects. Though usually triggered by pressure to the rear of the tongue, it is stimulated at a more shallow depth in the mouths of young infants (Wolf 1992). Some sensitive infants gag with touch pressure on the mid-tongue. The gag reflex is hyperactive in some infants. Constant activation of a noxious stimulus such as the gag reflex can contribute to the acquisition of feeding aversion. Those most at risk include the neurologically compromised infant whose mother has unusually long nipples, infants repeatedly subjected to invasive procedures or insensitive feeding practices, or infants coping with rapid milk ejection.

If the gag reflex is initiated mid-tongue or is hyperactive, the baby may refuse to draw the nipple in deeply enough. As a result of shallow latch, the baby may pinch the nipple, causing the mother pain. Milk intake and milk supply may be compromised. Because a shallow gag reflex may be a developmental issue, time and sensitive feeding practices may remedy the problem. Sometimes oral exercises are useful. These often consist of using pacifiers of increasingly longer length to help the baby tolerate deeper penetration of the oral cavity (see **Fig. 52**).

The Cough Reflex

The cough reflex protects the baby from aspiration of fluid into the airway (Wolf 1992). The cough reflex may be immature in preterm and even some term infants, leading to a phenomenon described as *silent aspiration*. Instead of coughing to clear fluids from the airway, the baby will hold his breath and attempt to swallow. Any cessation of breathing longer than 20 seconds is described as *apnea*. Brief apnea is protective, but prolonged apnea contributes to *bradycardia* (a slowing of the heart rate) and to oxygen desaturation and cyanosis. Chronic coughing can be an important clinical sign of illness or of a swallowing disorder. Coughing *during* feeding can be a sign of a swallowing disorder (dysphagia). Coughing *between* feeds may be in response to milk coming back up as reflux (as in GERD).

Looking Closely at the Baby

The baby in **Fig. 38** was born with a tooth. *Natal teeth* refers to tooth eruption present at birth (Venkatesh 2011). Considered to be common and typically benign, natal teeth may, however, be associated with genetic syndromes and conditions such as congenital hypothyroidism. The mother of the normal infant pictured in **Fig. 38** called the LC complaining of nipple pain and small sores on both nipples resulting from the tooth. Typically teething occurs later when the infant can learn to respond to the mother's instructions about not biting. In this case, management consisted of nipple cleansing and lubrication to prevent infection and brief use of a nipple shield until the nipple wounds healed. The LC suggested prone positioning to help the baby's tongue fall forward, providing more padding over the lower gum.

The baby in **Fig. 39** demonstrates normal lip rounding as she interacts with her mother in a quiet alert state. Note the robust facial tone, manifested by the well-defined philtrum and the bow in the upper lip. This infant has full, rounded cheeks that help stabilize the muscles of the lips. There is facial symmetry with no evidence of droop or weakness.

In contrast, **Fig. 40** pictures a 14 day-old infant with *hypertonic* (excessive tone), "purse string" lips. Note the excessive tension around her lips that is revealed by the pallor of the skin around the lips At the time of the consultation, this baby had never latched. The parents had difficulty inserting even a fingers or a bottle teat into the baby's mouth. This infant was not able to breastfeed in spite of numerous interventions. After several weeks of pumping and bottle-feeding, the discouraged mother discontinued trying to breastfeed.

Compare the hypertonic infant in **Fig. 40** with the infant in **Fig. 41** who demonstrates generalized low tone (*hypotonia*) in her facial features. This 17 day-old infant was still below birth weight and unable to sustain a latch at the breast. Note her thin cheeks (revealed in part by the deep creases under her eyes) and the lack of definition of both the upper lip and philtrum. Most strikingly, the baby is unable to bring her lips into a closed position. Her tongue protrudes. Because of her low facial tone, the baby was unable to form a seal at breast and could not generate suction. Pumped milk fed by bottle helped the baby gain weight, strength, and energy. Her mother elected to obtain Cranial Sacral Therapy (CST), a form of soft tissue massage therapy, to help improve the baby's facial tone. Additionally, the mother performed oral-motor strengthening exercises with the baby on a daily basis (see **Fig. 31**).

Fig. 42 shows the same infant at 5.5 weeks after receiving her fifth session of CST. She gained weight well with bottle-feeds, but still had never breastfed. **Fig. 42** shows the infant achieving lip closure for the first time. Increased weight gain and oral-motor exercise improved her cheek

tone. The lips and philtrum are now more defined. The baby experienced her first effective breastfeeding following massage therapy that day. From then on, the mother reported that each day the infant seemed to get stronger and was able to take more feedings from the breast, especially if the mother assisted by supporting her breast and using breast compression.

Breast compression while breastfeeding is demonstrated in **Fig. 43**. Breast compression helps weak babies obtain more milk and helps transfer higher calorie milk to the baby (Stutte 1988). Within 1 week, this baby was receiving all feeds from the breast.

It is especially important to note that hand expression of milk, breast compression during feeds, and cup feeding of expressed milk are the recommended methods of ensuring adequate milk intake for weak or compromised infants in environments lacking electricity for pumping. Cups may be boiled in hot water and cleaned more easily than bottles. These are life saving interventions during refugee situations, disasters or emergencies.

Lip, cheek, and jaw tone can be evaluated asleep or awake, on a bottle or at the breast. In **Fig. 44** a jaundiced, 4 day-old infant demonstrates poor facial tone during deep sleep. She cannot maintain lip closure. Note her elevated tongue tip and the sucking blister on the upper lip. Her habitual tongue-tip elevation blocked the nipple from entering her mouth each time her mother attempted to latch her to the breast. Due to the ineffective latch, the baby attempted to grab the nipple with her retracted lips, causing a friction callous (see **Figs. 29** and **30**). Lip retraction may be a compensation for low tone, or may reflect excessive tone that prevents the baby from comfortably flanging the lips.

Watching a baby feed from a bottle or feeding tube device may provide helpful clinical insights that explain why an infant cannot breastfeed. Lip retraction can be observed during bottle-feeding, as in **Fig. 45**. This infant is grimacing; a stress cue indicating that the experience is unpleasant.

The jaundiced preterm baby in **Fig. 46** manifests the general low tonality that is common in preterm infants. He leaks milk during bottle-feeding and has difficulty sustaining a latch at breast. Weak lip seal creates breast and bottle-feeding difficulties, and may result from immaturely developed subcutaneous cheek fat pads. Thin cheeks, weak lip seal, and low muscle tone are factors contributing to increased lactation risk among preterm and late-preterm infants (Meier 2007).

Jaw asymmetry is apparent in the infant pictured in **Fig. 47**. Note the droop on the left side of his face involving the lips and cheek as well as the jaw. This boy was never able to breastfeed but did receive pumped milk by bottle for several months He received CST for over a year, along with other forms of physical therapy. At 2 years old, his facial asymmetry was less apparent, although his parents were told he would eventually need orthodontia.

In the case of an infant with physical anomalies or structural deformities, early identification of the impact upon feeding is crucial. The mother, particularly, needs to know that the child's breastfeeding problems do not result from failure or lack of skill on her part. It is necessary, in such circumstances, to recommend more aggressive measures to protect the milk supply. Neglecting to begin pumping during the important milk calibration phase (the first few weeks postpartum) may contribute to what Woolridge (1992) calls an *acquired low milk supply*.

Jaw Support

The mother of the infant in **Fig. 48** has placed her finger under the baby's chin to help stabilize jaw excursions that are too wide. This infant loses the breast when his jaw swings too wide, causing a break in the lip seal. The firmly placed finger helps grade the width of the jaw excursion, preventing the baby from opening too wide. The LC should teach the mother to place the supporting finger forward under the bony part of the chin. If placed under the soft part of the baby's chin, it may choke the baby.

Depressed Reflexes

If a baby becomes apathetic only when the mother attempts to breastfeed, but has normal reflexes the rest of the time, the baby may be stressed about some aspect of feeding. Behavioral, respiratory, or swallowing issues should be investigated. However, a baby who consistently manifests low reflexive arousal may be ill, affected by medications, have CNS depression, injury, or have a sensory-based feeding problem (Palmer 1993b).

The 1 week-old infant in **Fig. 49** demonstrates a depressed rooting reflex. Taking her clothes off (**Fig. 50**) helped her rouse. Effective arousal following a minor intervention such as undressing is reassuring. It suggests that this is a normal baby who was merely in the wrong state for feeding (see the discussion of state behavior in Ch. 2).

Feeding Affect

Normal infants feed robustly. They go to the breast with open eyes and feed with apparent enjoyment. They suck in sustained bursts. Contrast that norm with the appearance of the distressed 37 week gestational age infant in

Fig. 51. This mother's large, long nipples triggered a gag reflex each time the baby tried to latch. This preterm baby needed 6 weeks of growth and maturation before she was able to comfortably latch to her mother's nipples. The mother, a busy physician, returned to work at 4 weeks postpartum. Once reassured that this "fit" problem would resolve over time, she pumped and bottle-fed the baby. As the mother described her situation, her nipples "competed well" with bottle teats. Once the baby grew big enough to accommodate the nipples, the mother continued to breast and bottle-feed until the baby was 18 months old (see Ch. 10 for a detailed discussion of the effect of nipple size on breastfeeding).

Oral Aversion

Repeated trauma to the oral and pharyngeal regions may alter an infant's sensory perceptions, creating avoidance behavior or aversion (Palmer 1993b). Swallowing dysfunction or an upper-airway obstruction may disrupt oral feeding and create aversive behaviors that interfere with establishing normal feeding (Miller 2007).

The 6 week-old infant born at term pictured in **Fig. 52** experienced a month-long stay in the NICU as the result of a serious lung infection. He was intubated for several weeks and developed sensory defensiveness. He refused the breast and was extremely difficult to bottle-feed as well. His parents were trained to gavage feed him during the night, and most of his milk intake occured while he slept. Because the original airway obstruction had since resolved, he can be described at this point as having a *non-organic*, behaviorally-based feeding problem.

The LC and an OT worked together with the parents to help this baby overcome his oral defensiveness. Here the LC shows the mother how to use a pacifier to play with the baby's lips. The pacifier (or a finger) is gradually penetrated to increasing depth, but only as the infant will permit it. Note the baby's interested, relaxed facial expression. The pacifier is removed if the infant begins to look or act stressed. Therapeutic exercises with a pacifier can be useful for infants with tone problems as well. This activity helps the baby grip with lips and tongue, and it gives the baby the opportunity to strengthen the muscles of the soft palate during non-nutritive sucking. The goal is to improve breastfeeding ability and resolve aversion (Lessen 2011).

Torticollis

Torticollis refers to a contracted state of the muscles of the neck, producing a twisting of the neck and unnatural position of the head (van Vlimmeren 2006). The 12 day-old, term infant pictured in **Fig. 53** developed torticollis, presumably from her breech position in the womb. Note the slight facial asymmetry, the pull of the head to the left, and the baby's general physical rigidity.

The baby was initially unable to breastfeed. She could not form lip seal because excessive muscle tension on the left side of her neck interfered with her jaw alignment. This is illustrated in **Fig. 54** where she is pictured bottle-feeding. Note the gape and break in seal at the corner of her mouth as her head pulls toward the affected side. Hip flexion is being used to improve postural stability at the neck, head, and lips. Over time, physical therapy helped reduce this child's muscle spasms and improved the range of motion of her head and neck. She was able to partially breastfeed by 4 weeks of age, assisted by a nipple shield that helped compensate for her weak ability to create seal and suction. By age 2, physical therapy had successfully resolved her problems, and her physical appearance normalized.

Other Unusual Presentations

The infant in **Fig. 55** has an ear tag. An isolated ear tag is a minor anomaly consisting of a rudimentary bud of ear tissue, often with a core of cartilage, usually located just in front of the ear. Isolated ear tags are felt to be benign. However, since the ears and the kidneys form at about the same period of intrauterine development, infants with ear tags are generally screened for renal anomalies (Kohelet 2000). The infant in **Fig. 55** was medically evaluated prior to discharge and the parents were relieved to learn that their baby did not have a kidney anomaly. The baby previously discussed in **Fig. 33** has an unusually shaped ear, and also was screened to rule out renal anomalies.

The presence of 2 or more minor anomalies in a child increases the probability of a major malformation. Patients with auricular (ear) anomalies should be assessed carefully for accompanying *dysmorphic* (abnormally formed) features, including facial asymmetry (Wang 2001). Whenever an infant has difficulty breastfeeding, underlying anomalies and illness must be ruled out.

The infant in **Fig 56**, who appears to be wearing a vest has a large hairy *nevus*. A nevus is a type of mole or birth-mark. Like a mole, it can become cancerous, so changes in appearance should be reported to a physician. This condition does not affect breastfeeding.

Congenital dermal melanocytosis is pictured in **Fig. 57**. Formerly called Mongolian spots, this type of birthmark is a benign bluish or bruised appearing mark, typically located on the lower back or buttocks. Sometimes mistaken for signs of abuse, it may fade over time, or may persist for

years. This type of birthmark is most often observed in infants with Asian or African ancestry.

Epstein's Pearls, seen in **Fig. 58**, are small white epithelial cysts usually found in the midline of the palate in newborn infants at the junction of the hard and soft palates (Genna 2013). Sometimes mistaken for oral thrush, these benign cysts do not spread and typically disappear a few weeks after birth. Oral thrush, in contrast, produces asymmetrical white plaques that rapidly spread.

The 6 week-old infant in **Fig. 59** has a hemangioma on her upper lip. Infantile hemangiomas are very common and consist of raised red or purple discolorations of the skin that develop shortly after birth, grow rapidly, and often involute. Most are localized, painless, benign, and will fade or disappear as the child grows. Others may require medical or surgical intervention if their size or location affects vision or feeding. Some infantile facial hemangiomas are associated with neurological, opthalmic, and cardiac anomalies. Hemangiomas involving the upper lip are generally limited to the philtrum or are unilateral (Haggstrom 2006). The infant pictured here is growing well, and her hemangioma, while it disfigures her lip, does not interfere with her breastfeeding ability.

Fig. 60 shows a mother engaged in skin-to-skin holding with her newborn. Skin-to-skin care facilitates bonding between the baby and all members of the family, and should be encouraged, particularly with mothers and fathers.

Hand Hygiene

We offer a brief note on the use of gloves by the authors (as seen in various photos throughout *The Breastfeeding Atlas*). The use of examination gloves remains somewhat controversial in the field of lactation. The argument revolves around the issue of whether use of gloves "medicalizes" breastfeeding assistance. In addition, wearing gloves is not a substitute for hand hygiene. Fuller (2011) observed that the rate of compliance with hand washing was significantly lower when gloves were worn by healthcare workers. The LC who wears gloves during infant oral examination or when touching the breasts of a woman with a suspected infection must wash their hands before and after gloving. Gloving is also advised during examination of the mother and baby if the LC has open cuts on her hands.

Proponents of evidence-based care have emphasized the importance of utilizing research to support clinical practice. Hand hygiene has been singled out as the most important measure in preventing *nosocomial infections*

(infections acquired in health care settings) (Lam 2004). And yet, research indicates that health care provider compliance with hand hygiene is poor (Harbath 2001). This issue is of special concern with regard to preterm and ill babies, who are particularly vulnerable to nosocomial infection (Hanrahan 2004). Whatever the gestational age of their baby, all new mothers have the right to know that their caregivers are scrupulous about hand hygiene.

During hospital, clinic, and home visits, the LC comes in contact with other children (often with respiratory symptoms) and with pets. It is easy to transmit organisms on the hands and under fingernails (Pittet 2001, CDC 2002). Scales, clip boards, pens, and other surfaces may also become contaminated with viruses or bacteria (Hanrahan 2004). These objects should be routinely cleaned with sterilizing wipes between patients. Observance of infection control practices has become even more critical with the spread of antibiotic-resistant strains of bacteria, including *Clostridium difficile* (*C difficile*) and Methicillin-resistant *Staphylococcus aureus* (MRSA). MRSA infections among postpartum women may manifest as mastitis, and are associated with increased risk of progression to breast abscess (Saiman 2003, Reddy 2007).

MRSA infections in hospitalized infant populations have been documented in neonatal special care units and pediatric departments (Kitajima 2003). Community acquired MRSA has also been documented with increasing frequency, resulting in hospital readmission of young infants (Fortunov 2007). Infants may be exposed by carrier medical staff, family members, and even pets. Therefore, it is best for mothers to hold and breastfeed immediately after birth in order to colonize their infants with normal bacteria; to room-in with their infants; and to minimize non-essential interventions by staff (Kitajima 2003). Mothers should remind caregivers to wash their hands prior to handling the infant.

LCs in all practice settings should wash their hands carefully before and after consultations. Alcohol-based hand cleansers may be used to clean the hands (Stone 2012). For infant oral exams and for examination of breasts or nipples when open sores are present, the LC should wash his or her hands before and after the consultation and wear non-latex gloves or finger cots (see **Fig. 32**).

Abadie U, Andre A, Zaouche A, et al. Early feeding resistance: a possible consequence of neonatal oro-oesophageal dyskinesia. *Acta Paediatrica* 2001; 90(7):738-745.

Alper M. Dysphagia in infants and children with oral-motor deficits: assessment and management. *Seminars in Speech and Language* 1996; 17(4):283-309.

Bamford O, Taciak V, Gewold IH. The relationship between rhythmic swallowing and breathing during suckle feeding in term neonates. *Pediatric Research* 1992; 31(6):619-624.

Baudon J, Renault F, Goutet J, et al. Assessment of dysphagia in infants with facial malformations. *European Journal of Pediatrics* 2009; 168(2):187-193.

Beals S, Joganic E. Form and function in craniofacial deformities. *Seminars in Pediatric Neurology* 2004; 11(4):238-242.

Bosma J. Structure and Function of the Infant Oral and Pharyngeal Mechanisms, in J Wilson, ed. *Oral-motor Function and Dysfunction in Children.* Chapel Hill, NC: University of North Carolina at Chapel Hill, 1977; May 25-28, p. 46.

Brake S, Fifer W, Alfasi G, et al. The first nutritive sucking responses of premature newborns. *Infant Behavior and Development* 1988; 11:1-9.

Burton P, Deng J, McDonald D, et al. Real-time 3D ultrasound imaging of infant tongue movements during breastfeeding. *Early Human Development* 2013; May 13, ahead of print.

Center for Disease Control (CDC). Guidelines for Hand Hygiene in Healthcare Settings. Recommendations and Reports 2002; 51(RR16):1-44. Available at: http://www.cdc.gov/handhygiene/Guidelines.html. Accessed July 2012.

Fortunov R, Hulten K, Hammerman W, et al. Evaluation and treatment of Community-Acquired *Staphylococcus aureus* infections in term and late-preterm previously healthy neonates. *Pediatrics* 2007; 120(5):937-945.

Fuller C, Savage J, Besser S, et al. "The dirty hand in the latex glove": a study of hand hygiene compliance when gloves are worn. *Infection Control Hospital Epidemiology* 2011; 32(12):1194-1199.

Geddes DT, Kent JC, Mitoulas LR, et al. Tongue movement and intraoral vacuum in breastfeeding infants. *Early Human Development* 2008; 84(7):471-477.

Geddes D, McClennen H, Kent J, et al. Patterns of respiration in infants during breastfeeding. Proceedings of the 13th International Conference of the International Society for Research in Human Milk and Lactation Sept. 22-26, 2006; Niagara-on-the-Lake, Ontario, Canada.

Genna CW. *Supporting Sucking Skills in Breastfeeding Infants.* Boston: Jones and Bartlett, 2013a; pp. 12; 334.

Genna CW. Infant Anatomy for Feeding, in R Mannel, P Martens, M Walker (editors), *Core Curriculum for Lactation Consultants 3rd ed.* Boston: Jones and Bartlett Learning, 2013b; p. 282.

Glass R, Wolf L. Incoordination of sucking, swallowing, and breathing as an etiology for breastfeeding difficulty. *Journal of Human Lactation* 1994; 10(3):185-189.

Goldfield E, Buonomo C, Fletcher K, et al. Premature infant swallowing: patterns of tongue-soft palate coordination based upon videofluoroscopy. *Infant Behavioral Development* 2010; 33(2):209-218.

Hall J. Importance of muscle movement for normal craniofacial development. *Journal of Craniofacial Surgery* 2010; 21(4):1336-1338.

Hafstrom M, Kjellmer I. Non-nutritive sucking in the healthy pre-term infant. *Early Human Development* 2000; 60(1):13-24.

Haggstrom A, Lammer E, Schneider R, et al. Patterns of infantile hemangiomas: new clues to hemangioma pathogenesis and embryonic facial development. *Pediatrics* 2006; 117(3):698-703.

Hanrahan K, Lofgren M. Evidence-based practice: examining the risk of toys in the microenvironment of infants in the neonatal intensive care unit. *Advances in Neonatal Care* 2004; 4(4):184-201.

Harbath S, Pittet D, Grady L, et al. Compliance with hand hygiene practice in pediatric intensive care. *Pediatric Critical Care Medicine* 2001; 2(4):311-314.

International Board of Lactation Consultant Examiners (IBLCE). *Principle 4, Code of Professional Conduct.* International Board Certified Lactation Consultants, Falls Church, VA, 2011. Accessed June 2012.

Kitajima H. Prevention of Methicillin-resistant *Staphylococcus aureus* infections in neonates. *Pediatrics International* 2003; 45:238-245.

Kohelet D, Arbel E. A prospective search for urinary tract abnormalities in infants with isolated preauricular tags. *Pediatrics* 2000; 105(5):e61.

Lam B, Lee J, Lau Y, et al. Hand hygiene practices in a neonatal intensive care unit: a multimodal intervention and impact on nosocomial infection. *Pediatrics* 2004; 114(5):e565-e571.

Lessen BS. Effect of the premature infant oral motor intervention on feeding progression and length of stay in preterm infants. *Advances in Neonatal Care* 2011; 11(2):129-139.

McBride M, Danner S. Sucking disorders in neurologically impaired infants: assessment and facilitation of breastfeeding. *Clinics in Perinatology* 1987; 14(1):109-130.

Meier P, Engstrom J, Crichton C, et al. A new scale for in-home test-weighing for mothers of preterm and high risk infants. *Journal of Human Lactation* 1994; 10(3):163-168.

Meier PP, Furman LM, Dengenhardt M. Increased lactation risk for late preterm infants and mothers: evidence and management strategies to protect breastfeeding. *Journal of Midwifery and Women's Health* 2007; 52(6):579-587.

Miller CK, Willging JP. The implications of upper-airway obstruction on successful infant feeding. *Seminars in Speech and Language* 2007; 28(3):190-203.

Morris S. Sensorimotor Prerequisites for Speech and the Influence of Cerebral Palsy, in I Wilson, ed. *Oral-motor Function and Dysfunction in Children.* Chapel Hill, NC: University of North Carolina at Chapel Hill, 1977; May 25-28, pp. 123-132.

Narayanan I, Mehta R, Choudhury D, et al. Sucking on the 'emptied' breast: non-nutritive sucking with a difference. *Archives of Disease in Childhood* 1991; 66(2):241-244.

Ogg L. Oral-pharyngeal development and evaluation. *Physical Therapy* 1975; 55(3):235-241.

Palmer M. Identification and management of the transitional suck pattern in premature infants. *Journal of Perinatal and Neonatal Nursing* 1993a; 7(1):66-75.

Palmer M, Heyman M. Assessment and treatment of sensory-versus motor-based feeding problems in very young children. *Infants and Young Children* 1993b; 6(2):67-73.

Phillipp BL. Teaching in Thirty: Tongue-tie. Presentation at Philadelphia Breastfeeding Promotion MotherBaby Summit -- Next Steps: Using your mPINC Score to Leverage Change. Philadelphia, PA. March 23, 2012.

Pinelli J, Symington A. Non-nutritive sucking for promoting physiologic stability and nutrition in preterm infants. *Cochrane Database System Review* 2005. 19(4):CD001071

Pittet D. Improving adherence to hand hygiene practice: a multidisciplinary approach. *Emerging Infectious Diseases* 2001; 7(2):234-240.

Premji S, Paes B. Gastrointestinal function and growth in premature infants: is non-nutritive sucking vital? *Journal of Perinatology* 2000; 20(1):46-53.

Ramsay D, Kent J, Owens R. Ultrasound imaging of milk ejection in the breast of lactating women. *Pediatrics* 2004a; 113(2):361-367.

Ramsay D, Mitoulas L, Kent J, et al. Ultrasound imaging of the sucking mechanics of the breastfeeding infants. Proceedings of the 12th International Conference of the International Society for Research in Human Milk and Lactation, Sept. 10-14, 2004b; Queen's College, Cambridge, UK.

Ranly D. Early orofacial development. *Journal of Clinical Pediatric Dentistry* 1998; 22(4):267-275.

Reddy P, Qi C, Zembower T, et al. Postpartum mastitis and Community-acquired Methicillin-resistant *Staphylococcus aureus.* *Emerging Infectious Diseases* 2007; 13(2):298-301.

Saiman L, O'Keefe M, Graham P, et al. Hospital transmission of Community-acquired Methicillin-resistant *Staphylococcus aureus* among postpartum women. *Clinical Infectious Diseases* 2003; 37(15 Nov):1313-1319.

Sachs M, Oddie S. Breastfeeding - weighing in the balance: reappraising the role of weighing babies in the early days. *MIDIRS Midwifery Digest* 2002; 12(3):296-300.

Sakalidis VS, Williams TM, Garbin CP. Ultrasound imaging of infant sucking dynamics during the establishment of lactation. *Journal of Human Lactation* 2013; 29(2):205-213.

Sapin S, Miller A, Bass H. Neonatal asymmetric crying facies: a new look at an old problem. *Clinical Pediatrics* 2005; 44(2):109-119.

Smith JD, Crumley RL, Harker LA. Facial paralysis in the newborn. *Otolaryngology, Head and Neck Surgery* 1981; 89(6):1021-1024.

Stone S, Fuller C, Savage J, et al. Evaluation of the national Cleanyourhands campaign to reduce *Staphylococcus aureus* bacteraemia and *Clostridium difficile* infection in hospitals in England and Wales by improved hand hygiene: four year study, prospective, ecological, interrupted time series study. *British Medical Journal* 2012; 3(344):e3005.

Stutte P, Bowles B, Morman G. The effects of breast massage on volume and fat content of milk. *Genesis* 1988; 10(2):22-25.

Taki M, Mizuno K, Murase M, et al. Maturational changes in the feeding behavior of infants - a comparison between breastfeeding and bottle feeding. *Acta Paediatrica* 2010; 99:61-67.

van Vlimmeren LA, Helders PJ, van Adrichem LN, et al. Torticollis and plagiocephaly in infancy: therapeutic strategies. *Pediatric Rehabilitation* 2006; 9(1):40-46.

Venkatesh C, Adhisivam B. Natal teeth in an infant with congenital hypothryoidism. *Indian Journal of Dental Research* 2011; 22(3):498.

Wall V. Mandibular asymmetry and breastfeeding problems: experience from 11 cases. *Journal of Human Lactation* 2006; 22(3):326-334.

Wang R, Earl D, Ruder R, et al. Syndromic ear anomalies and renal ultrasounds. *Pediatrics* 2001; 108(2):e32.

Wolf L, Glass R. *Feeding and Swallowing Disorders in Infancy.* Tucson, AZ: Therapy Skill Builders, 1992; pp. 25-29,106-108, 114-122.

Woolridge M. The 'anatomy' of infant sucking. *Midwifery* 1986; 2(4):164-167.

Woolridge M. The Analysis, Classification, Etiology of Diagnosed Low Milk Output. Conference Presentation, La Leche League of Texas Area Conference. Houston, TX. July, 1992.

Woolridge M. Nutritional, management and clinical implications of revised suckling physiology. Conference presentation, ILCA Conference, Orlando, FL. July 27, 2012.

Infant Stools, Urine, and Vaginal Discharge

The elimination patterns of breastfed infants help assess infant hydration status and risk for excessive weight loss and jaundice (Chen 2011, AAP 2012). The absence of daily bowel movements in the first weeks suggests inadequate milk intake, delayed onset of copious milk production, increased risk of hyperbilirubinemia, or bowel blockage (Dewey 2003, Shrago 2006, Nommsen-Rivers 2008, Ameh 2009).

Clinics and hospitals often provide parents with log forms to help them monitor the number of diapers changed each day in the first week postpartum. The rationale for recording diaper output is that it is a rough proxy for determining milk intake in the breastfeeding infant. Several infant stool reporting forms utilizing photographs have been developed (Hoover 2002, Bekkali 2009). Pollard (2011) concluded that such log forms "may be a valuable tool" to help parents and health workers assess newborn feeding.

Owing to a lack of education in normal stooling and voiding patterns, parents worry that their baby is constipated, has diarrhea, or they may fear that a normal vaginal discharge is a sign of illness. Breastfeeding mothers may conclude that changes in bowel or urine color indicate that their diet is adversely affecting the baby's digestion or that the baby has allergies. Anticipatory guidance should be provided to minimize such fears.

The most accurate way to determine adequate milk intake is to weigh the baby. The AAP recommends all breastfeeding infants be seen by a pediatrician at 3 to 5 days of age or within 48 to 72 hours after hospital discharge. Close follow-up may be required for infants whose stooling patterns deviate from the expected norms and whose mothers experience delays in the onset of adequate milk production.

Normal Appearance of Stools

A baby's first stools are black tar-like meconium (**Fig. 61**). Within a few days of birth, the stools lighten in color to greenish brown (**Fig. 62**). Early transition to yellow stool is associated with less infant weight loss and earlier weight gain (Shrago 2006). Long, stressful labor or cesarean delivery may delay lactogenesis stage II, the onset of copious milk production (Chen 1998, Dewey 2003). A delay in the onset of lactogenesis II is defined as >72 hours without signs of increased milk production. Fewer than 4 stools daily by Day 4 and delayed onset of lactogenesis II are risk factors for inadequate lactation (Nommsen-Rivers 2008). If an infant has low diaper counts and fails to

produce yellow stools by Day 7, a follow-up weight check should be obtained in the health care office.

Well-feeding breastfed infants typically stool frequently, often with each feeding. **Fig. 63** shows the 24-hour output of a term newborn on Day 3.

Research has demonstrated the validity of maternal perception of the timing of lactogenesis stage II, commonly referred to as the milk "coming in" (Chapman 2000). Because women can reliably identify whether or not this event has occurred, it is important to ask if a mother's milk has come in. This is a useful screening question with important public health implications because delayed lactogenesis II is a risk factor both for shorter breastfeeding duration and greater infant weight loss by Day 3 (Perez-Escamilla 2001). Sleepy infants, especially of first-time mothers, may understimulate early milk production, increasing their risk for hypernatremic dehydration with associated risk of seizure and even death (Ozdogan 2006). The first sign of these problems may be delayed transition to light colored stools or lack of stooling.

Lack of infant stooling in the first week postpartum is a problem parents should be instructed to discuss with their health care provider. In order to do this, parents need to know how to describe and evaluate stool color and output. Some parents fail to distinguish between small and substantial stooling. This can cause confusion, especially during telephone screening. Ideally, graphic verbal descriptions or photos can be provided to help parents better communicate with their health care providers.

Fig. 64 provides a graphic comparison of the sizes of 2 transitional-colored bowel movements. By Day 4, it is normal for babies to produce 4 or more stools in the course of 24 hours; some large and some small. Caregivers should request a weight check if a parent reports that a newborn fails to stool during any 24-hour period, or if all the daily bowel movements are small. **Fig. 65** shows a coin comparison to provide parents with a vocabulary to describe the size of bowel movements. In order for the stool to "count," it must be larger than 24 mm, about the size of a US quarter (Shrago 2006).

Quick passage of meconium is not only a marker for less weight loss, it is a marker for lower risk of developing jaundice (de Carvalho 1985, Yamauchi 1990). In a study of 358 Nigerian mothers exclusively breastfeeding their term infants, mothers averaged 13 feeds each 24 hours during the first 7 days. High frequency of breastfeeding was associated with rapid passage of meconium and lower neonatal serum bilirubin levels on Days 3 and 7 (Okechukwa 2006).

While it is important to avoid alarming the mother whose baby is feeding adequately in spite of slightly low diaper counts, it is also important not to falsely reassure the inexperienced mother whose baby may be breastfeeding poorly. The key public health message is that adequate intake in the healthy neonate typically is associated with frequent stooling (Nyhan 1952, Neifert 1996, AAP 2012). Breastfed newborns are seldom constipated. Scant stooling in the first month should be reported as a red flag for poor feeding (Caglar 2006). Rare causes of lack of stooling in a newborn infant include malrotation of the intestines, bowel blockage, constipation, and Hirschsprung's disease.

Exclusive Breastfeeding and Infant Gut Health

The most important determinants of infant gut microbe composition are the following: mode of delivery, gestational age, infant hospitalization, antibiotic treatment of the infant, and type of infant feeding. "Term infants who were born vaginally at home and were breastfed exclusively seemed to have the most 'beneficial' gut microbiota (highest numbers of bifidobacteria and lowest numbers of *C difficile* and *E coli*)" in their stools (Penders 2006). Exposure to maternal bacterial strains in the birth canal has been assumed to be the primary source of innoculation and colonization of the infant. However, breast milk and infant feces from mother-infant pairs share the same strains of bacteria. This suggests that breastfeeding contributes to the transfer of bacteria from mother to baby (Martin 2012).

In emergency situations, when neither own mother's milk nor donor human milk from a safe source is available, some infants must be stabilized on formula. However, exposure of the permeable infant gut to foreign proteins creates documented risk to the infant. Disruption of exclusive breastfeeding should never be done without a sound medical rationale. The mother's need to rest or the desire of a relative to bottle feed the baby are not valid reasons to risk damage to the newborn gut and disruption of the normal colonization of the intestinal tract conferred by exclusive breastfeeding. One thorough review of the risks of formula feeding is, *Supplementation of the Breastfed Baby: "Just One Bottle Won't Hurt --Or Will It?"* (Walker 2010).

Colic

While human milk fed infants have been shown to have healthy guts, colic still may affect them. Research into infant colic using molecular methods to evaluate gut colonization patterns in healthy versus control infants has identified coliform bacterias (such as *E coli*) and other pathogens such as *Helicobacter pylori (H pylori)* to be more abundant in colicky infants (Savino 2009, Ali 2012). Colic affects from 5 to 40 percent of infants and prevalence of colic is similar among exclusively breastfed, formula fed, and mixed fed infants. In Ali's 2012 study, antigen testing of stools revealed that 81.8 percent of case infants with colic tested positive for *H pylori* compared to 23.3 percent of the control infants. One study of 1,021 Turkish children observed that infants with colic in the first 2 months tended to have less frequent stooling during the first 2 years of life (Tunc 2008). Perhaps in the future, such research will establish treatments for colic.

The normal stools of breastmilk-fed babies occasionally look watery (**Fig. 66**). Constant watery, explosive stools may be a sign of milk oversupply.

Sometimes the stools of a breastfed baby resemble mustard mixed with sesame seeds (**Fig. 67**).

Some stools may appear to contain curds (**Fig. 68**) and will be bright yellow like the stool of this 6 day-old baby.

Maternal vitamins, medications, certain vegetables (notably, beets), flavored fruit drinks, *et cetera* can stain a mother's milk, causing temporary discoloration of the bowel movement and of urine (Lawrence 2011). **Fig. 69** pictures the diaper of a 3 week-old infant whose mother had just begun taking a new vitamin compound. A temporary appearance of green-colored stool in an otherwise healthy infant is not generally a cause for concern.

Anecdotal reports suggest that some infants older than 1 month stool infrequently. So long as general health and weight gain continue to track at reference standards, infrequent stooling in the totally breastfed older baby is not considered to be a problem. Most breastfeeding mothers continue to observe frequent stooling, often with each diaper change until solids are begun at around 6 months. The diapers in **Fig. 70** represent the 24-hour output of a 13 lb 4 oz (5999 g) 8 week-old male. His birth weight was 7 lb 11 oz (3480 g).

Fig. 71 shows the more formed, solid-appearing stools of a 7 month-old infant who began complimentary foods at 6 months of age. The addition of solid food, juice, or formula will cause both texture, odor, and color changes in the stool. Once solids are introduced, loose or foul smelling stools are typically symptoms of illness or infection and should be reported to the child's health care provider. Diarrhea can rapidly cause dehydration in infants.

Urination

Urination is an accepted marker for adequate hydration, but is less clinically accurate at predicting adequate lactation performance (Nommsen-Rivers 2008). In one study, infant weight loss of greater than 7 per cent was observed in the infants with significantly more total voids and higher breastfeeding frequency on day 2 (Mulder 2010). The researchers speculated that, in the absence of other indicators of suboptimal breastfeeding, some babies may be experiencing a physiologic diuresis after birth, unrelated to their feeding behavior.

Adequately hydrated newborns produce 1 or more wet diapers on day 1, 2 or more wet diapers on day 2, and on day 3 produce 3 or more urine soaked diapers (Lawrence 2011).

Parents using disposable diapers may have difficulty assessing the degree of wetness, although some new brands of disposable diapers have visible "wetness strips" that change color when the baby urinates. When instructing parents about monitoring wet diapers, some lactation consultants suggest putting a facial tissue or piece of toilet paper into the disposable diaper in order to better detect when the baby has urinated. Others advise using cloth diapers during the first week when diaper monitoring is more critical. Another tip is to encourage parents to pour 3 tablespoons (45 cc) of water into a diaper and compare its weight to that of a dry diaper. The baby should produce at least 6 wet diapers of this weight each day by Day 7.

Brick Dust Urine

It is not abnormal to see brick dust urine (indicative of the presence of uric acid crystals) in the diapers of some infants in the first 3 days after birth. It is sometimes mistaken for a blood stain. The persistence of uric acid crystals in the diapers past Day 3 or the onset of their appearance after Day 3 is a warning sign of poor milk transfer and dehydration (Neifert 1996, Caglar 2006).

Fig. 72 shows brick dust urine in a diaper. A diaper containing concentrated or dark urine is an indication that the baby is not taking in sufficient volumes of milk and requires further evaluation. Black (2001) observed that "...it is common for 3 day-old, breastfed infants to urinate only once in the 24 hours before the mother's milk 'comes in.'" Therefore, if diapers are scant during this time period, it is necessary to carefully assess for risk factors for delayed lactogenesis. If the mother and baby lack known risk factors, a wait-and-see policy can be adopted with regard to the necessity for introducing supplementation to protect against infant dehydration.

Excessive infant crying has been associated with urinary tract infection (UTI). Any newborn with a UTI due to *E coli* should have urine screening to rule out *galactosemia,* a condition which is a rare contraindication of breastfeeding (Merewood 2001). Galactosemia is an inherited disorder of galactose metabolism, an inability to digest the sugar in milk. In the US, infants are routinely screened for galactosemia at birth. Affected infants must receive specialized formulas in order to survive. Symptoms include jaundice, hypoglycemia, vomiting, failure to thrive and a susceptibility to *E coli* sepsis that may manifest as a UTI.

Abnormal Stools

Some breastfed infants stool each time they feed. Because of the frequent stooling pattern, parents need reassurance that diarrhea in the breastfed baby is accompanied by other signs of illness, such as fever and malaise, foul smell, or blood in the stool. Report such signs to medical care providers.

Human milk protects young infants from diarrhea. Risk increases when weaning foods are introduced at 6 months of age. Parents in some environments may need instruction about food safety when they begin complementary feeding in order to minimize their infant's exposure to food-borne pathogens (WHO 1993).

Breastfed babies older than 1 month may stool less frequently than newborns; however, their stools will remain loose and unformed (Tham 1996, Tunc 2008). One large study investigating the normal defecation pattern of healthy infants observed that stooling frequency in breastfeeding infants decreased significantly during the first 3 months from 3.65 to 1.88 times per day (den Hertog 2012). No significant changes in stooling frequency were observed in formula or mixed feeding infants. At every age, breastfed infants stooled more frequently, and their feces were softer and more yellow-colored. Green stool color was associated with formula feeding.

Parents may observe gradual changes in the appearance of the stool of their exclusively breastfed baby over time. Slightly thicker stools in the older baby may perhaps be connected to changes in the whey to casein ratio in human milk, which varies depending upon the stage of lactation (Kunz 1992). During early lactation, the whey to casein ratio is 90:10. It is 50:50 in late lactation. Whey proteins aide digestion and promote critical immunological functions. The whey factor of human milk contains many beneficial components, including 401 different enzymes, lactoferrin (which promotes growth of protective gut bacteria such as lactobacilli), and Secretory immunoglobulin A (SIgA), which coats mucosal surfaces, preventing penetration by pathogens. The whey to casein ratio is reversed in bovine milk, with casein predominating (Smith 2013). Sudden changes in stooling patterns can be a marker for illness. For example, one of the first signs of infant botulism is lack of stooling (Stiefel 1996). A sudden change in stooling should prompt questions about the baby. Is the baby active and alert? Diarrhea, changed feeding behavior, changes in tone, or increased crying should be reported to the medical care provider immediately.

Blood in the Stools

Blood in the stool (**Fig. 73**) can have multiple causes:

- small anal fissures
- infection
- sensitivity to something in the mother's diet
- a reaction triggered by a food or drug the baby is directly ingesting
- internal bleeding from another cause

The appropriate reaction to the discovery of blood in the stool is a referral to the primary care provider for evaluation. Modern tests are about 90 percent accurate in localizing the bleeding site. The most common reason for bright red blood that coats, but is not mixed with the stool, is bleeding in the anorectal area. Darker blood or blood more mixed in with the stools may indicate bleeding from a site higher in the intestinal tract (Silber 1990). While alarming to parents, blood in the stool often occurs in infants who are otherwise well and growing normally. Blood in the stool of the breastfed baby has been attributed to cow milk allergy. New research suggests that cow milk allergy may have been over diagnosed in the past. Rectal bleeding in infants often resolves without definitive diagnosis, leading some to describe it as a "benign and self-limiting disorder" (Arvola 2006).

Vaginal Discharge

A baby girl may have a bloody vaginal discharge (**Fig. 74**). This is caused by withdrawal of maternal hormones from the baby's system after birth and generally will subside within a few days. White vaginal discharges (**Fig. 75**) are also common. Persistent or foul-smelling discharge should be reported to the HCP, along with persistent diaper rashes that do not resolve with usual measures of airing, frequent diaper changes, and applications of non-irritating diaper ointments and creams.

Ali AM. *Heliocobacter pylori* and infantile colic. *Archives of Pediatric and Adolescent Medicine* 2012; 166(7):648-650.

American Academy of Pediatrics (AAP) Section on Breastfeeding. Breastfeeding and the use of human milk. *Pediatrics* 2012; 129(3): e827-e841.

Ameh N, Ameh EA. Timing of passage of first meconium and stooling pattern in normal Nigerian newborns. *Annals of Tropical Paediatrics* 2009; 29(2):129-133.

Arvola T, Ruuska R, Keranen J, et al. Rectal bleeding in infancy: clinical, allergological, and microbiological examination. *Pediatrics* 2006; 117(4):e760-768.

Bekkali N, Hamers SL, Reitsma JB, et al. Infant stool form scale: development and results. *Journal of Pediatrics* 2009; 154(4):521-526.

Black LS. Incorporating breastfeeding care into daily newborn rounds and pediatric office practice. in RJ Schanler. *Pediatric Clinics of North America: Breastfeeding 2001, Part II*. The Management of Breastfeeding; 48(2):299-319. p. 302.

Caglar MK, Ozer I, Altugan FS. Risk factors for excess weight loss and hypernatremia in exclusively breast-fed infants. *Brazilian Journal of Medical and Biological Research* 2006; 39(4):539-544.

Chapman D, Perez-Escamilla R. Maternal perception of the onset of lactation is a valid, public health indicator of lactogenesis stage II. *Journal of Nutrition* 2000; 130(12):2972-2980.

Chen CF, Hsu MC, Shen CH, et al. Influence of breastfeeding on weight loss, jaundice and waste elimination in neonates. *Pediatric Neonatology* 2011; 52(2):89-92.

Chen DC, Nommsen-Rivers L, Dewey KG, et al. Stress during labor and delivery and early lactation performance. *American Journal of Clinical Nutrition* 1998; 68(2):335-344.

de Carvalho M, Robertson S, Klaus M. Fecal bilirubin excretion and serum bilirubin concentrations in breast-fed and bottle-fed infants. *Journal of Pediatrics* 1985; 107(5):786-790.

den Hertog J, van Leengoed E. Kolk F, et al. The defecation pattern of healthy term infants up to the age of 3 months. *Archives of Disease in Childhood. Fetal and Neonatal Edition.* 2012; 97(6):F465-470.

Dewey K, Nommsen-Rivers M, Heinig MJ. Risk factors for suboptimal infant breastfeeding behavior, delayed onset of lactation, and excess neonatal weight loss. *Pediatrics* 2003; 112(3):607-619.

Hoover K, Wilson-Clay B. *Diapers of the Breastfed Baby*, Manchaca, TX:Lactnews Press, 2002. www.BreastfeedingMaterials.com.

Kunz C, Lonnerdal B. Re-evaluation of the whey protein/casein ratio of human milk. *Acta Paediatrica* 1992; 81(2):107-112.

Lawrence RA, Lawrence RM. *Breastfeeding: A Guide for the Medical Profession* (7th edition). Philadelphia, PA: Elsevier Mosby, 2011; pp. 276, 493.

Martin V, Maldonado-Barragan A, Moles L, et al. Sharing of bacterial strains between breast milk and infant feces. *Journal of Human Lactation* 2012; 28(1):36-44.

Merewood A, Philipp BL. *Breastfeeding: Conditions and Diseases*. Amarillo, TX: Pharmasoft Publishing, 2001; pp. 99-100.

Mulder PJ, Johnson TS, Baker LC. Excessive weight loss in breastfed infants during the postpartum hospitalization. *Journal of Obstetric Gynecological and Neonatal Nursing* 2010; 39(1):15-26.

Neifert M. Early assessment of the breastfeeding infant. *Contemporary Pediatrics* 1996; 13(10):142-166.

Nommsen-Rivers LA, Heinig MJ, Cohen RJ, et al. Newborn wet and soiled diaper counts and timing of onset of lactation as indicators of breastfeeding inadequacy. *Journal of Human Lactation* 2008; 24(1):27-33.

Nyhan WL. Stool frequency of normal infants in the first week of life. *Pediatrics* 1952; 10(4):414-425.

Okechukwu AA, Okolo AA. Exclusive breastfeeding frequency during the first seven days of life in term neonates. *Nigerian Postgraduate Medical Journal* 2006; 13(4):309-312.

Ozdogan T. Hypernatremic dehydration in breast-fed neonates (letter) *Archives of Disease in Children* 2006; 91(12):1041.

Penders J, Thijs C, Vink C, et al. Factors influencing the composition of the intestinal microbiota in early infancy. *Pediatrics* 2006; 118(2):511-521.

Perez-Escamilla R, Chapman D. Validity and public health implications of maternal perception of the onset of lactation: an international analytical overview. *Journal of Nutrition* 2001; 131(11):3021S-3024S.

Pollard DL. Impact of a feeding log on breastfeeding duration and exclusivity. *Maternal Child Health* 2011; 15(3): 395-400.

Savino F, Cordisco L, Tarasco V, et al. Molecular identification of coliform bacteria from colicky breastfed infants. *Acta Paediatrica* 2009; 98(10):1582-1588.

Shrago LC, Reifsnider E, Insel K. The neonatal bowel output study: indicators of adequate breast milk intake in neonates. *Pediatric Nursing* 2006; 32(3):195-201.

Silber G. Lower gastrointestinal bleeding. *Pediatrics in Review* 1990; 12(3):85-92.

Stiefel L. In Brief: Hypotonia in infants. *Pediatrics in Review* 1996; 17(3):104-105.

Smith L. Components of milk and their function. In *Core Curriculum for Lactation Consultant Practice 3rd Edition,* ed. R. Mannel, P. Martens, M. Walker. Burlington, MA: Jones & Bartlett Learning, 2013; pp. 357-359.

Tham EB, Nathan R, Davidson GP, et al. Bowel habits of healthy Australian children aged 1-2 years. *Journal of Paediatric Child Health* 1996; 32(6):504-507.

Tunc VT, Camurdan AD, Ilhan MN, et al. Factors associated with defectation patterns in 0-24-month-old children. *European Journal of Pediatrics* 2008; 167(12):357-1362.

Walker M. Supplementation of the Breastfed Baby: "Just one bottle won't hurt --- or will it? http://www.health-e-learning.com/ resources/articles. Accessed August 2012. Search words: *Walker one bottle*.

World Health Organization (WHO). Contaminated food: a major cause of diarrhoea and associated malnutrition among infants and young children. *Facts for Infant Feeding.* 1993; 3:1-4.

Yamauchi Y, Yamanouchi I. Breast-feeding frequency during the first 24 hours after birth in full-term neonates. *Pediatrics* 1990; 86(2):171-175.

Appearances of Human Milk

Lactogenesis describes the multiple-stage process during which the mammary gland prepares to secrete milk, begins copious milk production, maintains production over time, and involutes during weaning.

Lactogenesis stage I refers to the mid-pregnancy maturation of the gland. Small amounts of fluid produced during this phase may accumulate in the ducts. Some women may leak or be able to hand express during pregnancy. Collection of this colostrum is recommended by some LCs for use by mothers in case their infants require early supplementation, but this practice has not been well-studied.

Lactogenesis stage II, occurs 30-40 hours postpartum (Arthur 1989, Neville 2001). This is commonly described as the milk "coming in." When the onset of copious lactation has not occurred by 72 hours postpartum, lactogenesis stage II is characterized as "delayed" (Dewey 2003). Even in well-motivated populations, delays are common. Delays are associated with suboptimal neonatal breastfeeding behavior, and maternal factors such as primiparity, prolonged labor, instrumental delivery, cesarean birth, retained placenta, hypo-androgenism, hypertension, maternal diabetes, excessive blood loss, use of non-breast-milk fluids, obesity, and maternal insulin resistance (Hall 2002, Dewey 2003, Sert 2003, Rasmussen 2004, Nommsen-Rivers 2012, Lemay 2013). Dewey reported that 22 percent of mothers studied experienced delays >72 hours (33 percent of primiparas vs 8 percent of multiparas). Chapman (1999) found 35 percent of women experience delayed onset of lactogenesis II.

Women need accurate, careful guidance in milk supply calibration for the critically sensitive period during the first 2 weeks postpartum. Failure to stimulate sufficiently during this phase may prevent these mothers from establishing adequate lactation.

Delays in the onset of copious milk production increase risk for the infant, including the risk of greater newborn weight loss and longer periods for recovery of birth weight than is considered optimal (Nommsen-Rivers 2008). Brownell (2012) reported an association between delayed lactogenesis II (> 3 days postpartum) and cessation of both any and exclusive breastfeeding. Routine assessment of the timing of the onset of copious milk production is warranted at the baby's 3 to 5 day evaluation.

Women experiencing delayed onset may benefit from early postpartum interventions to support favorable outcomes. These might include evaluation of maternal hormone levels,

early initiation of breast pumping and hand expression, and assessment of infant latch and feeding frequency. In some rare cases, women report no postpartum breast changes or milk production. Failure to lactate is an important symptom for some conditions, such as Sheehan's syndrome, and signals the need for further medical evaluation of the mother (Sert 2003, Villaseca 2005).

Normal Milk Volumes

A Note to Readers: Researchers in the following studies report milk production volumes in both milliliters (ml) and grams (g). Grams, milliliters and cubic centimeters (cc) are essentially equivalent. One ounce (oz) equals 28.3 g, cc, or ml.

Volumes of colostrum are normally low on Day 1, especially in primiparous mothers. However, Wang (1994) described the physiological capacity of the newborn stomach as only 6 ml on the first day and 12 ml on the second day after birth. Wang states, "Although the amount of colostrum secreted is not voluminous, it can still meet the needs of the newborn."

Neville (1988) looked at milk production in a group of 13 multiparous women, following them longitudinally (over time) for 6 months. Her study describes low volumes of milk production on Days 1 and 2, with the mean total for Day 2 of about 175 ml/day (6 oz). Milk production in this group rose rapidly on days 3 and 4 to about 500 ml/day (17.6 oz), and reached levels of about 750 ml/day (26.5 oz) by the end of the first week postpartum. By 6 months these mothers averaged production levels of about 800 ml/day (28 oz).

Villalpando (1996) observed that Day 3 milk production averaged about 360 ml in a group of 30 women. All their infants regained birth weight within 74 hours post birth.

Hill (2005) observed greater challenges in establishing lactation in mothers pumping for preterm infants compared to mothers whose breastfeeding infants directly stimulated the breasts. The nursing mothers' milk output continuously increased over time, while milk output tended to decline or remain stable in mothers who were exclusively pumping. Other research suggests that women delivering preterm infants at less than 28 weeks may not experience full glandular development of the breast. Issues related to preterm birth, therefore, may impact milk production and delay the onset of lactogenesis II (Henderson 2004, Henderson 2008).

Hurst and Meier summarize issues regarding assisting mothers of preterm infants in the text *Breastfeeding and Human Lactation* (Riordan 2010). They recommend that mothers of nonnursing preterm infants establish a robust supply in early lactation (750-1000 ml/day). Frequent breast emptying during the so-called calibration phase of lactation may provide a hedge against observed decreases in production over time in pump-dependent mothers.

It is important, if possible, for mothers of preterm or other medically fragile infants to ensure a robust milk supply by the time of discharge of the infant from the special care nursery. A Cochrane review (Becker 2008) found that electric breast pumping produced a greater total volume of milk compared with hand expression. Simultaneous pumping was more efficient, but did not produce greater milk volumes. Morton (2009, 2012) found that a combination of hand expression and electric pumping increased milk production and increased the caloric content of milk in mothers of preterm infants.

Hill (2005) studied milk production in preterm and term mothers and observed that milk output on Days 6 and 7 is highly associated with Week 2 milk output, and moderately associated with Week 6 output. The same researchers identified similar predictors of term infant feeding outcomes in a longitudinal study of healthy singletons. Milk output during Weeks 1-6 was predictive of feeding type at Week 12 (Hill 2007). If mothers perceived their milk supply was low during the calibration phase, or if they stimulated their breasts fewer than 7.8 times daily, they were more likely to be supplementing their infants at Week 12.

Available research speaks strongly to the need for appropriate early support of mothers who are exclusively pumping. Similar levels of support must be provided for mothers with real or perceived insufficient milk supply.

A *galactagogue* is a medication or an herb believed to help initiate, maintain, or increase the rate of maternal milk synthesis. Many authorities suspect a placebo effect with regard to galactagogues. According to the Academy of Breastfeeding Medicine (ABM 2011) "...the case for using pharmaceutical galactogogues has grown weaker." Herbal galactagogues are unregulated in many countries, and there is insufficient evidence of their safety and efficacy, along with concerns about herb/drug interactions.

A Cochrane Review (Donovan 2012) showed a modest increase in expressed breast milk when the drug domperidone was prescribed to mothers of preterm infants with a dosage of 10 mg 3 times a day. Because prolactin normally spikes during breastfeeding, Hale (2012) recommends that maternal prolactin levels be measured 2 to 3 hours after breastfeeding when the blood prolactin levels are at baseline. This will help determine whether the baseline prolactin levels are within the normal range for lactation. Lawrence (2011) recommends obtaining a baseline level followed by a second value after 10 minutes of breastfeeding to capture the expected spike in prolactin elicited by infant sucking. Such an assessment should optimally be done before prescribing a prolactin-stimulating medication. If the mother is not deficient in prolactin, the medication will not assist her.

Metoclopramide, a medication known to increase prolactin levels has significant nervous system side effects (such as depression) when used to treat milk insufficiency for long periods of time. In 2011, the US Food and Drug Administration (FDA) approved use of domperidone as an "orphan drug" for breastfeeding mothers experiencing insufficient breastmilk. Domperidone has fewer side effects, although there is concern about cardiac arrhythmia at high dosages. The orphan drug designation is seen by some as a first step in obtaining FDA approval for use of domperidone to treat milk insufficiency in the US.

Patterns of Established Lactation

Kent (1999, 2006) confirmed earlier research findings that once established, milk production is relatively constant over the first 6 months of lactation. Using sophisticated imaging techniques, Kent observed that average 24 hour milk production from *each breast* in a group of 8 women was 453.6 ± 20.1 g (16 oz). This level of production is consistent with previous research by Hartmann (1995) describing 24 hour milk production of 798 ± 216 g at 1 month and 837 ± 190 g a day at 6 months. What is striking in all these studies is the wide range in milk production.

Individual milk production during established lactation in normal women appears to be fairly consistent over a 24 hour period. Based on pumping studies by Lai (2004), Hale reports this to be approximately 15 cc per breast each hour for 24 hours (2012), or 720 cc per day.

Available milk production averages and ranges suggest rough norms, but it is important to remember that there is great individuality in the feeding patterns of each mother-baby pair (Dewey 1986, Kent 2006). In general, healthy women appear to be able to produce adequate quantities of milk. Infant intake is also variable depending on the individual baby. After the first month postpartum, infant appetite is more significant in regulating the milk supply than is maternal production capacity (Woolridge 1982, Kent 1999). Night feeds are common in the early months and comprise a substantial proportion of the daily intake for most infants (Kent 2004, 2006).

Several researchers (Kent 2004, Engstrom 2004) report differences, sometimes dramatic, in milk volume production between left and right breasts.

Milk Nutrient Variations

Milk nutrients vary between women and in the same woman according to stage of gestation, stage of lactation, time of day, degree of breast fullness, and maternal diet (Czank 2007). Obtaining an adequate maternal health history screens for significant issues that may affect milk nutrient values. A maternal history of vegan diet or previous bariatric surgery, for example, may influence maternal levels of vitamin B12, creating deficiencies in the milk (Stefanski 2006). Vegan status and multiparity may result in zinc deficiencies that manifest in the infant as persistent infant diaper rashes and poor weight gain. The LC must screen clients adequately to identify such issues.

Preterm infants may require supplementation to permit normal bone mineralization. This supplementation may be done with fortification of mother's own or donor human milk. Mothers providing milk for their own preterm infants may also require assistance in learning to harvest hind milk to improve infant weight gain (Slusher 2003). Owing to variances between women in the caloric value of their milk, milk donated to milk banks should be tested for fat content. Targeted pooling of high calorie milk (rather than random pooling) may better ensure the growth of preterm infants receiving donor milk (Updegrove 2005).

Milk Color Variations

Human milk comes in a variety of colors. Colostrum may be clear (**Fig. 76**), bright yellow (**Figs. 77** and **80**), orange/pink (**Fig. 78**), light brown (**Fig. 79**), or even dark brown. Babies probably drink colored milk at their mothers' breasts fairly frequently, but we never see it unless the mother is pumping. Some foods, vitamins, medicines, and flavored drinks may color milk without doing harm (Lawrence 2011).

The orange/pink colored colostrum in **Fig. 78** is attributed to dried blood in the milk ducts that washes out as lactation begins. This is called "rusty pipe" syndrome and is well known in the dairy industry. Red coloration may also result from bleeding inside a milk duct, or from a cracked nipple. The temporary appearance of small amounts of blood are not harmful to the infant, although parents and professionals may find it disturbing and some prefer to discard the milk. Phelps (2009) found varying recommendations about the safety of feeding blood-tinged milk when surveying NICU professionals, and recommended

that evidence be assembled to document whether feeding blood-tinged milk is problematic.

Lawrence (2011) reports that pink milk observed while pumping may be the result of contamination of the breast or of a breast pump with *Serratia marcescens,* a drug-resistant human pathogen often found in hospitals. This bacteria causes significant infections and can spread rapidly, becoming epidemic. Transient carriage on the hands and on equipment is the likely mode of transmission (Dessi 2009, Maragakis 2008). Pumps of mothers pumping pink milk should be cultured and cleaned with bleach.

Hand expression can be an effective way to obtain colostrum to feed to a non-nursing newborn. Often mothers are able to express drops of colostrum into a spoon to offer to the infant (as in **Fig. 80**). Parents may need reassurance that the amounts of colostrum, although small, are physiologically normal and sufficient for Day 1.

Figures 76-80 show the first expressions of milk from mothers who are less than 24 hours postpartum. **Fig. 79** shows a mother's first 3 pumpings at 2-hour intervals. The milk yield decreased over the first 3 pumpings, and the light brown color became lighter each time. The lightening in color suggests that a flushing action is clearing accumulated debris from the ducts that has stained the colostrum. Over time, milk typically turns whiter and increases in volume.

Figures 76-79 represent rather large amounts of milk for expressions on Day 1. Many primiparous mothers may only obtain a few drops of milk at their first attempt at expression. Casey (1986) found the total volume of milk produced on the first postpartum day to range from 3 to 32 ml. When women express a large amount (7 ml or more) during the first expression attempt, anticipatory guidance is prudent because the next few times they may express less colostrum. They may need reassurance that the volume will increase gradually over the next few days.

Fig. 80 shows about 0.6 ml of colostrum, which is about the size of a newborn's swallow (Lawrence 2011). Eight to 10 swallows of this size would provide sufficient intake at a feeding during the first 24 hours for a full-term, medically stable newborn.

Fig. 81 documents the typical color change that occurs when milk matures. This mother has pumped in the middle of the night of Day 2. She obtained 32 ml of yellow-stained colostrum. By morning of Day 3, when she pumped off enough milk to help soften her engorged breast, the milk had assumed the whitish color typical of mature milk. Note the thin, transparent quality of this foremilk.

Fig. 82 shows 70.7 ml (2.5 oz) pumped by a primiparous woman on Day 3. The yellow color suggests that this is transitional milk. The color and volume of this pumped milk are consistent with typical Day 3 milk appearance.

Fig. 83 shows green pumped milk next to a bottle of normally colored milk. Yazgan (2012) reports a case of green milk. After physical examination and laboratory tests, it was revealed that the cause of the green milk in that case was related to multivitamin intake. The mother was reassured that it was safe to breastfeed. The authors of the case report state: "Although clinical specialists know that the color of breastmilk can change with the ingestion of certain medications and foods, mothers are usually unaware and may unnecessarily terminate breastfeeding."

Fig. 84 shows two containers of milk from a woman during *lactogenesis stage III*, the on-going maintenance of milk production over the course of lactation. The mother was asked to express a small amount of milk before breastfeeding her baby and another small amount once her baby had finished feeding. The milk has separated, with the cream rising to the top, providing a graphic illustration of the difference in the fat content of foremilk and hindmilk. Research suggests that when the breast is full, the volume of fluid dilutes the cream content of the milk (Daly 1993).

Academy of Breastfeeding Medicine. ABM Clinical Protocol #9: Use of galactogogues in initiating or augmenting the rate of maternal milk secretion (First Revision Jan. 2011). *Breastfeeding Medicine* 2011; 6(1):41-45.

Arthur P, Smith M, Hartmann P. Milk lactose, citrate and glucose as markers of lactogenesis in normal and diabetic women. *Journal of Pediatric Gastroenterology and Nutrition* 1989; 9(4):488-496.

Becker GE, McCormick FM, Renfrew MJ. Methods of milk expression for lactating women. *Cochrane Database System Review* 2008; Oct. 8(4): CD006170.

Brownell E, Howard CR, Lawrence RA, et al. Delayed onset lactogenesis II predicts the cessation of any or exclusive breastfeeding. *Journal of Pediatrics* 2012; 161(4):608-614.

Casey CE, Neifert MR, Seacat JM, et al. Nutrient intake by breastfed infants during the first five days after birth. *American Journal of Diseases of Children* 1986; 140(9):933-936.

Chapman DJ, Pérez-Escamilla R. Identification of risk factors for delayed onset of lactation. *Journal of the American Dietetic Association* 1999; 99(4):450-454.

Czank C, Mitoulas LR, Hartmann PE. Human Milk Composition - Fat. in *Hale & Hartmann's Textbook of Lactation*. Amarillo, TX: Hale Publishing 2007; pp. 56-58.

Daly S, Di Rosso A, Owens R, et al. Degree of breast emptying explains changes in the fat content, but not fatty acid composition, of human milk. *Experimental Physiology* 1993; 78(6):741-755.

Dessi A, Puddu M, Testa M, et al. *Serratia marcescens* infections and outbreaks in neonatal intensive care units. *Journal of Chemotherapy* 2009; 21(5):493-499.

Dewey K, Nommsen-Rivers L, Heinig MJ. Risk factors for suboptimal infant breastfeeding behavior, delayed onset of lactation, and excess neonatal weight loss. *Pediatrics* 2003; 112(3 Pt 1):607-619.

Dewey K, Lonnerdal B. Infant self-regulation of breast milk intake. *Acta Paediatrica Scandia* 1986; 75(6):893-898.

Donovan TJ, Buchanan K. Medications for increasing milk supply in mothers expressing breastmilk for their preterm hospitalized infants. *Cochrane Database System Review* 2012; Mar 14; 3:CD005544.

Engstrom J, Meier P, Zuleger J, et al. Comparison of volume of milk pumped from the right and left breasts in mothers of very low birthweight (VLBW) infants. (Poster) 12th International Conference of the International Society for Research in Human Milk and Lactation. Sept. 10-14, 2004; Queen's College, Cambridge, UK.

Hall R, Mercer A, Teasley S, et al: A breast-feeding assessment score to evaluate the risk for cessation of breast-feeding by 7 to 10 days of age. *Journal of Pediatrics* 2002; 141(5):659-64.

Hale T. Control and Production of Human Milk - Medications that Increase Milk Production (lecture). Hale, Newman, Wilson-Clay Conference, San Antonio, Texas. Sept 12, 2012.

Hartmann P, Sherriff J, Kent J. Maternal nutrition and the regulation of milk synthesis. *Proceedings of the Nutrition Society 1995*; 54:379-389.

Henderson JJ, Hartmann PE, Newnham JP, et al. Effect of preterm birth and antenatal corticosteroid treatment on lactogenesis II in women. *Pediatrics* 2008; 121(1):e92-e100.

Henderson JJ, Simmer K, Newnham PJ, et al. Impact of very preterm delivery on the timing of lactogensis II in women. *Proceedings of the 12th International Conference of the International Society for Research in Human Milk and Lactation.* Sept. 10-14, 2004; Queen's College, Cambridge, UK.

Hill P, Aldag J, Chatterton R, et al. Comparison of milk output between mothers of preterm and term infants: the first 6 weeks after birth. *Journal of Human Lactation* 2005; 21(1):22-30.

Hill PD, Aldag JC. Predictors of term infant feeding at week 12 postpartum. *Journal of Perinatal & Neonatal Nursing* 2007; 21(3):250-255.

Hurst N, Meier P. Breastfeeding the preterm infant. in J Riordan and K. Wambach. *Breastfeeding and Human Lactation* (4rd edition). Sudbury, MA: Jones and Bartlett. 2010; pp. 425-470.

Kent J, Cregan M, Mitoulas L, et al. Frequency, volume and milk fat content of breastfeeds of exclusively breastfed babies. (Poster)12th International Conference of the International Society for Research in Human Milk and Lactation. Sept. 10-14, 2004; Queen's College, Cambridge, UK.

Kent J, Mitoulas L, Cox D, et al. Breast volume and milk production during extended lactation in women. *Experimental Physiology* 1999; 84(2):435-447.

Kent JC, Mitoulas LR, Cregan MD, et al. Volume and frequency of breastfeedings and fat content of breast milk throughout the day. *Pediatrics* 2006; 117(3):e387-395.

Lai C, Hale T, Simmer K, et al. Hourly rate of milk synthesis in women. (Poster) 12th International Conference of the International Society for Research in Human Milk and Lactation. Sept.10-14, 2004; Queen's College, Cambridge, UK.

Lawrence RA, Lawrence RM. *Breastfeeding: A Guide for the Medical Profession* (7th edition). Maryland Heights, MO: Elsevier Mosby, 2011; pp. 236, 313-314, 352, 591.

Lemay DG, Ballard OA, Hughes MA, et al. RNA Sequencing of the human milk fat layer transcriptome reveals distinct gene expression profiles at three stages of lactation. *PLoS ONE* 2013; 8(7):e67531.

Maragakis LL, Winkler A, Tucker MG, et al. Outbreak of multidrug-resistant *Serratia marcescens* infection in a neonatal intensive care unit. *Infection Control Hospital Epidemiology* 2008; 29(5):418-423.

Morton J, Hall JY, Wong RJ, et al. Combining hand techniques with electric pumping increases milk production in mothers of preterm infants. *Journal of Perinatology* 2009; 87(11):757-764.

Morton J, Hall JY, Wong RJ, et al. Combining hand techniques with electric pumping increases the caloric content of milk in mothers of preterm infants. *Journal of Perinatology* 2012; 32(10):791-796.

Neville M. Anatomy and physiology of lactation. in Schanler R ed. *The Pediatric Clinics of North America.* Philadelphia: WB Saunders 2001; 48(1):13-34.

Neville M, Keller R, Seacat J, et al. Studies in human lactation: milk volumes in lactating women during the onset of lactation and full lactation. *American Journal Clinical Nutrition* 1988; 48(6):1375-86.

Nommsen-Rivers LA, Dolan LM, Huang B. Timing of stage II lactogenesis is predicted by antenatal metabolic health in a cohort of primiparas. *Breastfeeding Medicine* 2012; 7(1):43-49.

Nommsen-Rivers LA, Heinig MJ, Cohen RJ, et al. Newborn wet and soiled diaper counts and timing of onset of lactation as indicators of breastfeeding inadequacy. *Journal of Human Lactation* 2008; 24(1):27-33.

Phelps MM, Bedard WS, Henry E, et al. Attitudes of NICU professionals regarding feeding blood-tinged colostrums or milk. *Journal of Perinatology* 2009; 29(2):119-123.

Rasmussen K, Kjolhede C. Prepregnant overweight and obesity diminish the prolactin response to suckling in the first week postpartum. *Pediatrics* 2004; 113(5):e465-470.

Sert M, Tetiker T, Kirim S, et al. Clinical report of 28 patients with Sheehan's Syndrome. *Endocrine Journal* 2003; 50(3):297-301.

Slusher T, Hampton R, Bode-Thomas F, et al. Promoting the exclusive feeding of own mother's milk through the use of hindmilk and increased maternal milk volume for hospitalized, low birth weight infants (<1800 grams) in Nigeria: a feasibility study. *Journal of Human Lactation* 2003; 19(2):191-198.

Stefanski J. Breast-feeding after bariatric surgery. *Today's Dietitian* 2006; 8(1):e47.

Updegrove KK: Human milk banking in the United States. *Newborn Infant Nursing Review* 2005; 5(1):27-33.

Villalpando S, Flores-Huerta S, López-Alarcón M, et al. Social and biological determinants of lactation. *Food and Nutrition Bulletin* 1996; 17(4):328-335.

Villaseca P, Campino C, Oestreicher E, et al. Bilateral oophorectomy in a pregnant woman: hormonal profile from late gestation to postpartum: case report. *Human Reproduction* 2005; 20(2):397-401.

Wang YF, Shen YH, Wang JJ, et al. Preliminary study on the blood glucose level in the exclusively breastfed newborn. *Journal of Tropical Pediatrics* 1994; 40(3):187-188.

Woolridge M, Baum J, Drewett R. Individual patterns of milk intake during breast-feeding. *Early Human Development* 1982; 7(3):265-272.

Yazgan H, Demirdoven M, Yazgan Z, et al. A mother with green breastmilk due to multivitamin and mineral intake: a case report. *Breastfeeding Medicine* 2012; 7(4):310-312.

Positioning and Latch Technique

Latching onto the breast is an instinctive skill of the normal newborn. Most robust, term infants can eventually self-attach if placed skin-to-skin with their mothers in a conducive environment. Best practices for breastfeeding thus emphasize early and unrestricted contact for breastfeeding, rooming-in, and avoidance of artificial teats unless medically indicated.

Many experienced LCs view the demonstrated ability of a baby to latch to the breast with minimal assistance to be an important assessment criterion. Given the innate capabilities of newborns to self-attach, it is important to advise mothers to get comfortable and to wait until they request or appear to require help with positioning and attachment rather than offering such help routinely (Colson 2005). If the mother and baby appear to be managing well, the LC primarily encourages and provides anticipatory guidance. Such guidance may include tips on how to more optimally position the baby and care for tender nipples. It is useful to provide information on using diaper counts and timing of engorgement as markers for adequate feeding.

In the case of compromised dyads, especially when the baby cannot latch, more active assistance may be required to bring the baby to the breast and to protect the milk supply until breastfeeding normalizes.

All hospital and birthing personnel need to have a basic understanding of how to help mothers bring their infants to the breast. The lactation consultant requires a more sophisticated understanding of the anatomy and physiology of breastfeeding in order to effectively assist compromised dyads. The following overview is a synopsis of positioning and latch information from experts (Gunther 1945 and 1955, Newton 1967, Woolridge 1986a and 1986b, Savage-King 1992, Glass 1994, Neifert 1995, Wiessinger 1998, Royal College of Midwives 2000, Glover 2000, Smilie 2007, Colson 2008). Ultrasonographic studies have expanded our understanding of the mechanics of breastfeeding (Ramsay 2004, Ramsay 2005, Jacobs 2007, Geddes 2008).

The Mechanics of Sucking

The baby locates the breast guided by nipple coloration and scent (Varendi 1994, Prime 2007). Touch on the face stimulates the rooting reflex, causing the baby to seek the nipple, open wide and latch. With all of his lip surface in contact with the breast, the baby grasps and draws in the breast tissue.

Suction holds the breast in the mouth and elongates the breast tissue to form a "teat." This teat extends to within approximately 5 mm of the junction of the hard and soft palates (Ramsay 2004, Jacobs 2007). During normal, painless sucking, the position of the teat in the mouth has been observed to move (Jacobs 2007). The dropping of the posterior tongue creates negative pressure in the oral cavity. The strong vacuum generated when the tongue droups facilitates milk removal by the infant (Ramsay 2004, Geddes 2007). A wave-like peristaltic movement of the tongue appears to organize the milk bolus for safe swallowing (Woolridge 2012).

Less than 10 ml of milk is available to the infant prior to the milk ejection (Prime 2007). Nipple stimulation triggers the mother's milk ejection reflex (the *let-down*), facilitating milk transfer and thorough breast emptying. A mother experiencing significant distraction, pain, or stress may have inhibited milk ejection, and her infant may not receive full feeds (Newton 1948, 1967).

Because the infant must be able to draw in enough breast tissue to manipulate the teat, flat and inverted nipples, or severely engorged breasts may prove problematic especially for small, weak, or medically fragile infants. The infant must have a fully mobile tongue in order to suck and swallow normally; a tongue-tied infant may be challenged to breastfeed. Similarly, there may be problems when the mother has large diameter nipples, long nipples, or meaty, hard-to-manipulate nipples.

Primitive Neonatal Reflexes

There appears to be great variability in normal breastfeeding behavior. *Primitive neonatal reflexes* (PNRs) refer to reflex responses (rooting, sucking, swallowing), spontaneous behaviors, and reactions to environmental stimuli that may trigger normal breastfeeding responses in mothers and babies (Colson 2008). So-called biological nurturing methods emphasize skin-to-skin holding of newborns and semi-reclined feeding positions, activating PNRs and assisting infant-self attachment to the breast.

Normal infants cared for in this manner may need little help with positioning. Compromised dyads may need much more active assistance with positioning. Stable head position improves jaw control, influences swallowing, and reduces the risk of aspiration. Stability of the head is influenced by trunk alignment, particularly the stability of the pelvic area (Redstone 2004). Pelvic stability is the reason breastfeeding experts often emphasize hip flexion. Normal infants may be able to compensate for misalignment of body position during feeding. Children with birth injury, neurodisabilities or other weaknesses may not be able to overcome misalignment.

Visual Images of Positioning

Pulling on the baby's jaw or manipulating the baby's head to achieve correct positioning is ineffective and distracts the baby. Correctly orienting the baby to the breast can be more easily done by realigning the placement of the baby's body relative to the mother. At the start of the latching sequence in any position chosen, the baby's body is held close, with the mother's arms providing boundaries and support. The baby's head will tilt and the mouth will open wide in order to reach for the nipple. Extension of the head permits the receding lower jaw of the infant to fit tightly against the breast (see **Figs. 112** and **116**).

Mothers should ignore advice to push on the baby's head. Pushing the baby's head will flex the head forward, driving the nose into the breast. Burying the nose obstructs breathing and prevents the baby from looking at the mother. Additionally, if the upper jaw makes first contact with the breast, it is akin to biting an apple with your chin tucked into your neck. Hyperflexion at the neck inhibits jaw opening and prevents comfortable swallowing.

Women breastfeeding in the cradle position are often instructed to place the newborn's head in the crook of their arm. The crook of the arm naturally falls beside the body and may be too far to the side of the mother's body for a small baby. When the infant's head "over-shoots" the nipple target, the baby has to bend his head forward, tucking his chin into his chest in order to locate the nipple. Breathing, swallowing, and wide jaw excursions are inhibited.

Fig. 85 shows a poorly positioned baby, whose frustration has resulted in crying and breast rejection. The blankets are in the way, and the mother has resorted to "chasing" the baby with her breast, trying to push it into his mouth. Distortion of the shape of the breast may result in poor milk transfer by collapsing the easily compressible milk ducts (Ramsay 2005, Geddes 2007).

In **Fig. 86,** the same woman has made several changes resulting in a successful latch. The blankets have been removed, allowing the mother and baby to sense one another more acutely. The baby's body is rotated, so that he no longer has to struggle to turn his head in order to find the nipple. The mother has brought the baby's head onto her forearm, which orients the baby to the front of her breast.

This allows her to line up the baby so that her nipple touches his nose. Now the baby has to extend his head slightly during latch-on, so that he leads with his chin. This places the chin tightly against the breast. When the chin is tucked into the breast, the nose will be slightly tipped away from the breast, helping to maintain an open breathing passage. The mother's hand supports the weight of the breast.

Fig. 87 shows a baby lined up with the nose touching the nipple. As the baby roots in response to the stimulus, the head tilts back, the mouth opens, and the lower jaw is planted on the breast.

Note the uncomfortable looking position of the baby's lower arm in **Fig. 88**. When an infant begins to struggle at the breast, it could be that some part of his body is twisted or strained. Sometimes a baby suffers minor neck, shoulder or clavicle injury during birth, which influences how he responds to handling in the early postpartum period. Observe, also, how the mother's arm in **Fig. 88** does not adequately support the baby. The baby's body appears to be falling away. The mother's arm needs to be under the baby, providing sufficient postural support to stabilize the baby's position at the breast.

Positioning the infant's arm around the mother's side may be uncomfortable for some newborns. It can be useful, instead, to gently place the baby's lower arm across his chest before rolling him onto his side (**Fig. 89**). This will round the shoulder, placing it in a more comfortable position. Bringing the infant's upper torso into physiologic flexion may reduce the discomfort of torticollis. Note also that the infant in **Fig. 89** has a healing incision on her abdomen and is using a feeding tube device. She suffered a bowel rotation, which was corrected surgically. The baby needed supplementation with pumped milk until she grew stronger. Trapping her lower arm across her chest prevented her from grabbing the feeding tube.

When one arm is brought to the midline of the baby's body, the other hand seeks it. Improving physiologic flexion helps stabilize and calm disorganized infants (**Fig. 90**).

Fig. 91 emphasizes that some newborns may be too small to be placed in the crook of the mother's arm when the arm is held at the side of her body. Passive support of the head on the mother's forearm more correctly aligns the baby in front of the nipple. Additionally, notice that this woman has very long arms. In assisting a woman with comfortable positioning, the LC needs to take into consideration the size of the baby, the size (length, width, and weight) of the woman's breasts, the location of her nipples, the length of her arms, and the length of the mother's torso.

The 6 week-old baby pictured in **Fig. 92** is being breastfed in the cradle position. She has gained 3 pounds (1358 g) above her birth weight and is big enough to be comfortably positioned in the crook of her mother's arm. Careful attention to positioning technique generally is a concern of early breastfeeding. As time goes by, each dyad works out their own way of doing things. The hallmark of good positioning is simple: both mother and baby are comfortable, avoiding strain and exertion. Effective breastfeeding allows the newborn to self-regulate intake by efficiently emptying the breast (Daly 1993). The baby will release the breast spontaneously when satiated, and growth will be appropriate (Kent 2007).

The mother in **Fig. 93** is breastfeeding in the cradle position. This mother is using a nursing pillow to support the baby. Her 6 week-old baby needs less postural control and support from her mother than would a newborn. Laying a newborn baby directly on the pillow is generally not a good idea. As the baby sinks into the pillow he may slip off the breast. Sometimes a firm commercial breastfeeding pillow helps, but many pillows are the wrong height and interfere with good positioning. If the mother has a short waist, a pillow may place the baby above the level of the nipple. This forces the mother to lift her breast to the baby, putting strain on her shoulders. Remind the mother of a newborn that her arms support the baby and the pillow supports her arms.

Notice how the mother in **Fig. 93** turns the baby's body in toward her own. Pulling the hips close stabilizes the baby's body. When babies are well-positioned, face-to-face gazing can occur. This facilitates bonding and gives pleasure to both mother and baby.

The mother in **Fig. 94** has slightly over-rotated the body of her infant. Observe how this buries the baby's face so that the mother and baby are not able to see one another. The mother is putting too much pressure on the baby's top shoulder, causing the over-rotation. This will cause the "down" side cheek to back away from the breast. The nipple may emerge from the baby's mouth looking pinched.

Maternal overweight and obesity are associated with poor breastfeeding outcomes (Jevitt 2007). Poor outcomes in this population may result from difficulty in positioning caused by short arms relative to body mass, large breasts, no lap, and issues related to body image (Rassmussen 2006, Hoover 2008). In order to reduce the risk of early discontinuation of breastfeeding in overweight or obese mothers, the LC must assist with sensitive counseling and teach creative positioning (Hoover 2000). It is important

to chose positions that support both the baby and the breast. If the breast is heavy and the nipple ill-defined, some mothers may use a free hand to shape the breast to help the baby latch (as in **Fig. 96**, **Fig. 100** and **Fig. 101**).

The football hold is pictured in **Fig. 95**. Note how the baby's flexed hips enable the mother to position the baby's body in a relaxed fashion. If the baby's feet touch the back of the chair, he may reflexively push off, going stiff and arching away. Putting the baby's bottom against the back of the chair may be a solution.

Fig. 96 shows a slight variation of the football hold that is especially useful for preterm babies or hypotonic babies because it gives the mother good control of her baby's body (Tully 1991, Brodribb 1998). Once again, the mother uses active support at the nape of the baby's neck with her hand. She supports the baby's torso with her forearm. Her free hand supports her breast to perform deep breast compressions.

It is important when demonstrating the football position to caution the mother against placing her hand on the baby's head and pushing it toward the breast. The mother in **Fig. 97** was instructed to move her hand position and to support the baby at the neck and shoulders as shown in **Fig. 98**. Now she is less likely to hyperflex the baby's head, mashing the baby's nose into the breast and constricting the throat. If the baby's breathing and swallowing are inhibited by the mother's poor positioning technique, breastfeeding turns into a struggle as the baby attempts to communicate discomfort.

A modified cross-cradle position is useful for women with short arms, large breasts, or during engorgement because it helps the mother better support her breast. Note how the mother in **Fig. 99** rests the weight of the breast on her wrist. Her baby's head rests passively in the palm of her hand, but her other arm actively guides the baby and holds him close with support at the nape of the neck and along his torso. When the baby is well positioned, both cheeks will touch the breast and the nose will be clear to breathe.

Fig. 100 shows a mother with large breasts positioning her infant on a table in a modified cross-cradle position. The table stabilizes the baby and the weight of the breast. Using her free hand, the mother shapes and holds the breast in the baby's mouth.

Creative positioning may also assist a baby in a hip brace (See **Fig. 365**). Some babies when first placed in a brace for hip dysplasia do not feed well for a few days until they become accustomed to the restriction of their legs. The LC can teach the mother to use a breastfeeding pillow to help position the baby in a cross-cradle position.

The mother in **Fig. 101** is nursing in the side-lying position. An obvious advantage of side-lying is increased rest for the mother (Milligan 1996). Side-lying also protects the infant's ability to self-attach (Colson 2005). A mother recovering from an episiotomy, a painful perineal tear, or hemorrhoids may find side-lying more comfortable than a seated position. Lang (2002) states that this position may help the woman "who is disabled and cannot take the weight of the baby in her arms." The authors have found side-lying to be another useful feeding position for women with large breasts. The bed supports the weight of the breast. This frees up the mother's hands to guide the baby during latch if such help is required.

Hypertonic babies or babies who resist touch also may benefit from a side-lying nursing position. The baby may feel less constrained and more in control -- an important issue if previous breastfeeding experiences have resembled a wrestling match! Infants who previously experienced great difficulty breastfeeding often enjoy being placed in a side-lying position and allowed to discover the breast at their own pace. Observing her infant's capacity for self-attachment is an encouraging experience for a mother who feels she is struggling to establish breastfeeding.

Notice that the side-lying mother in **Fig. 101** has oriented the baby slightly below the level of her breast. The baby has to tip his head back to latch, clearing a breathing space for his nose and allowing the mother and baby to look at one another. Note how the mother is using her free hand to guide her breast. She could easily employ deep breast compressions to increase milk intake, if needed (see **Fig. 43**).

The infant's bottom arm may be drawn across the chest, rolling the bottom shoulder and hip toward the mother's body. The "edges" of the mother and baby come together in a "V." If the baby cannot look into his mother's eyes, his head is too close to her armpit, and he should be moved down her torso in the direction of his feet. A rolled-up cloth can be used at the baby's back to keep the baby slightly turned toward the mother.

Fig. 102 shows a 22 month-old toddler nursing to sleep in the side-lying position. This older child typically does not require asssistance from his mother to latch onto the breast. Moments before this photo was taken, the over-tired toddler began crying. Many mothers who breastfeed beyond infancy find that comfort nursing is an important aspect of calming and caring for their older children. Howard (2004) reported that "Nursing to comfort a crying infant was a highly effective calming method and a strong independent predictor of extended long-term breastfeeding duration." The mother in this photo remarked that she viewed breastfeeding as an essential mothering technique. The ability to comfort her toddler at the breast was even more important to her than the nutritional benefits of breastmilk.

The seated straddle position shown in **Fig. 103** may be helpful for the baby when the mother has a rapid milk ejection. It also may assist infants with clefts of the palate. Some infants with swallowing or breathing disorders may benefit from upright feeding positions that reduce choking. The head must be well-supported at the neck in an extended position to maintain airway patency (Wolf 1992).

The baby in **Fig. 104** has been struggling with his mother's forceful milk ejection reflex. Here the mother reclines in a chair with the baby lying on top of her. The baby is in a prone position. This is sometimes called *posture feeding*. *Laid back positioning* stimulates primitive neonatal reflexes (Colson 2008), especially if practiced skin-to-skin.

The mother in **Fig. 105** was injured during the repair of her episiotomy after delivery. Sitting was painful for over a year. Her LC (KH) mentioned this mother's problem to the late Chris Mulford, an IBCLC colleague. Chris had experienced back pain and found that standing and lying were the only positions in which she was comfortable. Chris suggested breastfeeding standing up. The mother was delighted with this suggestion. She wore a nursing pillow wrapped around her waist and rested it on the changing table. The height of this table worked well for her. The story illustrates the creative process that mothers and LCs employ to solve problems.

Fig. 106 illustrates that nipple placement on the breast may vary between mothers. When the nipple is placed on the "downhill slope" of the breast, it can be challenging for the mother to position the baby. Mothers worry when they are unable to see what the baby is doing during latch. Some mothers will temporarily tighten the straps on their nursing bras to help raise the breast, tipping the nipple up so it is visible. Other mothers find that all they need to do is lower the level at which they hold the baby. If the baby feels the chin touch the breast and the nipple stroke his nose, most normal babies can latch themselves without the mother needing to see what the baby is doing. The mother in **Fig. 106** demonstrates the technique in **Fig. 107**. In this position, the baby is almost lying flat on his back under the breast.

Breastfeeding texts often refer to ways of holding the breast. **Fig. 108** shows a mother holding her breast with the "scissors" hold. Many books discourage this hold; however, it is frequently seen in fine art depictions of breastfeeding. The scissors hold is clearly effective for this mother, perhaps because she has long fingers. LCs are not obligated to correct mothers if what they are doing works.

Fig. 109 and **Fig. 110** show a modification of the cradle hold that increases maternal control of the infant's body. This position is especially useful if the mother has short arms. The preterm infant shown in **Fig. 109** lacks good postural control. The LC removed the nursing pillow and showed the mother how to hold the baby more securely. The mother of the baby in **Fig. 110** has been encouraged by the LC to lie back and to support the weight of the baby on her semi-reclined body.

A final word on positioning. It is best to hold the baby at the breast in a way that feels comfortable to the mother and secure to the baby. Remember: the normal baby can latch him or herself on without much assistance. The skill of positioning may not be as instinctive to the mother initially as the skill of latching is to the baby. It helps to reassure mothers that their coordination will improve with practice. As the baby gets older, technique goes by the wayside. **Fig. 111** illustrates that this 5 month-old has her own ideas about breastfeeding!

Visual Images of Latch

Latching is an activity that relates more specifically to the infant drawing the breast into the mouth. Note how the mother in **Fig. 112** has positioned her newborn baby with his chin touching her breast. Observe how the baby uses his hand to grasp and guide the breast.

The mother in **Fig. 113** positions her breast so that baby's mouth is level with the round underside of the breast. The baby's nose is level with the nipple. As the mother's breast gently touches the baby's chin, the infant instinctively gapes and tips back the head (**Fig. 114**). Notice in this photo that the nipple is aimed toward the palate. In **Fig. 115** the baby is drawn in close by the mother with support at the shoulders.

When latched, we see in **Fig. 116** asymmetric attachment to the areola. Notice the nose is tipped away from the breast and the chin tight up against the globe of the breast. This orients the baby's head so that breathing, wide jaw excursions, and unrestricted swallowing are facilitated. The slight extension of the head that permits these activities also enables the baby to look into her mother's eyes. *En face* (face-to-face) gazing provides bonding opportunities.

Sometimes, the LC or the mother makes a breast "sandwich" (Wiessinger 1998) as shown in **Fig. 117** in order to assist a baby who is having difficulty latching -- especially to a flat nipple or to an engorged breast. Some weak infants may need the mother to continue to hold the wedged tissue for the duration of the feed. Other infants may only require such assistance until successfully latched.

Helping parents read the body language of their infant can be useful in reassuring them that their baby is well-latched and taking a good feeding. Note the baby's open eyes, alert affect, and wide gape in **Fig. 118**. After several minutes of robust, rhythmic sucking with few pauses, the baby may briefly rest. Generally, another milk release stimulates another round or 2 of active sucking, after which the baby's eyes may close. Some babies will detach, others will suck until falling asleep. Providing the infant is growing well, the mother should allow the baby to set the pace.

In **Fig. 119** the baby has closed his eyes. His fist is beginning to relax, a sign that Springuel (1994) points to as an indication that the baby is getting full.

In **Fig. 120**, the baby's hand is even more relaxed. The parents may note longer pauses between sucking bursts. Some mothers may be tempted to end the feed at this point. However, this is an important phase of the feeding. As the breast softens, the fat concentration of the milk rises. The baby may be more satiated and "settled" after the feeding if allowed to self-terminate the feed.

Fig. 121 beautifully illustrates a completed breastfeeding. The infant has released the breast and appears totally relaxed, with an open hand resting gently on the mother's breast. Note the round shape of the nipple. The shape demonstrates no evidence of compression injury. After such a feeding, both mother and infant typically appear mutually satisfied with the experience.

Fig. 122 illustrates a baby who is poorly latched to the breast. Her nose is pushed into the breast, her chin rests on her chest, and her view of her mother is inhibited. It may be that the mother's hand, unseen in this photo, is pushing on the back the baby's head. Pressure on the back of the head flexes the neck, inhibiting both breathing and swallowing. The baby may begin to struggle to protect the airway.

The infant pictured in **Fig. 123** has been rolled slightly to the side to allow a view of a poor latch. Note that the infant's chin is too far away from the breast. Poor proximity between the lower jaw and the breast will result in the jaw closing on the shaft of the nipple. This may result in painful breastfeeding and compromised milk transfer. The nipple will emerge from the baby's mouth looking pinched or flattened into a shape resembling an "orthodontic" pacifier or a new tube of lipstick.

The mother in **Fig. 123** has a large areola. She may have been following the advice to "get all the areola into the baby's mouth." Helpers must remember that the mother's view of the baby at breast is limited to the top half of the areola. If the mother is attempting to follow instructions to cover up as much areola as possible, she should be reminded that it is lower jaw coverage that matters. Since areolae come in many sizes, telling women to cover the areola is an inappropriate description and may result in incorrect lower jaw positioning. It may also instill doubt in a mother whose baby is actually well latched.

The poorly gaining infant in **Fig. 124** has a shallow latch on a long nipple. Priority was given to placement of the upper rather than the lower jaw. However, to compound the problem, the nipple may be marginally too long to fit in the baby's mouth without triggering a gag reflex. Notice how the nipple is bent at an angle.

Bending the nipple in a way that constricts the easily compressed milk ducts may obstruct milk flow (Morton 1992, Geddes 2007). The baby in **Fig. 124** closed his eyes almost immediately after latching. Flat or depressed feeding affect early in the feed may indicate poor milk transfer. It is important for the LC to confirm this impression with a test weight. Rather than allow ineffective sucking to proceed indefinitely, a mother in this situation should be encouraged to relatch the baby, and to employ stimulation techniques such as breast compressions to improve milk transfer. Or, she may need to discontinue the breastfeeding session to allow enough time to express milk. Appropriate interventions such as pumping and alternate feeding protect the milk supply and provide milk for supplementation.

When the mother of the baby in **Fig. 124** was taught to draw the baby's entire body in closer, jaw closure occurred over breast tissue, not just on the nipple shaft. Despite the long nipple, this positioning change effectively improved the infant's latch. When optimally latched, the baby took in more milk (confirmed by a test weight). The mother observed changes in the infant's feeding behavior. He opened his eyes and appeared more engaged in the activity. He breastfed with audible swallows. His diaper output increased. Within a few days, he recovered his birth weight and continued to grow well.

The infant in **Fig. 125** is not gaining weight and her mother has cracked nipples. Notice how the baby's upper lip retracts (rolls in). The angle at the corner of her mouth is very narrow - a clue that incorrect latch is part of the problem.

Rolling in the lips can be abrasive to breast tissue and may be a marker for poor oral stability. During feeding, the lips help hold the breast in the mouth to form an effective seal. Normally, the lips should shape to the breast in a relaxed manner, neither too loose (spilling milk), nor too tight.

If a baby is preterm, weak, or thin, the lack of sufficient fat pads in the cheeks will decrease ability to maintain the shape of the mouth. Thus, the infant may struggle to hold the breast. The baby may compensate by putting too much pressure on the lips. Decreased or increased lip tone should be noted when evaluating poorly feeding infants (Wolf 1992). Maturation and growth will help resolve many such problems. The mother can assist the baby by supporting the breast so the infant does not have to work so hard to hold the breast in his mouth. Temporary pumping and supplementation may be needed to protect the milk supply and the baby's intake until the infant matures.

The infant in **Fig. 126** is grasping only the nipple. The narrow angle at the corner of the baby's mouth indicates that the baby's jaw compressions will fall on the shaft of the nipple, resulting in pinching. The mother will experience pain, and milk flow will be limited. Note the distance between cheek and chin, and the breast. The cheeks and chin should be in direct contact with the breast.

In **Fig. 127** the nipple appears pinched. **Fig. 128** shows a pinched nipple that resembles the shape of an "orthodontic" pacifier or a new tube of lipstick. When babies grasp only the shaft of the nipple, jaw and tongue compression form a characteristic creased shape. Looking at the nipple as it emerges from the baby's mouth may provide information about the latch.

When an infant is well latched, as is the 24 hour-old baby in **Fig. 129**, the angle at the corners of the mouth will be very wide; this one is 150°. Note how the chin touches the breast, and the nasal passages are clear. Proof of a good latch is verified by lack of pain during the feed. The nipple will emerge from the baby's mouth looking undistorted as in **Fig. 130**. Notice that the baby ends the feed right where she started, with the nose opposite the nipple.

Brodribb W (Editor). *Breastfeeding Management in Australia*, 3rd ed. East Malvern: Merrily Merrily Enterprises, 1998; pp. 52-53, Fig. B 2.5.

Daly S, DiRosso A, Owens R, et al. Degree of breast emptying explains changes in the fat content, but not fatty acid composition, of human milk. *Experimental Physiology* 1993; 78(6):741-0755.

Colson S. Maternal breastfeeding positions: have we got it right? *The Practising Midwife* 2005; 8(11):29-32.

Colson SD, Meek JH, Hawdon JM. Optimal positions for the release of primitive neonatal reflexes stimulating breastfeeding. *Early Human Development* 2008; 84(7):441-449.

Geddes DT. Gross Anatomy of the Human Breast, in *Hale & Hartmann's Textbook of Human Lactation*. Amarillo, TX: Hale Publishing, 2007; pp. 19-34.

Geddes DT, Kent JC, Mitoulas LR, et al. Tongue movement and intra-oral vacuum in breastfeeding infants. *Early Human Devlopment* 2008; 84(7):471-477.

Glass R, Wolf L. Incoordination of sucking, swallowing, and breathing as an etiology for breastfeeding difficulty. *Journal of Human Lactation* 1994; 10(3):185-189.

Glover R. *Follow Me Mum* (video). Perth, Australia, 2000. Contact: reblact@rebeccaglover.com.au

Gunther M. Instinct and the nursing couple. *Lancet* March 15, 1955; 575-578.

Gunther M. Sore nipples, causes and prevention. *Lancet* ii 1945; 590-593.

Hoover K. Latch-on difficulties: a clinical observation. *Journal of Human Lactation* 2000; 16(1):6-10.

Hoover KL. Maternal obesity: problems of breastfeeding with large breasts. *Women's Health Report: A dietetic practice group of the American Dietetic Association* 2008; 6:10.

Howard C, Lanphear N, Lanphear B, et al. Variations in parental comforting practices and breastfeeding duration. Abstract for the 9th Annual Meeting of the Academy of Breastfeeding Medicine, Oct 20-25, 2004, in *ABM News and Views* 2004; 10(S):31-32.

Jacobs LA, Dickinson JE, Hart PD, et al. Normal nipple position in term infants measured on breastfeeding ultrasound. *Journal of Human Lactation* 2007; 23(1):52-59.

Jevitt C, Hernandez I, Groer M. Lactation complicated by overweight and obesity: supporting the mother and newborn. *Journal of Midwifery and Womens Health* 2007; 52(6):606-613.

Kent JC. How breastfeeding works. *Journal of Midwifery and Womens Health* 2007; 52(6):564-570.

Lang S. *Breastfeeding Special Care Babies*, 2nd Ed. Philadelphia: Bailliere Tindall, 2002; p. 49.

Milligan RA, Flenniken PM, Pugh LC. Positioning intervention to minimize fatigue in breastfeeding women. *Applied Nursing Research* 1996; 9(2):67-70.

Morton J. Ineffective suckling: a possible consequence of obstructive positioning. *Journal of Human Lactation* 1992; 8(2):83-85.

Neifert M, Lawrence R, Seacat J. Nipple confusion: toward a formal definition. *Journal of Pediatrics* 1995; 126(6):S125-129.

Newton M, Newton N. The let-down reflex in human lactation. *Journal of Pediatrics* 1948;33(6):698-704.

Newton N, Newton M. Psychologic aspects of lactation. *New England Journal of Medicine* 1967; 277:1179-88.

Prime D, Geddes D, Hartmann P. Oxytocin: Milk Ejection and Maternal-Infant Well-being, in *Hale & Hartmann's Textbook of Human Lactation*. Amarillo, TX: Hale Publishing, 2007; p. 150.

Ramsay D, Mitoulas L, Kent J, et al. Ultrasound imaging of the sucking mechanics of infant feeding from the breast and an experimental teat. *Proceedings of the 12th International Conference of the International Society for Research in Human Milk and Lactation*. Queen's College, Cambridge, UK. Sept. 10-14, 2004

Ramsay DT, Kent JC, Hartmann RA. Anatomy of the lactating human breast redefined with ultrasound imaging. *Journal of Anatomy* 2005; 206(6):525-534.

Rassmussen KM, Lee VE, Ledkovsky TB, et al. A description of lactation counseling practices that are used with obese mothers. *Journal of Human Lactation* 2006; 22(3):322-327.

Redstone F, West J. The importance of postural control for feeding. *Pediatric Nursing* 2004; 30(2):97-100.

Royal College of Midwives. *Successful Breastfeeding*, 3rd ed. London: Churchill Livingstone, 2002.

Savage-King F. *Helping Mothers to Breastfeed*. Nairobi: African Medical and Research Foundation, 1992.

Smilie C. Baby-Led Breastfeeding: *The Mother-Baby Dance* (video). Los Angeles, CA: Geddes Productions, 2007.

Springuel E. Empowering parents while you educate them about breastfeeding. Conference presentation. The Lactation Consultant in Private Practice Workshop, Philadelphia. PA, 1994.

Tully MR, Overfield M. *Breastfeeding: A Special Relationship* (video). Raleigh, NC: Eagle Video Productions, 1991.

Varendi H, Porter R, Winberg J. Does the newborn baby find the nipple by smell? *Lancet* 1994; 344(8928):989-990.

Wiessinger D. A breastfeeding teaching tool using a sandwich analogy for latch-on. *Journal of Human Lactation* 1998; 14(1):51-56.

Wolf R, Glass L. *Feeding and Swallowing Disorders in Infancy*. Tucson, AZ: Therapy Skill Builders, 1992; pp. 120-21.

Woolridge M. Aetiology of sore nipples. *Midwifery* 1986a; 2(4):172-176.

Woolridge M. The 'anatomy' of infant sucking. *Midwifery* 1986b; 2(4):164-171.

Woolridge M. The mechanics of infant feeding revisited: Fresh ultrasound studies of breastfeeding and bottle-feeding. Conference presentation, ILCA Conference, Orlando, Florida. July 27, 2012.

Flat and Inverted Nipples

In the 1950's, pioneering lactation physiologist, Mavis Gunther, described women with flat and inverted nipples whose infants became "apathetic" when put to breast. She speculated that baby humans (like other young animals) have an inborn receptivity to certain qualities and patterns of stimuli that evoke responses important to survival. These responses are not merely reflexive; they are behavioral triggers set in motion by certain physical signals. Normal feeding will be interrupted if the baby does not receive these signals. Gunther theorized that babies expect protractile nipple tissue that is sufficiently elastic to pull deeply into the oral cavity. (See **Fig. 130** to view a just-released nipple which a nursing infant has pulled into a fully protractile position.) Ultrasound research confirms that normal nipples extend during sucking to within approximately 5 mm of the infant's hard/soft palate junction (Ramsay 2004, 2005, Jacobs 2007, Geddes 2008).

Clinicians have observed that when babies are presented with breast tissue that is problematic to manipulate, it is as if a short-circuit occurs. The baby acts bewildered, shaking his head back and forth, bumping against the breast, or batting at the nipple with his fists. Some babies scream, others simply tune out and fall asleep. The mother may say, "It is as if he cannot figure out how to close his mouth around my breast." She may complain that the baby does not like breastfeeding, her milk, or her.

There may be several reasons why some infants struggle with flat or inverted nipples. Ramsay's ultrasound studies of breast anatomy (2005) identified that nipple ducts are easily compressed and collapse with gentle pressure. When infants encounter flat or inverted nipples, they may exert such high suction trying to draw in the teat that they collapse and occlude milk ducts. The resultant poor milk flow may frustrate the infant, and contribute to increasing levels of engorgement. Engorgement, itself, contributes to further flattening of the nipples, creating a cycle of frustration. To break this cycle, the LC must help the mother manage both engorgement and excess edema.

Several papers explore a massage technique used to redistribute fluid edema that accumulates close to the nipple. Shifting some of the edema back away from the nipple-areola complex results in briefly improved nipple protractility (Miller 2004). Cotterman (2004) names this technique Reverse Pressure Softening (RPS). The technique only provides a momentary shift of edema, but sometimes the baby, if put to breast immediately, can latch on and soften the breast. Also a pump can be used to drain off excess milk. However, pumping appears to pull the edema into the nipple-areolar complex, so the mother may have to pause frequently to massage until the engorgement decreases.

The LC assessing the mother must be aware that the presence of flat or inverted nipples is an indication of elevated risk for serious breastfeeding problems and influences the level of lactation acuity. Cooper (1995) identified 5 infants with severe breastfeeding dehydration and malnutrition. The mothers of 3 of the 5 infants had inverted nipples. Even in populations of well-educated and highly-motivated mothers, the presence of flat or inverted nipples is associated with suboptimal breastfeeding behavior on Days 0, 3, and 7, and with resulting delayed onset of lactation (Dewey 2003). Infants of mothers with flat or inverted nipples should therefore be closely followed for adequate weight gain. Mothers should receive special assistance until their infants are latching effectively.

Nipple Elasticity and Nipple Confusion

Infants whose mothers have difficult-to-manipulate breast tissue may react with relief when presented with a bottle teat. Possessing far greater proprioceptive stimulus than a flat or inverted nipple, a bottle teat elicits the full feeding response. Gunther (1955) called such substitution a "super-sign" and Woolridge (1996) called it a "supernormal stimulus."

Once exposed to the super-sign of a bottle teat, the baby may refuse the breast if there has been no improvement in the protractility of the maternal nipple or softening of the breast tissue. In such cases, the breast cannot "compete." The quick, easy milk flow rate of the bottle, combined with the stimulating effect of the artificial teat, overwhelms the signals the baby is receiving from the flat or inverting nipple and partially explains the condition called "nipple confusion." It may also explain why some studies show that many newborns can easily go back and forth between bottle and breast with no apparent difficulty (Cronenwett 1992), and why other experts connect early bottle teat exposure with breastfeeding failure (Newman 1993).

The unexamined, confounding factor in studies of nipple confusion may be the nipple protractility of the mothers involved. If women have erectile nipples with good elasticity, their babies may not be as vulnerable to what is termed nipple confusion. Thus, women with normal nipple elasticity may have less difficulty resuming breastfeeding after their babies have been exposed to bottle teats.

Much debate surrounds the definition and even the existence of what is termed "nipple confusion" (Dowling 2001). Some breastfeeding experts have attempted to clarify the discussion about nipple confusion by proposing a clinical definition (Neifert 1995). They make the point that it is important to distinguish between preference and dysfunction. Many skilled practitioners find that it is not especially difficult to coax babies back to the breast who have merely become too familiar with bottles. "Confusion" is not an appropriate term to ascribe to a baby who is functionally incapable of breastfeeding, either temporarily or enduringly.

Flat Nipples

Nipple protractility cannot simply be visually assessed. The mother or LC must manually compress the tissue about 2 cm behind the base of the nipple. Either the nipple will evert, it will flatten, or it will collapse inward in a telescoping fashion (see also **Figs. 210** and **211**). Drawing up any part of the areolar tissue between the thumb and forefinger assesses elasticity. Ideally there is some degree of "stretch" to the areolar tissue.

In addition to having larger breasts, excess periareolar adipose tissue may flatten the nipples of obese women (Jevitt 2007). Engorgement also dramatically reduces the elasticity and protractility of the nipple-areolar complex, sometimes creating a temporary flattening.

Hand expression, pumping, reverse pressure softening, and brief application of cold compresses help reduce swelling and soften the breast, making it easier for the baby to grasp. Recommendations to use cold compresses must take into account cultural beliefs about avoidance of cold in the postpartum period. Use of cold may restrict milk duct diameter, so brief warming of the pump flange prior to pumping assists milk flow (Kent 2011).

Fig. 131 shows a flat nipple. There is poor definition of the nipple, even when the mother compresses the breast. Large, robust babies typically suck so effectively that they can often manage to pull out a somewhat non-elastic nipple. If the baby is weak, small, preterm, ill, tongue-tied, or compromised in some other way, the combination of impaired stamina and flat or inverted nipples frequently leads to breastfeeding problems.

In **Fig. 132** a woman pulls back on her breast tissue to create more definition of her nipple. This is a variation of the sandwich technique. Thinning the breast in the same

dimension as the corners of the baby's mouth sometimes helps the baby sense the nipple more effectively. If the mother can plant a wedge of breast deeply in the baby's mouth, this action will often trigger sucking (see **Fig. 117**).

Fig. 133 shows a woman shaping her flat nipple into what is colloquially called the "teacup" or inverted nipple hold. Sometimes a mother can wedge enough tissue to help the baby latch. The mother or LC continues to hold the nipple in a pinched-up shape until the baby is sucking well before releasing the hold.

Inverted Nipples

The nipple contains milk ducts, sensory nerve endings, and smooth muscle fiber (Lawrence 2011). These tissues are normally capable of elastic stretch, and ultrasonographic photographs taken during breastfeeding document nipple elongation (Smith 1988). Ramsay (2005) observed changes in the length of the nipple relative to the hard/soft palate junction depending upon whether the posterior tongue was in an elevated or dropped position. Ultrasound images suggest that sucking is an active process that moves and expands the nipple. The effect of nipple inversion upon sucking has not been well-studied.

According to Lawrence (2011), severe nipple inversion may be viewed as a congenital defect, and is rare; however, Alexander (1992) estimated that as many as 10 percent of pregnant women have non-protractile nipples. These women may possess nipple tissue that is functionally inadequate to be optimally manipulated by their breastfeeding newborns.

Devices such as breast shells were commonly suggested in the past to pregnant mothers when flat or inverted nipples were identified. However, Alexander failed to find any significant value in prenatal therapies to stretch the nipples, such as the use of breast shells or Hoffman's exercises. McGeorge (1994) examined devices to stretch nipples prenatally and found some clinical benefits. Both commercial and home-made nipple everters have been used to assist women with inverted nipples, but aggressive nipple stimulation to stretch flat or inverted nipples has been associated with prepartum mastitis (Lawrence 2011). Mothers should be cautioned to avoid painful, repeated nipple manipulation.

Postpartum nipple protractility appears to increase in response to both sucking and pumping. Over time, many women with flat or inverted nipples report increased elasticity. On rare occasions a women can have a type of congenital nipple inversion that is not remedied by stretching. Lawrence (2011) reports that microscopic pathologic examination of severely inverted nipples reveals abnormal ducts and, in some cases, a reduced number of ducts. Surgical procedures are performed to correct the cosmetic appearance of inverted nipples and to relieve chronic pockets of inflammation that can form in places where the nipple folds upon itself. Reports of these surgical procedures do not describe the effects on breastfeeding.

Some women have nipples that appear to invert at rest, but that evert well upon compression. Others have apparently protruberant nipples that flatten upon compression (see **Figs. 210** and **211**). If the baby grasps and compresses the areolar tissue and the nipple retracts, the baby may be frustrated and uncertain about how to latch.

Figs. 134, **135**, and **136** show an inverted nipple at rest, during compression, and pulled back so the nipple protrudes. This mother was not able to breastfeed her first 2 children, but pumped her milk for many months for them. With the help of an IBCLC, she was able to breastfeed her third child. Women find that nipple protractility changes with more months of breastfeeding or pumping, thus providing opportunity for the tissues to stretch. This information may prove encouraging to affected women.

Dimpled Nipples

A dimpled nipple is a form of nipple inversion in which the tissue inside the fold can become adhered. Such a variation of nipple configuration can result in painful breastfeeding. The woman in **Fig. 137** has just finished pumping her breasts. **Fig. 138** shows the same nipple 2 minutes later when the nipple has resumed its dimpled shape.

In this woman's case, breastfeeding and pumping have pulled the adhered nipple tissue apart for the first time. The adhered skin is very fragile compared to skin that receives a normal amount of light, air, and friction from clothing. When the nipple folds back on itself after breastfeeding or pumping, moisture can remain trapped in the dimple, causing maceration and bleeding. After breastfeeding or pumping, it is important to instruct the mother to manually retract and rinse off the nipple. It is helpful to hold the nipple in a position that allows it to air dry for a few minutes. She should be instructed to perform the same manipulating during and after bathing. Keeping mascerated dimpled nipples clean is important to prevent infection. Applications of topical antiseptics or antibiotic creams may be used briefly during early lactation to protect the skin from infection, or to treat infection if it occurs. With repeated exposure to light and air, the tissue can heal.

Using Nipple Shields to Help Bring the Breast-Refusing Infant to Breast

Since breastfeeding is the natural culmination of the birth process, it is safe to assert that the baby who will not breastfeed is a baby who *cannot* breastfeed. The LC must determine what barriers prevent the baby from breastfeeding. If the infant cannot overcome the confusion caused by flat or inverted nipples, the LC must consider 3 issues:

- How is the baby to be fed while nipple remediation takes place?
- How long will it take before the baby can manage the nipples?
- Can the baby be kept at breast until the nipples evert?

Pumping and breastfeeding (if the baby will accept the breast) will usually pull out flat and inverted nipples. This can take a few days, a few weeks, or even months depending on the severity of the nipple inversion and the elasticity of the breast tissue. If the baby is never put to the breast during the remediation period, it may become more difficult to transition the baby to the breast. This is true no matter how the baby has been fed in the interim.

Thin Silicone Nipple Shields

A chart review by Wilson-Clay (1996) identified 32 women who were given thin silicone nipple shields as an intervention to correct breast refusal, latch problems, or sore nipples. All the mothers identified themselves as being in danger of imminent weaning and viewed the shield intervention as a final attempt to bring their babies to the breast. Of these women, 38 percent weaned prior to 6 weeks, but 51 percent, a significant number of this high risk group, continued to breastfeed beyond 6 weeks. The results suggest that use of a thin silicone nipple shield can successfully remediate some cases of infant breast refusal. In this case series, 15 of the mothers presented with flat or inverted nipples. They were significantly more likely to wean.

Based primarily on clinical experience, Powers and Tapia (2012) described various uses of thin silicone nipple shields in lactation support, including protection of sore nipples, improvement of milk transfer in compromised infants, extending the protractility of flat and inverted nipples, and using the shield to block overly-strong milk ejection.

Although widely used to provide barrier protection for sore nipples, there is little in the lactation literature to document the safety or efficacy of thin silicone nipple shield with regard to contact with damaged nipples. Some

LCs have voiced concern about infection risk when nipple shields are worn over broken skin. Writing in a plastic surgery journal, Weissman, et al. (2010), describe a novel use of thin silicone nipple shields to protect the hyper-sensitive tissue of non-breastfeeding patients recovering from nipple reconstruction. The authors described newly reconstructed nipples as subject to "mechanical pressure and shearing forces that can cause flap necrosis and sloughing of the skin, eventually promoting infection." Current available post-surgical dressings were described as inadequate or cumbersome, leading to poor patient compliance. Ten surgical patients were instructed to wear breastfeeding nipple shields to cover their healing nipples. Shields were washed with soap and water daily, and topical antibiotic ointment was applied to the scar for several days or as needed. The patients experienced reduced pain, no complications, and "reported full adherence to the postoperative dressing regimen as well as ease of use, availability, cost and pleasing aesthetic appearance under garments."

This study, while not specifically relating to breastfeeding per se, offers some reassurance concerning the use of nipple shields in the care of breastfeeding-related sore nipples. Similar nipple sensitivity exists in postpartum women and the same shearing forces and infection risk exist when new mothers experience nipple cracking. So long as shields are kept clean, the Weissman study suggests that even if worn continually, infection did not occur. Further, the authors describe several mechanisms that describe the efficacy of topical silicone in the treatment of scar prevention. Broader understanding of these issues that are more commonly described in the plastic surgery literature may be helpful in developing guidelines for the use of nipple shields in breastfeeding patients.

At present, there is scarce evidence to guide practice with regard to use of thin silicone nipple shields. Despite this fact, Eglash (2010) surveyed US health professionals about their use of nipple shields and found that 92 percent of the 490 respondents had used nipple shields in their practices. In a follow-up study, McKechnie (2010) stated that use of nipple shields has become "commonplace in the US for a wide range of breastfeeding problems." The authors conclude that more research is needed.

In the absence of clear clinical guidelines on thin silicone nipple shields, clinicians must explore the literature for insights from related fields and must rely on experience and case reports to guide practice. The biggest risk many practitioners identify is that nipple shields can disguise poor infant milk intake and result in an understimulated milk supply. If a nipple shield is provided, close follow-up care is vital, and infant growth outcomes should be monitored.

The Clinical Importance of Nipple Shield Design

Nipple shields have a remarkably persistent longevity as a tool. Written descriptions of the device appeared over 500 years ago, and they have been constructed of various materials (some toxic, such as nipple shields made of lead that were sold in Victorian England.) Most of the materials used to make nipple shields have been so rigid that they undoubtedly contributed to impaired milk intake and poor breast stimulation. This basic design problem has been improved upon with the use of thin silicone as the teat fabric. While allergy to silicone can be an issue, silicone is widely used in medicine, and topical silicone has been used as a treatment for keloid scars as well as for scar prevention (Weissman 2010).

Fig. 139 illustrates the lack of elasticity in the nipple of a first-time mother with a non-nursing infant. Her nipple is pictured moments later (**Fig. 144**) after her infant took his first effective breastfeeding at 2 weeks old using a nipple shield. A test weight performed before and after the breastfeeding confirmed that the infant consumed 79 ml. The infant continued to breastfeed with the shield for several weeks, and continued to gain > 1oz/day (30g). The nipples gradually became more elastic, and the mother experienced no difficulty in transitioning the baby to direct breastfeeding.

Mothers may purchase a nipple shield without appropriate guidance. The nipple shield in **Fig. 140** was purchased at a pharmacy (chemist's shop) in London, UK in 2002. This device has a design similar to antique models of nipple shields, and is likely to contribute to poor milk transfer and inadequate breast stimulation owing to the fact that it does not fit closely to the breast. Thick, latex shields sat directly on the breast, but they, too, were associated with decreased milk transfer and infants who failed to thrive. Shields of these designs should be avoided. Thin silicone nipple shields do not appear to alter infant sucking patterns (Woolridge 1980). In a small subset of 5 women, Chertok (2006) found no significant change in the level of prolactin stimulation during breastfeeding sessions when a nipple shield was worn. Larger, better controlled studies are needed to validate this finding.

Shield thickness is not the only issue to consider. For a nipple shield to be an effective therapeutic tool, the teat height must not be so long that it triggers the infant's gag reflex, or causes jaw closure and tongue compression to fall on the shaft of the teat. Using a too-long nipple shield creates a real risk that the baby will be unable to extract milk effectively, setting up a cascade of events including poor infant growth and decreased milk supply. These considerations relating to nipple shield height may not be fully appreciated unless one considers that the heights of commercially available nipple shields range from 1.9 cm to 6.4 cm (Drazin 1998).

Fig. 141 demonstrates graduating sizes of 3 Medela nipple shields. Sizes pictured are 16 mm, 20 mm, and 24 mm. The diameter of nipple shields also can vary widely (Frantz 1994). This variability appears to be an attempt by manufacturers to accommodate the wide ranges of human nipple diameters. Several researchers have looked at the variability in size of human nipples. The average nipple diameter appears to be 15-16 mm (Zeimer 1993, Stark 1994, Zeimer 1995, Ramsay 2005). Wilson-Clay and Hoover first presented similar findings on ranges and averages of nipple sizes in the second edition of *The Breastfeeding Atlas* (2002), and expand the discussion in the current edition (see Ch. 10). Infants have been observed to have difficulty grasping, sealing off, and manipulating large nipples. Large nipple shields can cause similar problems for some babies.

It may be that the wide variability in responses and outcomes reported in shield use is related to inappropriate choices in shield sizes. The LC must calculate the effect of the height and base diameter of the shield on the infant's response to its use. There are differences in opinion between experienced practitioners with regard to fitting the shield. Both authors prefer to use the shortest available teat with the smallest base diameter. Inevitably, some of the small size shields are not wide enough at the base to accommodate larger diameter nipples.

Powers and Tapia (2012) recommend fitting the shield to the nipple, and assert that even preterm infants can open wide enough to accommodate the 24 mm shields. However, the ability to sustain a seal around such a large diameter object can be an issue for the infant whether the mother with large nipples is wearing a shield or not. For women with wide diameter nipples, their breastfeeding problem may be related to large nipple diameter in the first place. Issues of "fit" must be factored into clinical observations, and there will always be some degree of experimentation involved regarding choice of equipment.

Applying a Nipple Shield

LCs have devised various ways to apply a nipple shield and use different vocabularies to describe these methods. Some center the shield on the nipple with the "brim" turned up like a sombrero. They then smooth down the brim onto the breast. This helps it stay in place. Other LCs stretch the part of the shield where the "nipple" joins the "areola." They place the stretched shield over the mother's nipple, release the tension and withdraw their

fingers. As the stretched shield returns to its normal shape, it will draw the mother's nipple into the teat cavity before the baby begins to suck. This trick not only helps the shield stay in place better, it also reduces the initial work the baby must exert in order to draw the nipple into the teat cavity.

Some LCs turn all but the top half of the teat portion inside out before placing it over the nipple as demonstrated in **Fig. 142**. Others warm the shield with hot water to make it more pliable.

Fig. 143 shows a newborn infant breastfeeding with a thin silicone nipple shield placed over his mother's nipple. This 6 day-old infant screamed whenever he was put to the breast. He was exclusively bottle-feeding when first evaluated by the LC. His mother was ready to wean. With the nipple shield mimicking the familiar sensation of the bottle teat, the infant went to the breast easily, sucked with good rhythm, swallowed audibly, and perceptibly softened the breast. Test weights confirmed that the infant consumed 74 ml. Note how the baby's lips are flanged on the breast, suggesting that the baby has a good latch.

Fig. 144 demonstrates how the baby has drawn the mother's nipple into the shield. This woman had flat nipples with poor definition, but her baby was healthy and vigorous. Within a few days of such stretching, nipple elasticity dramatically improved. After the baby had breastfed for a few minutes, and was not as hungry, the mother removed the shield, thus beginning the process of weaning the infant from the shield. When babies are not too hungry, tired or frustrated, they are more willing to latch without a shield. As this baby grew more confident that he would be able to satisfy his hunger at the breast, he became more patient when latching without the shield. His mother gradually used the shield less and less, and the baby came to trust and love breastfeeding.

Some small infants and infants with neuromuscular issues (for example, infants with Prader-Willi Syndrome, Down Syndrome, and other genetic disorders) appear to feed better with a nipple shield. They may need to rely on the nipple shield intervention for longer periods of time than would a more robust infant.

Preterm infants seem to especially benefit from nipple shields. Meier studied a group of 34 premature babies who averaged 31.9 weeks gestational age. These babies were able to take in 14 ml more milk when at the breast using a nipple shield than when at breast without a nipple shield (Meier 2000). On average they took in approximately 75 percent more milk (3.9 ml without the nipple shield and 18.4 ml with the nipple shield). This represents a statistically and clinically significant increase in intake. The researchers further observed that use of the shield helped correct problems like "slipping off the nipple" and "falling asleep" at breast.

The data from the Meier (2000) study indicate that "for preterm infants who demonstrate insufficient milk intake during breastfeeding, the nipple shield can serve as an effective, temporary milk transfer device without adversely affecting the total duration of breastfeeding." Most of the babies were off the nipple shield in 2 to 3 weeks. Duration of breastfeeding was longer for the babies whose mothers used the nipple shields compared to those who did not.

Fig. 144 is of special interest when discussing the findings of Meier. In this photograph, the nipple remains in an extended position even though the baby has come off the breast. After the first suck, the baby is relieved of the work necessary to keep the nipple elongated. Additionally, the pooled milk in the tip of the shield serves as a reservoir that provides the baby with an encouraging milk reward when nutritive sucking resumes. These observations may identify the shield mechanisms that assist the weak or preterm infant to sustain more stable feeding behavior.

Nipple shields are imperfect devices, and some mothers become concerned when the base of the shield curls up to cover the baby's nose. Generally, the baby can still breathe. Several companies manufacture shields with a cutout or a butterfly space. Some people prefer this design because these nipple shields do not roll over the baby's nose. Others feel the traditional design stays in place better and slips less owing to its greater surface area.

Fig. 145 pictures a 7 day-old infant who is poorly latched to a nipple shield. This baby had latch difficulties in the hospital following a traumatic delivery and little milk transfer was occurring. Note how the baby's mouth is positioned on the shaft of the shield. The baby had lost more than 9 percent of his birth weight, and was still losing weight. This picture and case illustrate the pitfalls of unsupervised nipple shield use. The need for the shield implies that an infant is feeding dysfunctionally. Such infants need close follow-up and their mothers require additional support to ensure good latch.

When repositioned and appropriately latched with the shield in place, test weights showed that the baby consumed 52 ml of milk from the breast in approximately 15 minutes. The LC recommended weight checks every other day until the baby recovered his birth weight, which occurred within 4 days. As the baby gained strength and recovered from the traumatic birth, the mother was able

to withdraw the use of the shield. By the middle of the third week after birth, the baby nursed well directly from the breast, and was gaining slightly over 1 ounce a day (35 g).

Anyone who provides a mother with a nipple shield must also provide follow-up. Positioning and latch should be directly assessed to make sure the baby is not sucking only on the shaft of the shield. Many mothers with well established milk supplies find it unnecessary to pump when they are using a shield. However, until milk transfer is assessed and found to be adequate with the shield in place, the mother should pump after most feedings to insure a robust milk supply. Weight checks provide the information needed to decide whether the baby is able to maintain the milk supply during the period of nipple shield use.

Many clinicians have concluded that keeping the baby at breast with a simple, inexpensive device such as a shield is reasonable when measured against the work of pumping, bottle-feeding, and the risks of weaning. While breastfeeding without any paraphernalia is optimal, mothers whose infants are finally brought to the breast with nipple shields are usually grateful the tool exists.

Note: To access an on-line module reviewing the history and design of nipple shields and management rationales for using a thin silicone nipple shield, see Wilson-Clay/Hoover: Clinical Use of Nipple Shields at **www.BreastfeedingMaterials.com**. *Photos and videos demonstrate how to apply a thin silicone nipple shield and how to assess latch when a shield is in place. 1 L CERP provided by IBLCE.*

Alexander J, Grant A, Campbell M. Randomised controlled trial of breast shells and Hoffman's exercises for inverted and non-protractile nipples. *British Medical Journal* 1992; 304(6833):1030-1032.

Chertok IR, Schneider J, Blackburn S. A pilot study of maternal and term infant outcomes associated with ultrathin nipple shield use. *Journal of Obstetrics, Gynecologic and Neonatal Nursing* 2006; 35(2):265-172.

Cooper W, Atherton H, Kahana M. Increased incidence of severe breast-feeding malnutrition and hypernatremia in a metropolotan area. *Pediatrics* 1995; 96(5):957-960.

Cotterman K. Reverse pressure softening: a simple tool to prepare areola for easier latching during engorgement. *Journal of Human Lactation* 2004; 20(2):227-237.

Cronenwett L, Stukei T, Kearney M. Single daily bottle use in the early weeks post-partum and breastfeeding outcome. *Pediatrics* 1992; 90(5):760-66.

Dewey K, Nommsen-Rivers L, Heinig M. Risk factors for suboptimal infant breastfeeding behavior, delayed onset of lactation, and excess neonatal weight loss. *Pediatrics* 2003; 112(3):607-619.

Dowling D, Thanattherakul W. Nipple confusion, alternative feeding methods, and breast-feeding supplementation: state of the science. *Newborn and Infant Nursing Reviews* 2001; 1(4):217-223.

Drazin P. Taking nipple shields out of the closet. *Birth Issues* 1998; 7(2):41-47.

Eglash A, Ziemer AL, Chevalier A. Health professionals' attitudes and use of nipple shields for breastfeeding women. *Breastfeeding Medicine* 2010; 5(4):147-151.

Frantz K. *Breastfeeding Product Guide*. Sunland, CA: Geddes Productions, 1994; pp. 45-46.

Gunther M. Instinct and the nursing couple. *Lancet*, March 19, 1955; 575-578.

Jacobs LA, Dickinson JE, Hart PD, et al. Normal nipple position in term infants measured on breastfeeding ultrasound. *Journal of Human Lactation* 2007; 23(1):52-59.

Jevitt C, Hernandez I, Groer M. Lactation complicated by overweight and obesity: supporting the mother and newborn. *Journal of Midwifery and Women's Health* 2007; 52(6):606-613.

Kent JC, Geddess DT, Hepworth AR, et al. Effect of warm breastshields on breast milk pumping. *Journal of Human Lactation* 2011; 27(4):331-338.

Lawrence RA, Lawrence RM. *Breastfeeding: A Guide for the Medical Profession,* 7th ed. Maryland Heights, MO: Elsevier Mosby, 2011, p. 46-50, 240-244.

McGeorge D. The "Niplette:" an instrument for the non-surgical correction of inverted nipples. *British Journal of Plastic Surgery* 1994; 47(1):46-49.

McKechnie AC, Eglash A. Nipple shields: a review of the literature. *Breasrtfeeding Medicine* 2010; 5(6):309-314.

Meier P, Brown L, Hurst N, et al. Nipple shields for preterm infants: effect on milk transfer and duration of breastfeeding. *Journal of Human Lactation* 2000; 16(2):106-114.

Miller V, Riordan J. Treating postpartum breast edema with areolar compression. *Journal of Human Lactation* 2004; 20(2):223-226.

Neifert M, Lawrence R, Seacat J. Nipple confusion: toward a formal definition. *Journal of Pediatrics* 1995; 12(6):125-129.

Newman J. Nipple confusion (letter). *Pediatrics* 1993; 92(2):297.

Powers DC, Tapia VB. Clinical decision making: When to consider using a nipple shield. *Clinical Lactation* 2012; 3(1):26-28.

Geddes DT, Lanton DB, Gollow I, et al. Frenulotomy for breastfeeding infants with ankyloglossia: effect on milk removal and sucking mechanism as imaged by ultrasound. *Pediatrics* 2008; 122(1):e188-194.

Ramsay D, Mitoulas L, Kent J, et al. Ultrasound imaging of the sucking mechanics of infant feeding from the breast and an experimental teat. Abstract of the 12th International Conference of the International Society for Research in Human Milk and Lactation. Sept. 10-14, 2004; Queen's College, Cambridge, UK.

Ramsay DT, Kent JC, Hartmann RA. Anatomy of the lactating human breast redefined with ultrasound imaging. *Journal of Anatomy* 2005; 206(6):525-534.

Smith W, Erenberg A, Nowak A. Imaging evaluation of the human nipple during breastfeeding. *American Journal of Diseases of Children* 1988; 142(1):76-78.

Stark Y. *Human Nipples: Function and Anatomical Variations in Relationship to Breastfeeding*. Master's Thesis, Pasadena. CA: Pacific Oaks College, 1994.

Weissman O, Tessone A, Liran A, et al. Silicone nipple shields: an innovative postoperative dressing technique after nipple reconstruction. *Aesthetic Plactic Surgery* 2010; 34(1):48-51.

Wilson-Clay B. Clinical use of silicone nipple shields. *Journal of Human Lactation* 1996; 12(4):279-285.

Wilson-Clay B, Hoover K. *Clinical Use of Nipple Shields* (learning module). www.BreastfeedingMaterials.com. 2012.

Woolridge M, Baum J, Drewett R. Effects of a traditional and of a new nipple shield on sucking patterns and milk flow. *Early Human Development* 1980; 4(4):357-364.

Woolridge MW. Problems of establishing lactation. *Food and Nutrition Bulletin* 1996; 17(4):316-327.

Ziemer M, Cooper D, Pigeon J. Evaluation of a dressing to reduce nipple pain and improve nipple skin condition in breastfeeding women. *Nursing Research* 1995; 44(6):347-351.

Zeimer M, Pigeon J. Skin changes and pain in the nipple during the first week of lactation. *Journal of Obstetric, Gynogologic, and Neonatal Nursing* 1993; 22(3):247-256.

Sore Nipples

Many factors and conditions contribute to sore nipples. Evidence-based protocols identifying best practices for treating sore nipples have not been developed. The lack of clear protocols to treat sore nipples has contributed to a wide variety of nipple remedies, many having no evidence of efficacy, and some with the potential to worsen symptoms.

The diagram below clarifies the terminology employed to describe the location of nipple trauma:

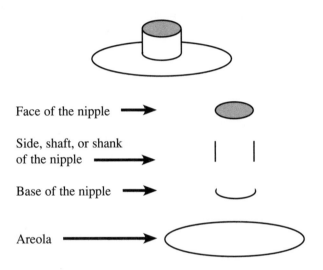

Face of the nipple ⟶

Side, shaft, or shank of the nipple ⟶

Base of the nipple ⟶

Areola ⟶

The Incidence and Significance of Nipple Pain

Studies of sore nipples during the first 2 weeks postpartum suggest that the height of nipple soreness occurs between Days 3 and 7, with peak levels occurring on Day 3 (*Best Practice* 2003). Some mothers report pain for as long as 6 weeks (Zeimer 1990). Gunther (1945) observed that nipple pain occurred in a majority (64 percent) of nursing mothers. In Ziemer's 1990 sample of 100 mothers, 96 reported nipple pain at some point in the study. Foxman, in a personal communication, (2002a) noted "nearly universal" nipple tenderness during the first week postpartum in a cohort of 946 women in a prospective mastitis study. "Nipple cracks and sores were reported by more than a third of all participants in the first week postpartum" (Foxman 2002b). Wagner, et al. (2012) reported that 44 percent of first-time mothers reported pain with breastfeeding on Day 3. These women had a >2-fold risk of early breastfeeding cessastion.

It is estimated that about one-third of breastfeeding women wean because of nipple or breast pain (Witt 2012).

Persistent nipple pain is associated with maternal depression that resolves when the pain resolves (Amir 1996). Women find this information to be reassuring, as they may otherwise interpret breastfeeding, itself, to be the cause of their depression. Indeed, family members and even health workers may suggest weaning to relieve maternal depression, rather than identifying it as a result of unmanaged nipple pain. Women's pain should be rated on a pain scale, and they should be observed for signs of visible nipple trauma. Mothers with visible nipple trauma are more likely to report higher levels of pain, and should be monitored for infection (McClellan 2012).

During Emergencies

Breastfeeding best protects infant survival. It is critical to protect newly delivered mothers who have sore nipples from developing infections during emergency situations when access to medical care or alternative sources of infant nutrition may be disrupted, such as in natural disasters or in regions where there is conflict. Basic, consistant strategies to manage new mothers with nipple pain should be developed and disseminated to aid workers, first responders, and to health care personnel. In the early postpartum, when the nipple tissue commonly experiences some degree of irritation, nipple skin should be kept clean, dry, and lightly lubricated (Page 2003).

Early Postpartum Nipple Sensitivity

There are a number of plausible theories that attempt to explain early nipple sensitivity. Normal physiological changes may contribute to postpartum nipple tenderness. Breast sensitivity increases significantly following birth (Prime 2007). Increased sensitivity provides a benefit by enhancing nipple responsiveness to the tactile stimulation necessary to release oxytocin and trigger the milk ejection response. As the milk ejection reflex becomes better conditioned, enhanced nipple sensitivity may become less critical and thus decline.

Early breast and nipple pain may be associated with other normal hormonal changes. Cox (1999) observed a relationship between nipple growth and prolactin levels, noting that nipple sensitivity at 20 weeks gestation coincides with rising levels of serum prolactin. Most women can recall a time during pregnancy when their nipples became extremely sensitive. This extreme sensitivity typically subsides as the pregnancy continues. The dramatic rise in prolactin levels after birth may contribute to a similar transient period of increased nipple tenderness during the first weeks.

While not formally quantified, there appears to be a wide range of individual variations in nipple sensitivity. Some women describe having nipples that are always hypersensitive to certain kinds of touch or to cold. Sometimes these women have had previous breast surgery and may have nerve injury, or circulation problems (as with Raynaud's phenomenon). But for most mothers, it is comforting to learn that early postpartum tenderness typically resolves.

During the early postpartum period, many women report pain only when the baby first latches on, lasting about 20 to 30 seconds. Such pain may result from a kind of *low load muscle strain* as nipple tissue adjusts to stretching. Having plausible explanations for discomfort assists women in dealing with the psychological stress associated with painful experiences. Mothers are reassured when the LC compares nipple stretching discomfort to other familiar activities such as muscle soreness after exercising.

Some LCs suggest that mothers apply the "30 second rule." If nipple pain subsides once the baby is well latched, the mother can safely ignore it. If discomfort persists, the mother should remove the baby and re-latch. If tissue breakdown occurs, mothers need to know this is a sign they need extra lactation assistance. In such cases, the LC should also carefully assess the infant's oral and facial anatomy to rule out tongue-tie, receding chin, or small mouth as potential reasons for maternal nipple pain.

Early postpartum latch discomfort usually resolves within several weeks and is typically not associated with skin damage. Nipples do not "toughen up" but simply gain elasticity and return to normal levels of sensitivity over time. Anticipatory guidance helps the mother view early nipple sensitivity as a temporary inconvenience.

Degrees of Tissue Damage

Women breastfeeding their first infant often need help distinguishing between common, temporary tenderness and acute pain with resultant nipple damage. Because so many women initially seek lactation help via telephone consultation, health workers must ask specific questions about nipple appearance in order to elicit information about whether or not the nipple skin is broken. It is important to know the duration of the problem, and whether or not the mother is self-treating with preparations that may worsen her symptoms. Nipple pain resulting from trauma may be associated with skin changes including *erythema* (redness), *edema* (swelling), fissures (cracks), blisters, inflamed areas with associated swelling and pain, skin color changes, scabs, peeling, pus, and delayed healing.

Wounds tend to occur on the nipple face, although some (notably those caused by a too-tight pump flange) may occur at the base of the nipple. Some early skin changes on the nipple face appear to be caused by suction damage due to overly strong suction, perhaps before the milk comes in (Zeimer 1993). A second characteristic wound commonly seen on the nipple face in early breastfeeding is the compression stripe, caused when some aspect of sucking distorts the nipple. Woolridge (1986) described suction damage and compression damage as two *primary* physical causes of nipple pain. *Secondary* causes such as infection or dermatitis may occur once the skin integrity is breached.

Mohrbacher (2004) proposed consistency in describing nipple trauma and developed a staging system to identify the degree and intensity of nipple damage.

- **Stage I** -- superficial pain, intact skin (redness, bruising, swelling)
- **Stage II** -- superficial pain, tissue breakdown (abrasion, shallow fissure, compression stripe, blistering)
- **Stage III** -- partial thickness erosion (skin breakdown to the lower layers of the dermis; deep fissure)
- **Stage IV** -- full thickness erosion (full erosion through the dermis)

Suction Lesions Related to Low Milk Flow Rate

Woolridge explains that when milk flows freely, the need to exert suction pressure diminishes. Hence "… if little milk issues from the nipple, or the baby's appetite has not been assuaged after milk flow has ceased, then unrelieved suction will be applied to the nipple surface and this may lead to suction trauma" (Woolridge 1986). Sakalidis (2012) used ultrasound to identify differences in sucking action between NS and NNS, and observed an altered sucking action when milk flow is absent.

In the first days of breastfeeding, perhaps the typically low volumes of available colostrum cause some babies to apply unrelieved suction in an attempt to access more milk. Certainly, many mothers report that breastfeeding feels more comfortable after their milk comes in. BWC has observed that mothers with chronic low milk supply often complain of sore nipples. Infants confronted with a low milk supply, engorgement, or blocked ducts may exert higher levels of suction to try to access available milk, traumatizing the nipples. Similarly, mothers report that so-called *dry pumping* (pumping in the absence of a milk ejection) feels uncomfortable. These observations support those of Woolridge that low milk flow contributes to nipple pain and to the potential for the nipples to become traumatized.

Variant Sucking Dynamics

In spite of apparently normal milk flow, some mothers report on going nipple pain that fails to resolve. They describe painful or "strong" infant sucking in spite of attentive positioning and careful latch technique. Using ultrasound and pressure transducers, researchers have observed that some infants appear to generate unusually high levels of suction, causing significant nipple distortion while breastfeeding (McClellan 2008).

BWC has worked with mothers whose babies and breasts seemed unremarkable except for reports of persistent pain while breastfeeding. Ultra thin silicone nipple shields helped some of these mothers manage discomfort; others were not assisted by shield use. Pumping with hospital grade breast pumps permitted protection of the milk supply; however, if these mothers attempted to breastfed more than a few times a day, their nipple tissue began to break down again. Over the course of 3 to 4 months, some of the mothers reported being able to drop pumping sessions and resume increaseingly more daily breastfeedings without pain or tissue breakdown. Some were eventually able to discontinue pumping altogether.

These cases may provide clinical support for McClellan's ultrasound observations. Perhaps these babies begin to suck differently over time, or their mothers tolerate the sensation better as nipple sensitivity decreases. Perhaps as their mouths grow bigger and their bottom jaws move forward something changes in the latch. When the LC is able to share information about this phenomenon, some mothers may decide to continue pumping in hopes of eventual improvement. In the meantime, their babies continue to benefit from human milk feeds.

Breast Engorgement and Nipple Pain

Unrelieved engorgement flattens nipples and makes them difficult for the infant to grasp. Geddes (2007) speculates that engorged women may experience transient decrease in milk production owing to increased intra-alveolar pressure that (in animal models) flattens *lactocytes* (milk-making cells). The infant may compensate for the harder-to-grasp nipples and try to generate better milk flow by exerting higher levels of negative pressure (see **Ch. 7**).

A Relationship Between Infant Pain, Comfort Sucking, and Nipple Pain?

Sucking is analgesic in infants (Gray 2002). Perhaps infants recovering from difficult deliveries and birth trauma suck more aggressively at the breast in an attempt to regulate state behavior and cope with pain. Because the nipple sensitivity is markedly increased in the first 24 hours postpartum (Geddes 2007), mothers of injured infants may experience more nipple pain.

Images of Nipple Trauma

Marmet describes *raspberry nipples,* seen in **Fig. 146**. Hoover (2013) proposes naming the individual sections *druplets*. The cracks between the druplets create a risk for sore nipples.

Engorged women whose milk flow is inhibited by breast edema may exhibit starburst-shaped lesions on the center of the nipple face. In these cases, the baby appears to have sucked so hard that the fragile, hyperstretched nipple tissue tears.

The baby may exert excessive negative pressure because:
- engorgement prevents easy teat formation
- flat nipples are difficult to grasp with normal levels of suction
- engorgement reduces milk production and flow
- nipple pain may inhibit milk release (let-down)

Fig. 147 shows the engorged breast of a woman with Stage I nipple damage. Note the venous engorgement apparent on her breast and areola. The face of her nipple appears as a collection of inflamed, swollen vesicles producing Stage I nipple damage. The woman's nipples developed suction lesions on Day 2 prior to hospital discharge. The nipple trauma became more pronounced over time, and she developed mastitis that required oral antibiotic treatment.

Fig. 148 shows an engorged breast on Day 4 with a flat nipple and Stage II damage. Note the asymmetrical distribution of the tissue damage on the nipple face. It suggests suction damage caused by the infant sucking too hard to form a teat from the flat nipple and engorged breast tissue.

Nipple lesions often have a characteristic appearance that may provide clues as to the cause of the damage. A nipple (when viewed in profile) may appear pinched, distorted into a shape resembling a new tube of lipstick, or an "orthodontic" pacifier. A cut or scab in the shape of a compression stripe forms across the face of the nipple, running parallel to an imaginary moustache on the baby's upper lip as the baby nurses. If the infant is being nursed in cradle hold, the stripe runs from 12 o'clock to 6 o'clock; if in football hold, the stripe appears from 3 o'clock to 9 o'clock.

The LC and the mother should observe the shape of the nipple immediately after the baby comes off the breast.

Distortion of the shape of the nipple is especially traumatic during breast engorgement, because swelling causes the nipple tissue to become more fragile as it stretches and thins. The skin rapidly breaks down, owing to repeated trauma.

Compression lesions may result from shallow latch, behavioral adaptations, anatomic anomalies of the infant's mouth or the mother's nipples, or variant sucking dynamics. For instance, a baby might pull off, compress or crimp the nipple to slow the milk flow, especially if the mother has a forceful milk ejection reflex. Certain infant anatomical problems may contribute to nipple distortion such as tongue-tie, short tongue, small mouth, receding chin, or high palate. Large or long maternal nipples may prevent a good latch, causing the baby to pinch the nipple shaft.

Fig. 149 shows a pinched nipple seconds after the baby came off the breast. The orientation of the nipple wound suggests the baby was being breastfed in the cradle hold. Note the characteristic misshaping of the nipple, and Stage II trauma.

Fig. 150 shows Stage II trauma on Day 4 postpartum when scabs have formed over the broken skin. The orientation of the stripe indicates the baby was held in the cradle position. Having corrected the latch, the LC may want to direct the mother to use another feeding position while the wounds heal. The LC must evaluate both the mother and the infant for anatomic or behavioral issues that may further explain nipple trauma. If all relevant issues are not managed, repeated trauma creates the risk of breast infection and untimely weaning.

Deep fissures can appear on the face of the nipple, as in **Figs. 151-152** where Stage III damage is observed. The mother in **Fig. 151** is 4 weeks postpartum. She breastfed 2 older children without difficulty, but her youngest baby was born with a tongue-tie. The mother developed fissures on both nipples that became infected and required oral antibiotics. The LC explained that taking a break from breastfeeding might speed recovery. "Resting on a pump" removed the source of the trauma and allowed her nipples to heal. She elected not to seek a frenotomy for the infant, and primarily bottle-fed pumped milk for 4 months and then weaned to formula.

Fig. 152 demonstrates a partial thickness wound where the dermis has been breached to the moist, underlying capillary bed. The wound appears to be in the healing phase when new cell proliferation occurs. This skin is very fragile and prone to re-injury and infection. The mother was told to wean so the fissure would heal. Determined to breastfeed, the woman persevered. The woman's physician was treating her nipples with nystatin, having assumed that the damage was the result of a yeast infection, when the LC (KH) evaluated her.

In the case of the woman in **Fig. 152**, KH speculated that rapid milk ejection and oversupply contributed significantly to the nipple damage. KH explained to the mother that the infant may have been deliberately pinching off the nipple in an attempt to regulate the force of the milk flow. Milk oversupply finally was brought under control at 10 weeks, and the infant discontinued the compensatory sucking behavior. Eliminating the source of the nipple trauma helped heal the mother's nipples while the baby continued to breastfeed. Perhaps significantly, this family's 2 dogs had fungal skin infections. Animals may serve as a reservoir for *Candida* infections that are communicable to humans (Edelmann 2005). It is possible that the mother had become infected with *Candida* by exposure to her pets, although no cultures were taken. and nystatin, alone, had failed to improve the condition of her nipples.

Fig. 153 shows a badly eroded nipple before and during treatment, illustrating Stage III damage. The reddened area and the mother's complaints of severe pain prompted the midwife to prescribe antibiotic cream and antifungal creams. Within 5 days, partial regeneration of the tissue can be observed. If a mother with such nipple damage cannot tolerate breastfeeding, an alternate method of milk expression must be employed to keep the breasts draining and protect the milk supply while the nipples heal. This mother is at high risk for mastitis and breast abscess.

Fig. 154 shows a mother with Stage IV nipple damage. The woman is holding a flat toothpick next to the fissure to help illustrate the 7 mm depth of the wound.

Negative Pressure Wound Debridement

Negative pressure therapy is used to treat pressure and diabetic ulcers (Enoch 2003, Kirby 2007). It is possible that both pumping and breastfeeding offer the mother's nipples some protection from infection by constantly removing exudate from any wounds that form. The effect of pressure debridement on the healing of nipple wounds may be an unexamined issue in breastfeeding. It may help explain why many mothers with nipple fissures do not develop infections in spite of inconsistent wound care practices and constant re-exposure to oral pathogens in the mouths of infants.

Sore Nipple Treatment Controversies

It is disappointing that research has not yet provided consistent guidance on the most effective methods to manage nipple tissue damage. Various methods have been promoted, many of them part of cultural traditions. These include the application of the mother's own milk, peppermint water soaks, lubrication with olive oil, applications of wet tea bags, lanolin, hydrogel pads, various herbal remedies (Riordan 1985, Hewatt 1987, Spangler 1993, Buchko 1994, Pugh 1996, Lavergne 1997, Beauchamp 2005, Sayyah 2007). The apparent efficacy of some of these preparations may stem from placebo effect or unexplored antiseptic and anti-inflammatory properties, or other issues unique to breastfeeding. (See above for discussion of negative pressure wound debridement.)

Fetherston (1998) supported the use of nipple creams to help heal sore nipples and identified this method of nipple care as a protective factor against development of mastitis. However, she identified wearing a nipple airer (breast shell or tea strainer) as a risk factor for breast infection. She speculated that such devices may become contaminated as a result of poor hygiene or ineffective sterilization practices, or they may indent the areola and cause blockage of ducts and bruising of engorged tissues. Ramsay (2004) identified that milk ducts "readily collapsed under slight pressure similar to that required to compress a superficial vein on the back of the hand." It may be that devices such as shells, strainers, and even improperly held pump flanges cause blockages by collapsing ducts. Poor breast drainage and nipple fissures are risk factors for mastitis, and care should be taken to avoid behaviors that increase risk of infection.

While it is important to base practice on evidence, it is difficult to achieve accurate and consistent comparisons between sore nipple treatment methods (Page 2003). A Cochrane review looked at intervention treatments to prevent mastitis after childbirth (Crepinsek 2010). It concluded that owing to small sample sizes and wide variations in the types of interventions tried, there is insufficient evidence to show effectiveness of any of the interventions. These included breastfeeding education, pharmacological treatments, and alternative therapies.

Perhaps different types and degrees of nipple trauma respond to different methods of treatment. Some cases of sore nipples resolve on their own simply by improving breastfeeding technique and improving the volume of milk transfer. Women with compromised immune systems however, including those with IgA deficiency may be at high risk for breast infections (Fetherston 2006). Additionally, hospital transmission rates of Methicillin Resistant *Staphylococcus aureus* (MRSA) have increased in recent years (Rutala 2006). Close follow-up of postpartum women with nipple fissures is critical, as MRSA cannot be treated with ordinary antibiotics and is highly contagious (Saiman 2003, Beam 2006). (See **Ch. 11**.)

A comparative study assessed sore nipple treatment in 90 primiparous mothers of term infants (Akkuzu 2000). Three techniques were examined for effectiveness in preventing or reducing nipple pain and cracked nipples in the first 10 days postpartum. Subjects were randomized into 3 groups with one group applying warm compresses, one group applying expressed breast milk (EBM), and one group using no treatment other than keeping the nipples clean and dry. The warm compress group had the most cracks. The expressed milk group had the fewest complaints of pain and the fastest healing of cracks. On the final day of assessment, the clean and dry group had the fewest cracked nipples. The authors concluded that mothers should be instructed to keep nipples clean and dry following the recommendations of WHO/UNICEF.

Keeping the nipples dry should not be interpreted to mean "dried out." Light lubrication promotes moist wound healing. Purified lanolin creates an air-permeable temporary skin barrier, and has been demonstrated to have anti-inflammatory, antimicrobial, skin-protecting, and barrier repair properties (Abou-Dakn 2011). In a study that compared 87 mothers who applied either highly purified anhydrous (HPA) lanolin or EBM to their cracked nipples, Abou-Kakn observed faster healing and reduced pain in the lanolin group.

Hydrogel Dressings

Hydrogel dressings have been proposed as a treatment for cracked nipples, based on moist wound healing theory. However, there is a difference between surface wetness and the preservation of internal moisture (the basis for moist wound healing theory). Wet breast pads and wet, dirty dressings cause maceration, expose fissures to pathogens, and do not speed healing. Hydrogel dressings that have begun to appear cloudy due to accumulation of fluids may pose an infection risk (Page 2003). Zeimer (1995) reported that the use of an occlusive dressing during the first week postpartum appeared to have limited influence on improvement in damaged skin condition; however, use of the dressing did significantly reduce reports of pain during the study period.

Brent (1998) compared use of a hydrogel wound dressing with lanolin and breast shells in a sample of 42 breastfeeding women with sore nipples. She reported significantly more infections in the hydrogel group, which resulted in early discontinuation of the study. Dodd (2003) found significantly greater reduction in pain scores in mothers who used hydrogel pads. The study protocol emphasized maternal handwashing before handling the dressings. Additionally, after removing them, mothers were instructed to wash the dressings with warm water, pat them dry, and advised to place the dressings on a clean surface. After feeding, the mothers were asked to rinse their breasts with warm water and pat themselves dry before re-applying the cleaned dressings. Whenever the hydrogels turned cloudy, the mothers were instructed to discard them and open a new dressing. Using this protocol, no mother using hydrogels experienced infection.

In essence, participants in the Dodd study were keeping their nipples clean while receiving the pain reduction benefit associated with use of hydrogels. This model is worth further consideration. Clearly, the emphasis on hygiene is an important factor in the lack of reported infections in this study of women using hydrogels.

Immediate Wound Care for Cracked Nipples

Acute (newly acquired) skin wounds elsewhere on the body are routinely cleansed in order to remove contaminants that could impede healing and cause infection. Generally mild soap and water are used (Potter 2001, Page 2003).

It can be difficult to delineate between wounds that are colonized and those that are infected. Host factors (the strength of the maternal immune system) play an important role in the rate of wound healing. Postpartum women have somewhat depressed immune response and thus increased vulnerability to infection.

Bacteria have the ability to generate a protective coating: a sticky goo called a *biofilm*, which they form over bacteria colonies growing in a wound. Biofilms are increasingly being recognized as a factor in delayed wound healing. Saliva potently stimulates biofilm production (Hale 2006). Repeated exposure to infant saliva may make nipple wound infections harder to eradicate because biofilms prevent both topical and oral antibiotics from penetrating to the wound. Antiseptic measures and gentle debridement (wound cleansing) may be helpful in removing biofilms so the immune system can manage the infection or so that antibiotics can do their work (Ryan 2007).

Since breastfeeding books have traditionally discouraged nipple cleansing, new mothers may need clear and specific explanation about why it is important to gently cleanse fissured nipples. The LC should explain that while it is unnecessary to engage in elaborate routines to clean intact nipple skin, cracked nipples require the same first aid attention normally followed when taking care of a bite wound on a finger.

Cleanse nipple wounds once a day with warm, soapy water. Following each breastfeeding, mothers should flush the nipple wounds with normal saline solution or tap water (Fernandez 2002). This reduces the likelihood that pathogens from the baby's mouth will re-colonize open nipple

fissures. Handle injured nipples with clean hands. Air or gently pat dry before applying expressed milk, purified lanolin, topical antibiotic cream, or a clean hydrogel dressing.

Non-healing Cracked Nipples

The LC may encounter a mother who reports a nipple wound that has been present for days, weeks, or even months in spite of various treatments. Enoch (2003) states that *chronic wounds* have several distinctive factors. They fail to heal in a timely, orderly manner, and remain stuck in the inflammation or proliferative phase. The main barriers to healing in chronic wounds appear to be:

- accumulation of necrotic (dead) tissue
- pathogen imbalance
- altered exudate levels

Chronic wounds appear to have underlying pathogenic abnormalities that cause constant accumulation of *necrotic* (dead) tissue, prolonging the inflammatory response, and mechanically obstructing the process of healing. The baby's sucking or the pump may continually remove the most visible accumulations of necrotic tissue and hide the fact that the wound is manifesting *altered exudate levels* (in other words, is oozing fluid.)

The terms *local infection* and *critical colonization* refer to wounds that will not heal but which may not display classic signs of infection (Enoch 2003).

The mix of microorganisms within a wound may also be an issue with regard to healing. The microflora present may include fungi as well as bacteria. Giandoni (1994) identified *cutaneous candidiasis* as a cause of delayed wound healing.

Identifying best practices for the management of cracked nipples awaits more conclusive evidence (Kvist 2007). To prevent infection, the LC focuses on correcting primary sources of nipple trauma and providing appropriate first aid care for damaged nipples. Close follow-up is required to identify progression to mastitis, which requires medical evaluation and treatment.

Bacterial Nipple Infections

Nipple trauma that does not heal after latch-on and positioning have been corrected may be an important sign of infection. The risk of constant re-exposure to pathogens via contact with the infant's mouth is a factor that may distinguish nipple injury from other types of wounds. *Staphylococcus aureus* (including also MRSA) may be carried on the hands, objects, and clothing. Owing to nasal colonization, it may be communicated orally from the baby to the nipple. MRSA is associated with mastitis and a high risk of abscess formation in breastfeeding women (Amir 2006, Kim 2007).

The majority of cracked nipples and breast infections occur during the first 2 weeks postpartum, when pathogens from the hospital environment may be present (Kitajima 2003). Livingstone (1999) states that, "Contaminated wounds are often slow to heal and can lead to widespread infections. *Staphylococcus aureus* ascends lactiferous ducts [causing] infections, mastitis, and breast abscess." Ramsay's ultrasound detection of milk backflow when the let-down subsides serves to provide a plausible explanation for migration of pathogens into the ductal system (Ramsay 2004).

Once pathogens have migrated into the milk ducts, topical cream or ointment are ineffective to resolve mastitis. Oral antibiotics must be considered (Livingstone 1999). However, it may be possible to prevent ascending pathogens by preventing cracked nipples from becoming infected.

Over-the-counter medications such as Polysporin™ (bacitracin and polymyxin B) and Neosporin™ (bacitracin, polymyxin and neomycin) are available in a number of countries worldwide. They are used to prevent infection and speed wound healing, and physicians often advise applying such medications to damaged nipples. However, neomycin has been noted to provoke allergic skin reactions in sensitive individuals, and some strains of MRSA have become resistant to both bacitracin and neosporin (Suzuki 2011).

Mupirocin (Bactroban™) is an antibiotic ointment available by prescription in the US and is highly active against *staphylococci* and most *streptococci*. There also is evidence to suggest it has anti-*candida* activity *in vivo* (Nicholas 1999, de Wet 1999). Mupirocin is minimally absorbed topically and is rapidly metabolized when ingested orally, so it is unlikely to produce side effects in infants, making it useful as a nipple cream (Hale 2012). However, as with all antibiotics, there is danger of overuse leading to bacterial resistance. Rash and skin irritation are possible side effects of mupirocin.

Mupiricin is the antibiotic agent included in the so-called all-purpose nipple ointment (APNO), a topical preparation also containing a steroid and an anti-fungal agent. Typically available from compounding pharmacies, APNO has been promoted to prevent the negative outcomes associated with painful, damaged nipples. However, the only available study evaluating the effectiveness of this preparation found no differences in outcomes at 1 week and 12 weeks between women using lanolin and APNO. Outcomes examined included nipple yeast symptoms and/ or mastitis. The authors concluded that APNO was not superior to lanolin in the treatment of damaged nipples (Dennis 2012).

Fig. 155 shows an infected, cracked nipple. The appearance of pus indicates the potential for the spread of the infection to underlying tissue and subsequent systemic symptoms. This situation requires medical attention. It is not appropriate to use hydrogel dressings on infected skin. Protocols for treating breast infections are reviewed in **Ch. 11**.

Fungal Infection

Two terms refer to fungal infections involving *Candida* species: candidiasis and candidosis. These terms are used interchangeably.

Using accurate assay methods, Hale (2009) designed an experiment to demonstrate that *Candida* can be detected in human milk using the proper assay methods. Using a novel assay, Hale succeeded in detecting *Candida albicans* in human milk seeded with yeast cultures. However, using the same assay technique, he was unable to detect *Candida* in milk pumped from women presenting with "classic" symptoms of "ductal yeast" infections, including deep breast pain and burning nipples. Hale's experiment suggests that yeast infections do not occur within the ducts of the breast.

Diagnoses of yeast infections of the breast have often been made without culture, based only on reported symptoms. This has resulted in the overuse of powerful systemic antifungal medications such as fluconazole. Aggressive overtreatment has also resulted in creating extra work for mothers who are often instructed to undertake radical dietary changes and to assume extra laundry and house cleaning chores in order to erradicate "resistant yeast" infections of the breast. Nipple vasospasm, dermatitis, and bacterial infection may be more common than previously believed, and create symptoms that have often been attributed to candidiasis (Thomassen 1998, Huggins 1993, Amir 1993, Livingstone 1999, Anderson 2004, Morino 2007).

Some common "yeast" treatments probably exert a therapeutic effect upon bacterial infections and dermatitis, adding to the confusion about whether a mother has "yeast" or not. For instance, topical gentian violet has antiseptic and antibacterial properties as well as being an antifungal agent. Oral fluconazole exerts anti-inflammatory activity common to other azole drugs (Gupta 1978). The anti-inflammatory activity of fluconazole is amplified when used in combination with ibuprofen (Arai 2005). Fluconazole also has been demonstrated to exert protective effect against sepsis (Khan 2005). Full or partial resolution of breast pain following the use of topical and oral yeast medications may create a mistaken impression that they have cured a *candida* infection when other factors may be the cause of the resolution of pain.

Further research is required to investigate the micro-organisms involved in the breast pain of breastfeeding women. The CASTLE study (a longitudinal evaluation of the roles played by *Staphylococcus* and *Candida* species in breast pain) will hopefully help resolve the controversy about the primary organism in the condition known as "breast thrush" or "yeast infections of the breast" (Amir 2011).

Superficial Candida Infection of the Nipple

Topical skin infections of *Candida*, particularly *comorbid* infection (combinations of bacterial and fungal organisms) have been identified on the nipple.

Yeast infection of the nipple presents as the onset of pain *after* early postpartum nipple discomfort has resolved. If untreated, superficial fungal infections may cause skin breakdown. Early nipple skin breakdown in the first few weeks postpartum is more likely to result from sucking trauma or bacterial infection. Late onset pain, a renewal of nipple tenderness, and progressive skin breakdown are important signs of superficial fungal infection.

Yeast infection of the nipple generally coincides with the appearance of a fungal infection in the infant's mouth (called *thrush)*, a fungal diaper rash, or *Candida* infection in another family member or pet. Handwashing for at least 15 seconds duration is important in preventing cross-infections. Cross-infection should be investigated if yeast infections recur. Treat any family member or pet with symptoms of fungal infection such as athlete's foot, diaper rash, vaginal yeast infection, finger or toenail fungus, jock itch, dandruff, ringworm, etc. Fungal infections of the skin can be persistent and take weeks to clear up, especially during hot, humid weather, and are particularly difficult to eradicate in people with immunosuppression, especially from HIV/AIDS.

Most infants have a white, milky coating on their tongues. Thrush appears as a fuzzy white plaque that spreads to cover the oral mucosa. White on the tongue is not thrush unless it becomes progressively thicker and spreads to other oral surfaces. Other causes may alter the appearance of the infant's oral mucosa, such as viral infections. **Fig. 156** shows a white tongue.

Untreated oral *Candida* infection rapidly spreads to the lips and to the oral mucosa. The infant in **Fig. 157** has fungal lesions on the inside of the cheeks on the buccal pads. The infant with thrush in **Fig. 158** has fuzzy white lesions covering much of her oral cavity.

Oral nystatin is the front line medication to treat infant thrush in the US, and miconazole oral gel is widely used-outside the US. Maternal treatment involves use of topical ointments or creams containing nystatin, miconazole, mupiricin, or clotrimazole. Breastfeeding can continue and these medications do not have to be washed off the breast. They are reapplied sparingly after each feeding.

Gentian violet is an antifungal agent that some doctors recommend as an over-the-counter treatment for thrush, providing care is taken to avoid infant swallowing too much of it. Gentian violet (0.5 percent) is typically applied to the baby's mouth and the mother's nipples once a day for 3 to 4 days (**Figs. 159** and **160**). After coating the baby's mouth with gentian violet, place the infant face down on a disposable pad so that excess medication is drooled out rather than swallowed. Over-use of gentian violet has been associated with ulceration of the mouth and throat (Utter 1990). Mothers often use purified lanolin to coat the skin around the baby's mouth to prevent the purple dye from staining the baby's face.

Yeast diaper rashes typically do not respond to standard care, but improve when treated with antifungal creams or ointments. Care must be taken, especially in populations of preterm infants, to rule out zinc deficiency and skin infection caused by *Staphylococcus* species as the cause of persistent diaper rash.

Fig. 161 shows a nipple that is becoming tender and inflamed. Note the accumulations of white material on the nipple face.

Fig. 162 shows an infected nipple that required treatment with both antifungal and antibiotic ointment.

Fig. 163 shows extreme tissue breakdown in a woman with a persistent, untreated infection. Her story demonstrates the limitations of telephone consultation. The woman had a dimpled nipple, the tip of which folds in on itself, (see **Figs. 137** and **138**). This type of nipple configuration traps moisture in the crevice, creating a hospitable environment for bacterial and fungal overgrowth. Unless women are shown how to retract the skin to rinse and air dry the nipple after feeding, the unexposed area can become colonized, macerated and infected. The woman had phone contacts with nurses in her pediatrician and obstetrician's offices and with a lay counselor, but no one directly examined her nipples.

At 5 weeks postpartum, BWC saw the mother in person. Deep fissures had opened on both nipples. The infant had normal oral anatomy and there was no obvious evidence of breast infection. The mother expressed concern about her cracked nipples, but surprisingly did not find them painful enough to prevent her from breastfeeding. The LC referred the mother to her obstetrician and he prescribed APNO (triple nipple cream). It took an additional 2 months for the nipples to completely heal. The woman never developed symptoms of mastitis.

Until the fissures closed, the mother was advised by her doctor to reduce the risk of infection by avoiding swimming pools, to maintain careful skin hygiene, and to wear clean cotton brassieres. Shortly before her nipples healed completely, they became exquisitely tender. The LC speculated that after such extensive tissue damage, nerve endings that had been destroyed were now regenerating. The woman maintained lactation throughout the experience and breastfed until her baby was 18 months old.

Allergic Reactions

Any condition that affects the skin elsewhere on the body can also affect the skin of the breasts and nipples. Allergic reactions (dermatitis) can occur on the breasts. Postpartum women have an enhanced sensitivity to contact with chemicals, irritants, or allergens (Pray 2000). Dermatitis often is mistaken for fungal infection. Women may phone an LC and complain about weeks of pain from unresolved nipple "yeast" in spite of complicated treatments. It is reasonable to suspect that the problem results from something else. Referral to a dermatologist is appropriate.

Possible Triggers of Allergic Dermatitis on the Breast

- Detergent, soap, shampoos, or spray deodorants
- Creams, ointments, herbal remedies, or medications
- Reaction to the material of breast shells, nipple shields, or pump flanges
- Introduction of solid foods (exposure via infant saliva)
- Baby receiving medication or using teething gels
- Salivary changes owing to teething
- Previous maternal history of atopic dermatitis in other areas of the body prone to maceration.

When the mother in **Fig. 164** stopped using the medicated cream she had been applying to her nipples, her allergic reaction resolved.

The mother in **Fig. 165** has itchy, red-raised *uticaria* (hives) on her breast caused by an allergic reaction to topical applications of nystatin, an antifungal drug. She chroni-

cally suffered from mild outbreaks of eczema, but did not associate her chronic skin condition with the irritated area that developed on her areola. After talking with friends, she became convinced that she had a yeast infection. She requested nystatin to treat it. Her pediatrician called in a prescription without evaluating the breast lesions in person. Over the course of 4 days, the mother treated the baby's mouth with nystatin and applied the drug directly to her nipple.

After taking a history and discovering patches of eczema on the woman's elbows, the LC suspected an allergic reaction to nystatin. The LC consulted with the obstetrician by phone. The doctor advised the mother to discontinue applying nystatin and suggested an over-the-counter topical corticosteroid cream to control the itching. She directed the mother to take 2 doses of oral Benadryl™ (diphenhydramine) elixir per package directions to control the allergic reaction. Within 12 hours the mother's symptoms cleared, and she required no additional care. This story illustrates the importance of direct examination, and the danger of assuming that every red or itchy patch of skin on the breast indicates a yeast infection. Exacerbation of symptoms after medication use begins should prompt evaluation for allergic reaction to the drug.

Eczema

The woman in **Fig. 166** has eczema on her nipple and areola. Note the dry, scaly appearance of the reddened skin. Eczema is common in people with a family history of hay fever and asthma, and is revealed by skin breakdown behind the knees, on the hands and feet, or on any area where the skin is exposed to stress.

LCs should ask women with breast lesions whether they have similar patches of irritated skin elsewhere on their bodies. This question helps determine if the breast condition is directly related to lactation or involves a pre-existing skin condition that has been exacerbated by the wet-dry, wet-dry nature of breastfeeding. Eczema also may develop when infants begin to eat solid foods if food residue acts as an allergen on the mother's nipples (Amir 1993). **Ch. 12** also contains a discussion of contact allergic reaction triggered by food.

Prolonged exposure to hot water, chlorine, and synthetic clothing may aggravate eczema. Mothers should be advised to take quick, warm showers, avoid swimming pools, and wear cotton clothes so the breast skin can "breathe."

Often a woman who develops eczema on the nipple or breast has an existing relationship with a dermatologist, and may have appropriate topical medications on hand. A physician or pharmacist can determine if the medication is safe for use on the nipples (Huggins 1993). Sometimes skin that is damaged and broken from eczema becomes infected. A combination of a topical antibiotic and a topical steroid is usually effective in this case (Hale 2002).

Prolonged use of steroids can cause health problems for the baby (Amir 1993). The pediatrician should be informed of ongoing steroid treatment of the mother's nipples in order to monitor the baby. If breastfeeding the infant is too painful for the mother, pumping protects the milk supply. Friction from the pump flange may further irritate eczematous skin. The mother can lubricate the plastic pump flange to help prevent friction trauma to fragile skin.

The woman pictured in **Fig. 166** did not have a previous history of eczema. No factor to explain the sudden onset of eczema was discovered. At 11 months postpartum, she called her midwife to report burning nipple pain and shooting, burning breast pain, and was given a prescription for a topical antifungal for 2 weeks. Her baby was treated with oral nystatin even though the baby showed no signs or symptoms of thrush. When treatment did not resolve her symptoms, the mother was given oral fluconazole for 2 weeks, but her condition did not improve.

The woman called KH to request assistance. KH suggested that the woman ask for a referral to a dermatologist, who diagnosed eczema and prescribed a steroid cream. Over the next month, the eczema gradually improved. The mother continued to breastfeed throughout the treatment.

Paget's Disease of the Nipple

A type of breast cancer called Paget's disease resembles nipple eczema (see also **Ch. 12**). Paget's disease of the breast accounts for approximately 2 to 3 percent of breast cancers. Clinical features include bloody nipple discharge, erythema and scaling of the nipple, nipple erosion or ulceration, nipple retraction, and a palpable mass or thickening in the breast with or without nipple changes (Burke 1998). It appears unilaterally (on one side) and progresses steadily. When eczema does not resolve with appropriate treatment, further investigation including biopsy may be required. See **Figs. 290-292** for photographs of a nipple biopsy to rule out Paget's disease of the nipple.

Psoriasis

Some women with psoriasis experience outbreaks on their nipples and areolae that have not significantly impacted

breastfeeding. In other cases, breastfeeding has been interrupted. **Fig. 167** shows psoriasis on the nipple and areola. This woman had salmon-colored patches covered with silvery scales on many parts of her body. After the birth of each of her 2 sons, psoriasis spread to her nipples. Breastfeeding was too painful to continue, and this mother opted to wean.

There are few prospective, randomized trials to guide treatment of psoriasis in pregnant and lactating women, but treatment with low- to moderate-potency topical steroids is considered to be the front-line therapy, followed by narrowband ultraviolet B phototherapy (Bae 2012).

Poison Ivy

Fig. 168 shows a woman with poison ivy on her breasts. After skin is washed, the oils from the plant that cause the allergic reaction are gone. Thus, there is no risk that the baby will develop poison ivy from contact with the nipple or breast. However, continued nursing poses the typical risks of secondary infection of the nipple and of excessive pain. If better tolerated than breastfeeding, the mother can pump milk until the lesions heal (Lawrence 2011). Hydrocortisone creams and short-term use of oral corticosteroids are considered safe for breastfeeding mothers who develop poison ivy (Hale and Berens 2002, Hale 2012).

White Spots on the Nipple: Blebs, Caked Ducts

Fig. 169 shows a white spot on the nipple face associated with a painful blockage of the milk duct openings (milk pores). Such white spots are often referred to as *blebs* (bubbles). Research has only just begun to describe why blebs may form. It may be that when the nipple is traumatized, a blister forms over a milk duct opening (see **Fig. 174**).

Whenever a duct opening is obstructed, the resulting backup creates a ropy, tender mass that extends into the interior of the breast. Dried material, the end of which is visible at the nipple pore, blocks milk from that lobe of the breast from draining freely. The experience of a nipple bleb and resultant plugged duct is so painful that some women seek to have blebs opened by a health care provider. Other women try to open blebs by lancing them with a sterilized needle; however, they may be at increased risk for infiltrating infection of the breast.

Ultrasound anatomy studies identify about 9 patent ductal openings at the surface of the nipple. Obstruction of any of the ductal openings significantly affect the drainage of the breast, causes pain, and may impair lactation (Ramsay 2005).

One mother described her experience with a blocked nipple pore as follows: "Blocking the pore "...was a small chunk (about the size of a mustard seed) that had a cheese curd consistency. I flicked it with my fingernail and dug in a bit and it came partially out. Then I used sterilized tweezers to grab and pull it the rest of the way out. Milk came shooting out of the pore and gushed for a good minute before slowing to a trickle. After the next feeding my nipple still felt a bit sore with a smaller bump under the skin. After the next feeding the bump was completely gone. No discomfort or swelling left at all."

O'Hara (2012) described histology studies that revealed a lack of bacteria or fungi in the material removed from a bleb. The rubbery tissue consisted of "histiocytes with foamy cytoplasmic vacuoles and fibrin deposition. These immune cells indicated a tissue reaction to milk that has leaked from ducts into surrounding tissues." Based on the finding that blebs may form as the result of an inflammatory reaction, a short daily course of a thin layer of mid-potency steroid was applied to the inflamed, fibrotic tissue. Treatment with topical steroid ointment resolved symptoms in the study population. The researcher recommended that women with blebs be evaluated carefully so that any underlying causes of recurrent trauma can be treated.

Not every white spot on the nipple causes pain, and some may result from issues unconnected with blockages of the ducts. For example, some white spots may be accumulations of dead skin, similar to cradle cap. The mother can lubricate her nipple and gently rub off dry skin. **Fig. 170** illustrates a white spot on the nipple that was not painful. It is more asymmetrical than a bleb. Because nothing in the breast feels blocked, it does not cover a ductal opening.

Sometimes a bite from a teething baby produces a ragged tear in the nipple skin. As moisture accumulates under the skin edges, the skin may turn white (similar to the edges of a cut on the finger that look white after bathing or washing dishes). The mother should cleanse a bite wound with warm water and mild soap, apply one application of a topical antibiotic ointment to prevent infection, and report any increase in pain or inflammation to a physician. Bites are often associated with ascending ductal infection and mastitis.

Cysts

Sore nipples may have unusual causes. Sometimes the fact that the woman is lactating is coincidental. The woman in **Fig. 171** phoned KH to describe a painful "plugged duct." She stated that "white, stringy" material could be squeezed from the white spot on her nipple, and she was unable to drain it thoroughly. When the LC observed the nipple,

she discovered that the white spot was on the shaft, not the face of the nipple (as would be the case with a blocked pore). The breast was soft, with no evidence of engorgement or masses. The stringy material exuded from the white spot more closely resembled a sebaceous secretion than dried milk. These clues led the LC to conclude that the condition was unrelated to lactation and appeared to be a kind of pimple. When the woman consulted a physician the next day, he confirmed the LC's suspicion and identified the problem as a sebaceous cyst. The doctor excised a quantity of the oily matter. Removal of the material brought relief from the pain, and the condition resolved.

Vasospasm

Nipple vasospasm is a constriction of the blood vessels with resultant color changes to the face of the nipple (Anderson 2004). The constriction causes a shooting pain or cramping (Page 2006). In describing normal wound healing processes, Enoch (2003) states that "Vasoconstriction...occurs in response to initial injury." Thus, previous nipple trauma may result in a tendency to experience vasospasm. Vasospasm is currently recognized as an important source of nipple pain in breastfeeding women. Descriptions of deep breast pain resulting from vasospasm have caused many women to be mistakenly diagnosed with 'yeast" infections (Morino 2007). **Fig. 172** shows a nipple in the blanching phase of vasospasm.

Cold stress may trigger vasospasm of the nipple, especially to a traumatized nipple. Keeping the nipples warm and applying dry heat immediately after breastfeeding relieves the stabbing, shooting pain of vasospasm. Wet compresses should be avoided as evaporative cooling may trigger resumption of vasospasm.

Lactation consultant, Diana West (personal communication 2005) shares the following: "Some women report that they can stop the vasospasm if they massage blood into the nipple. This is done by gently squeezing the base of the nipple and pushing forward" (**Fig. 173**). In West's opinion, restoration of blood flow to the nipple seems to stop the painful, burning sensation.

Mothers experiencing vasospasm should eliminate or reduce their exposure to nicotine and caffeine (which has a rebound vasoconstrictive effect). Consultation with a prescribing physician can determine how a mother might reduce her exposure to vasoconstrictive drugs such as theophylline, terbutaline, epinephrine, norepinephrine, serotonin, prostaglandin, and birth control pills. In Lawlor-Smith's case studies of 5 women with nipple vasospasm, each described severe, debilitating nipple pain (1996, 1997). Blanching of the nipple occured during and immediately after the feeds, and also somewhat randomly, between feeds. Exposure to cold precipitated nipple blanching and pain in all patients observed.

As has been previously emphasized, unexplained pain alarms women. It is helpful to explain that vasospasm, while annoying, is essentially a benign condition that cannot damage the breast. Some women observe nipple blanching without pain. One mother who experienced nipple blanching told BWC that it did not cause her pain.

If gently massaging the base of the nipple and applying dry heat fail to significantly relieve pain, a physician may prescribe oral nifedipine to treat nipple vasospasm (Eglash 1996, Anderson 2004).

Raynaud's Phenomenon

Nipple vasospasm can occur without an individual having *Raynaud's phenomenon*, a condition which includes lack of blood flow to the extremities of the body (such as the toes, fingers, nipples, ears, and nose). Raynaud's phenomenon is found in approximately 20 percent of women of childbearing age (Anderson 2004) and is known to cause vasospasm of the nipple (Morino 2007). Raynaud's phenomenon produces a biphasic or triphasic color change in the affected extremity (Lawlor-Smith 1996, Lawlor-Smith 1998). First the body part turns white. In some instances, it then turns blue. Finally, it reddens. Raynaud's phenomenon has been associated with other medical conditions including lupus erythematosus or rheumatoid arthritis, hypothyroidism, and with certain medications. There is an association (poorly described at present) between breast surgery and Raynaud's phenomenon affecting the nipple (Anderson 2004).

Blisters on the Nipple

The woman in **Fig. 174** had been using a breast pump uneventfully for many weeks. She suddenly developed a blister on her nipple after expressing her milk with a hospital grade electric breast pump using a too-high pressure setting. (The white material on her nipple is milk.) Such blisters can also result when a pump flange is too small or is not properly centered. Sometimes a baby causes a similar blister to form when the milk supply is low or blocked. In such situations, the baby compensates by sucking extra hard in an effort to obtain more milk. The mother in **Fig. 174** was encouraged to keep her nipple clean, dry, and lightly lubricated. She purchased a larger pump flange and used the highest *comfortable* pumping pressure. These measures resolved the problem and the blister disappeared without complications. It is especially important to protect engorged nipple tissue from pumping trauma.

Montgomery Glands

Montgomery glands (or tubercules) are scattered over the areolar surface. Great variation exists in the number observed, but the average is 9 (range 0-38). These areolar skin glands appear to function as scent organs and play a role in helping the baby find the breast (Schaal 2006). Montgomery glands enlarge during pregnancy and become less noticeable after weaning.

These glands have a small ductal subsystem almost like a miniature mammary system (Lawrence 2011). The small ducts that secrete sebaceous material sometimes merge with the ducts that secrete milk. It is common to see drops of moisture on these pimple-like structures. BWC worked with a mother who reported that her Montgomery glands significantly enlarged during her engorgement phase and appeared inflamed. They were tender before feedings. The discomfort resolved after feedings when the glands returned to a more normal (less swollen) appearance. She could express drops of milk from her Montgomery glands.

Occasionally a mother will report that a Montgomery gland gets plugged and may become inflamed (**Fig. 175**). This is typically a self-limiting condition. Applications of moist heat and gentle manipulation may help open the duct. A one-time application of topical antibiotic cream may prevent infection. The woman in **Fig. 175** phoned KH complaining of a "plugged duct." As they were concluding their conversation, the mother added an aside: "It has been interesting watching this 'second nipple' grow today." The LC asked the mother to describe the location of this "second nipple" and made an appointment to see the mother in person. Visual assessment confirmed the LC's suspicion that the problem was an infected Montgomery gland, rather than a plugged milk duct on the nipple face and within the breast.

The mother used warm soaks and attempted to squeeze the lump without success. The LC instructed the woman to call her obstetrician, who phoned in a prescription for an oral antibiotic. Within hours after starting the antibiotic, the woman felt better. The following day there was a white head on the infected area. The woman was then able to squeeze out white, thickened milk, followed by pus, then blood, and then clear serous fluid. The mother washed the area with warm soapy water, rinsed well, and applied a topical antibiotic cream. The area quickly healed. This woman frequently saw milk coming from her Montgomery glands.

Occasionally an infected Montgomery gland becomes a problem for a woman using a breast pump, especially if the inflammation is located where the breast flange rests. A notch can be cut in the flange if necessary. The cut out area is placed to avoid the sore area. Using a cutout flange is also useful to avoid causing friction or placing painful pressure on an areolar abscess while pumping. Be aware that the edges of the cut plastic may be sharp.

Occasionally, irregular thickening of the nipples and areola can occur with no sign of infection or other explanation such as was experienced by the mother in **Fig. 176** whose areolar tissue, starting with her 5th pregnancy, became inflamed with every subsequent pregnancy, but returned to normal several months after the births of her next 3 children. The tissue appears discolored and "warty."

One case study describes a benign but disfiguring condition called *nevoid hyperkeratosis* of the nipple and areola (Fenniche 2010). The cause of this condition is unknown and 80 percent of cases occur in women and manifest during puberty or pregnancy. There is no known treatment that is uniformly effective, and the condition may persist indefinitely.

Skin Tags

The mother in **Fig. 177** has a skin tag on the tip of her nipple. She worried that it might affect breastfeeding or cause nipple pain. In her case it did not. Breastfeeding was only slightly less comfortable on the affected breast. Occasionally skin tags tear off and bleed during breastfeeding. A dermatologist can easily remove them. While the procedure can be done during lactation, it is probably best performed during pregnancy in order to give the nipple time to heal.

The mother in **Fig. 178** has a skin tag on her areola, located a distance from the nipple. While this will not directly interfere with breastfeeding, some infants like to manipulate skin tags, causing irritation and potential risk of infection. If a mother chooses not to remove the skin tag from her breast, she may wish to keep it covered to discourage the baby from playing with the tag while feeding.

Proper Removal of The Baby From The Breast

The cause of sore nipples sometimes is related to lack of attention to unlatching the baby. Often mothers remove their babies from the breast without first breaking suction. This can be traumatic and can create abrasions on the nipple shaft as the baby tries to grab it back or bites down reflexively. **Fig. 179** demonstrates insertion of the mother's finger between the gums (not just between the lips). If the

baby becomes slightly startled and bites down, the bite will occur on the mother's finger rather than the nipple. Poor technique in removing a baby from the breast may be a significant contributing factor and help to explain a mother's complaint of persistent nipple pain.

Biting

Older babies, such as the 5 month-old in **Fig. 180** often present a new set of breastfeeding challenges. Easily distracted by noise or changes in the feeding environment, the baby may tug at the breast while trying to look around, or may bite down as the result of teething discomfort. Mothers should make eye contact and use simple language to tell the baby: "Don't bite! " Repeat the same phrase, especially at times during the feeding when the baby typically bites. If the baby ignores the verbal and visual commands, some mothers find it effective to remove the baby from the breast, put the baby down briefly, and repeat the verbal command firmly. Yelling at the baby is discouraged since it may precipitate a *nursing strike* (sudden breast refusal). Babies learn from repetition, and if the mother is consistent in her response, it generally does not take long before biting ceases. Sometimes toddlers leave teeth marks on the breast (as in **Fig. 181**). This is not a problem unless the skin is broken or the mother complains of bruising. If the baby bites the nipples and breaks the skin, it is important to prevent infection with basic first aid measures, including cleansing with warm soapy water. If infection occurs, consult a physician.

Hormonal Changes

Hormonal changes unrelated to breastfeeding may cause nipple pain. Occasionally, a woman who has resumed menstruation will notice nipple tenderness prior to the onset of her period. Changes in breast and nipple sensitivity may be the first indication of pregnancy, even before a woman misses a period. A woman who becomes pregnant may notice persistent nipple discomfort while breastfeeding. Along with heightened sensisivity, some of this pain may result from diminished milk production and compensatory strong suction by a toddler.

Abou-Dakn M, Fluhr JW, Gensch M, et al. Positive effect of HPA lanolin versus expressed breastmilk on painful and damaged nipples during lactation. *Skin Pharmacology and Physiology* 2011; 24; 27-35.

Akkuzu G, Taskin L. Impacts of breast-care techniques on prevention of possible postpartum nipple problems. *Professional Care of Mother and Child* 2000; 10(2):38-39, 41.

Amir L. Eczema of the nipple and breast: a case report. *Journal of Human Lactation* 1993; 9(3):173-5.

Amir LH, Cullinane M, Garland SM, et al. The role of micro-organisms (*Staphylococcus aureus* and *Candid albicans*) in the pathogenesis of breast pain and infection in lactating women: a study protocol. *BMC Pregnancy and Childbirth* 2011; 11:54.

Amir LH, Dennerstein L, Garland SM, et al. Psychological aspects of nipple pain in lactating women. *Journal of Psychosomatic Obstetrics and Gynecology* 1996; 17(1):53-58.

Amir LH, Garland S, Lumley J. A case-control study of mastitis: nasal carriage of *Staphylococcus aureus*. *BMC Family Practice* 2006; 7:57.

Anderson J, Held N, Wright K. Raynaud's phenomenon of the nipple: a treatable cause of painful breastfeeding. *Pediatrics* 2004; 113(4):e360-e364.

Arai R, Sugita T, Nishikawa A. Reassessment of the in vitro synergistic effect of fluconazole with the non-steroidal anti-inflammatory agent ibuprofen against *Candida albicans*. *Mycoses* 2005; 48(1):38-41.

Bae YS, Van voorhees AS, Hsu S, et al. Review of treatment options for psoriasis in pregnant or lactating women: From the Medical Board of the National Psoriasis Foundation. *Journal of the American Academy of Dermatology* 2012; 67(3):459-477.

Beauchamp GK, Keast RS, Morel D, et al. Phyto-chemistry: ibuprofen like activity in extra-virgin olive oil. *Nature* 2005; 437(7055):45-46.

Best Practice 2003. The management of nipple pain and/or trauma associated with breastfeeding. 2003; 7(3):1-7.

Beam JW, Buckley B. Community-acquired Methicillin-Resistant *Staphylococcus aureus*: prevalence and risk factors. *Journal of Athletic Traning* 2006; 41(3):337-340.

Brent N, Rudy S, Redd B, et al. A clinical trial of wound dressings vs. conventional care. *Archives of Pediatric and Adolescent Medicine* 1998; 152(11):1077-1082.

Buchko BL, Pugh LC, Bishop BA, et al. Comfort measures in breastfeeding primiparous women. *Journal of Obstetric, Gynocologic, and Neonatal Nursing* 1994; 23(1):46-52.

Burke E, Braeuning M, McLelland R, Pisano E, et al. Paget's disease of the breast: a pictorial essay. *Radiographics* 1998; 18(6):1459-1464.

Cox D, Kent J, Casey T, et al. Breast growth and the urinary excretion of lactose during human pregnancy and early lactation: endocrine relationships. *Experimental Physiology* 1999; 84(2):421-434.

Crepinsek MA, Crowe L, Michener K, et al. Interventions for preventing mastitis after childbirth. *Cochrane Database System Review* 2010; Aug 4:8:CD007239.

Dennis CL, Schottle N, Hodnett E, et al. An all-purpose nipple ointment versus lanolin in treating painful damaged nipples in breastfeeding women: a randomized controlled trial. *Breastfeeding Medicine* 2012; 7(6):473-479.

de Wet P, Rode H, van Dyk A, et al. Perianal candidosis — a comparative study with mupirocin and nystatin. *International Journal of Dermatology* 1999; 38(8):618-22.

Dodd V, Chalmers C. Comparing the use of hydrogel dressings to lanolin ointment with lactating mothers. *Journal of Obstetric, Gynecologic, and Neonatal Nursing* 2003; 32(4):486-494.

Edelmann A, Kruger M, Schmid J. Genetic relationship between human and animal isolates of *Candida albicans*. *Journal of Clinical Microbiology* 2005; 43(12):6164-6166.

Eglash A. Case report. *ABM News and Views* 1996; 2(1):4.

Enoch S, Harding K. Wound bed preparation: the science behind the removal of barriers to healing. *Wounds* 2003; 15(7):213-229.

Fernandez R, Griffiths R. Water for wound cleansing. *Cochrane Database of Systematic Reviews* 2002; 4(CD003861). Update: Nov. 2, 2007.

Fenniche S, Badri T. Nevoid hyperkeratosis of the nipple and areola. *New England Journal of Medicine* 2010; 362(17):1618.

Fetherston C. Risk factors for lactation mastitis. *Journal of Human Lactation* 1998; 14(2):102-109.

Fetherston C, Lai CT, Hartmann PE. Relationships between symptoms and changes in breast physiology during lactation mastitis. *Breastfeeding Medicine* 2006; 1(3):136-145.

Foxman B. Personal communication, March. 19, 2002a.

Foxman B, D'Arcy H, Gillespie B, et al. Lactation mastitis: occurrence and medical management among 946 breastfeeding women in the United States. *American Journal of Epidemiology* 2002b; 15(2):103-114.

Geddes DT. Gross Anatomy of the Human Breast, in *Hale & Hartmann's Textbook of Human Lactation*, Amarillo, TX: Hale Publishing, 2007, pp. 19-34.

Giandoni M, Grabski W. Cutaneous candidiasis as a cause of delayed surgical wound healing. *Journal of the American Academy of Dermatology* 1994; 30(6):981-984.

Gray L, Miller L, Philipp B, et al. Breastfeeding is analgesic in healthy newborns. *Pediatrics* 2002; 109(4):590-593.

Gunther M. Sore nipples, causes and prevention. *Lancet* ii 1945; 590-593.

Gupta AK, Bhargava KP. Some triazole analogs as anti-inflammatory agents. *Pharmazie* 1978; 33(7):430-431.

Hale TW. *Candida* infections: all the "NEW" details. Conference Presentation. Hale/Hartmann Human Lactation Research Conference. Richmond, VA. Spet. 28-29, 2006.

Hale TW, Bateman TL, Finkelman MA, et al. The absence of *Candida albicans* in milk samples of women with clinical symtoms of ductal candiadiasis. *Breastfeeding Medicine* 2009; 4(2):57-61.

Hale T. *Medications and Mothers' Milk 2012*, 15th ed. Amarillo, TX: Hale Publishing, 2012; pp. 805, 1212-1213.

Hale T, Berens P. *Clinical Therapy in Breastfeeding Patients*, 2nd ed. Amarillo, TX: Pharmasoft Medical Publishing, 2002; pp. 208-212.

Hewat RJ, Ellis DJ. A comparison of the effectiveness of two methods of nipple care. *Birth* 1987; 14(1):41-45.

Hoover K. Proposing a new term: drupelet. *Clinical Lactation* 2013; 4(1):36.

Huggins K, Billon S. Twenty cases of persistent sore nipples: collaboration between lactation consultant and dermatologist. *Journal of Human Lactation* 1993; 9(3):155-160.

Khan HA. Effect of fluconazole on phagocytic response of polymorphonuclear leukocytes in a rat model of acute sepsis. *Mediators of Inflammation* 2005; 1:9-15.

Kim YH, Chang SS, Kim YS, et al. Clinical outcomes in Methicillin-resistant *Staphylococcus aureus*-colonized neonates in the neonatal intensive care unit. *Neonatology* 2007; 91(4):241-247.

Kirby M. Negative pressure wound therapy. *British Journal of Diabetes and Vascular Diseases* 2007; 7(5):230-234.

Kitajima H. Prevention of methicillin-resistant *Staphylococcus aureus* infections in neonates. *Pediatrics International* 2003; 45(2):238-45.

Kvist L, Hall-Lord M, Larsson B. A descriptive study of Swedish women with symptoms of breast inflammation during lactation and their perceptions of the quality of care given at a breastfeeding clinic. *International Breastfeeding Journal* 2007; 2(2).

Lavergne NA. Does application of tea bags to sore nipples while breastfeeding provide effective relief? *Journal of Obstetric, Gynecologic, and Neonatal Nursing* 1997; 26(1):53-58.

Lawlor-Smith LS, Lawlor-Smith CL. Raynaud's phenomenon of the nipple: a preventable cause of breastfeeding failure? *Medical Journal of Australia* 1997; 166(8):448.

Lawlor-Smith L, Lawlor-Smith CL. Nipple vasospasm in the breastfeeding woman. *Breastfeeding Review* 1996; 4(1):37-39.

Lawlor-Smith C. Nipple Vasospasm, Conference and annual meeting of the International Lactation Consultants Association, July 15-19, 1998, Boca Raton, FL, US.

Lawlor-Smith LS, Lawlor-Smith CL. Vasospasm of the nipple -- a manifestation of Raynaud's phenomenon: case reports. *British Medical Journal* 1997; 314(7081):644-645.

Lawrence RA, Lawrence RM. *Breastfeeding: A Guide for the Medical Profession,* 7th ed. Philadelphia, PA: Elsevier Mosby, 2011; pp. 48, 600.

Livingstone V, Stringer J. The treatment of *Staphylococcus aureus* infected sore nipples: a randomized comparative study. *Journal of Human Lactation* 1999; 15(3):241-246.

McClellan H, Geddes D, Kent J, et al. Infants of mothers with persistent nipple pain exert strong sucking vacuums. *Acta Paediatrica* 2008; 97(9):1205-1209.

McClellan H, Hepworth AR, Garbin CP, et al. Nipple pain during breastfeeding with or without visible trauma. *Journal of Human Lactation* 2012; 28(4):511-521.

Mohrbacher N. Nipple pain and trauma: causes and treatments, Conference presentation, North Austin Medical Center, Austin, Texas, 2004.

Morino C, Winn S. Raynaud's phenomenon of the nipples: an elusive diagnosis. *Journal of Human Lactation* 2007; 23(2):191-192.

Nicholas R, Berry V, Hunter P, et al. The antifungal activity of mupirocin. *Journal of Antimicrobial Chemotherapy* 1999; 43(4):579-582.

O'Hara MA. Bleb histology reveals inflammatory infiltrate that regresses with topical steroids: a case series. *Breastfeeding Medicine* 2012; 7(Supp 1):S1.

Page SM, McKenna DS. Vasospasm of the nipple presenting as painful lactation. *Obstetrics and Gynecology* 2006; 108(3 Part 2):806-808.

Page T, Lockwood C, Guest K. Management of nipple pain and/or trauma associated with breastfeeding. *International Journal of Evidence-based Healthcare* 2003; 1(4):127-147.

Potter P, Perry A. *Fundamentals of Nursing,* 5th ed. Philadelphia: Mosby, 2001; pp. 1597-1599.

Pray W. Consult your pharmacist: dermatitis causes are diverse. *U.S. Pharmacist* 2000; 25(8):14-24.

Prime D, Geddes D, Hartmann P. Oxytocin: Milk Ejection and Maternal-Infant Well-being, in *Hale & Hartmann's Textbook of Human Lactation,* Amarillo, TX: Hale Publishing, 2007; p. 147.

Pugh L, Buchko B, Bishop B, et al. A comparison of topical agents to relieve nipple pain and enhance breastfeeding. *Birth* 1996; 23(2):88-93.

Ramsay D, Kent JC, Hartmann RA, et al. Anatomy of the lactating human breast redefined with ultrasound imaging. *Journal of Anatomy* 2005; 206(6):525-534.

Ramsay D, Kent J, Owens R, et al. Ultrasound imaging of milk ejection in the breast of lactating women. *Pediatrics* 2004; 113(2):361-367.

Riordan J. The effectiveness of topical agents in reducing nipple soreness of breastfeeding mothers. *Journal of Human Lactation* 1985; 1(3):36-41.

Rutala W, White M, Gergen M, et al. Bacterial contamination of keyboards: efficacy and functional impact of disinfectants. *Infection Control Hospital Epidemiology* 2006; 27(4):372-377.

Ryan TJ. Infection following soft tissue injury: its role in wound healing. *Current Opinions in Infectious Disease* 2007; 20(2):124-128.

Saiman L, O'Keefe M, Graham P, et al. Hospital transmission of Community-Acquired Methicillin-Resistant *Staphylococcus aureus* among postpartum women. *Clinical Infectious Disease*s 2003; 37:1313-1319.

Sayyah MM, Rashidi MR, Delazar A, et al. Effect of peppermint water on prevention of nipple cracks in lactating primiparous women: a randomized controlled trial. *International Breastfeeding Journal* 2007; 2:7.

Schaal B, Doucet S, Sagot P, et al. Human breast areolae as scent organs: morphological data and possible involvement in maternal-neonatal coadaptation. *Developmental Psychobiology* 2006; 48:100-110.

Spangler A, Hildebrandt E. The effect of modified lanolin on nipple pain/damage during the first ten days of breastfeeding. *International Journal of Childbirth Educators* 1993; 8(3):15-19.

Suzuki M, Yamada K, Nagao M, et al. Antimicrobial ointments and Methicillin-resistant *Staphylococcus aureus* USA300. *Emerging Infectious Diseases* 2011. 17(10):1917-1920.

Thomassen P, Johansson VA, Wassberg C, et al. Breastfeeding, pain and infection. *Gynecologic and Obstetric Investigation* 1998; 46(2):73-74.

Utter A. Case report. *Journal of Human Lactation* 1990; 6(2):178-189.

Wagner EA, Chantry CJ, Dewey KG, et al. Among first-time mothers in a diverse U.S. cohort, breastfeeding problems are highly prevalent and contribute to early breastfeeding cessation. *Breastfeeding Medicine* 2012; 7 (Supp 1):S2.

West D. Personal communication. 2005. Used with permission.

Witt A, Mason MJ, Smith S, et al. Bacterial species and colony count growth in breastfeeding women with chronic breast pain as compared to controls. *Breastfeeding Medicine* 2012; 7(Supp 1): S-1.

Witt A. Breastfeeding women with chronic breast pain who fail conservative therapy: is there a role for oral antibiotics? Conference presentation, American Academy of Family Physicians, Philadelphia, PA. 2012.

Woolridge M. Aetiology of sore nipples. *Midwifery* 1986; 2(4):173-6.

Ziemer M, Cooper D, Pigeon J. Evaluation of a dressing to reduce nipple pain and improve nipple skin condition in breastfeeding women. *Nursing Research* 1995; 44(6):347-351.

Ziemer M, Paone J, Schupay J, et al. Methods to prevent and manage nipple pain in breastfeeding women. *Western Journal of Nursing Research* 1990; 12(6):732-744.

Ziemer M, Pigeon J. Skin changes and pain in the nipple during the 1st week of lactation. *Journal of Obstetric, Gynecologic, and Neonatal Nursing* 1993; 22(3):247-256.

Unusual Presentations of the Breast and Nipple

Sensitivity, tact, and concern for the mother's self-image are important whenever the lactation consultant performs a breast assessment because women are often self-conscious about the appearance of their breasts. Occasionally, the LC observes variations of the breast or nipple that may impact lactation. The mother needs honest feedback from the assessment in order to make informed decisions, yet information should always be presented in a supportive manner. This chapter reviews breast variations and discusses their significance for lactation.

Engorgement in the Tail of Spence

Mammary glandular tissue extends into the *axillary* region (the armpit) known as the *tail of Spence* (Lawrence 2011). Milk produced in mammary tissue in the tail of Spence usually drains through the central ductal system. Women may experience significant, uncomfortable engorgement in this area. Plugged ducts, mastitis, and breast cancer may occur in the tail of Spence.

The woman in **Fig. 182** was worried about the swelling under her arm that occurred on Day 3 postpartum. She was relieved to learn that engorgement in the tail of Spence is common. Cold compresses and ibuprofen eased her discomfort. Within a few days, the engorgement resolved.

The breast is a vascular organ; it is sensitive to bruising and swelling. When engorgement occurs, it impairs normal blood circulation and lymphatic drainage, contributing to pain and interfering with thorough drainage of milk. Pooled fluids of any kind that accumulate anywhere in the body trigger host defences that cause localized inflammation. As the milk volume in a poorly drained breast exceeds the storage capacity of the lobes, milk pushes against the cells that line the ductal walls and leaks into spaces where milk is not supposed to be. When milk leakage triggers the immune response, producing breast reddening and pain, the phenomenon is described as *inflammatory mastitis*. It can occur in any breast tissue, no matter where it is located. For this reason, it is important for women with axillary breast tissue to avoid constricting clothing and brassieres that might bruise the tissue and interfere with drainage, especially during the earliest phase of lactation when engorgement is commonly observed.

Accessory Breast and Nipple Tissue

Fig. 183 pictures a woman at one month postpartum with *hypermastia* (also referred to as *polymastia*) in her axilla. These terms refer to the presence of *accessory* (extra) mammary tissue. Accessory tissue is different from mammary tissue that is part of the tail of Spence. Also referred to as *supernumerary* tissue, these accessory ducts, nipples, and glandular tissue can occur anywhere along the *mammary ridge*. This is the so-called "milk line" that extends down the body from the armpit to the groin and labia. Accessory tissue may appear in other places on the body, including the thighs and buttocks. Polymastia may not appear until enhanced by sex hormones during puberty or early pregnancy. *Polythelia* (supernumerary nipples) is associated with renal anomalies. Pediatricians generally screen infants who present with accessory nipples for renal and other organ abnormalities. While both polymastia and polythelia can occur randomly, there appears to be a familial link (Grossl 2000).

Accessory tissue is capable of producing milk (Lawrence 2011). The same conditions that affect the breasts can affect accessory tissue, including engorgement, development of cysts and abscesses, and cancer.

When mammography is used to study accessory breast tissue, the tissue resembles normal glandular tissue, but is separate from it and does not drain into the central ductal system. It should be recognized as a common developmental variant. Using radiographic studies to distinguish hypermastia from malignant masses can eliminate the need for unnecessary biopsy (Adler 1987).

Note the side of the breast of the woman in **Fig. 184**. She has accessory breast tissue with no nipple.

The woman pictured in **Fig. 185** has accessory breast tissue in the axilla, but no nipple. This area became engorged on Day 3 following the birth of her third child The engorgement took several days to resolve. Interestingly, she did not experience this swelling with her first 2 children. Unlike glandular tissue in the tail of Spence that drains into the central ductal system of the breast, accessory breast tissue is a separate system. Because there was no outlet for the milk, the unrelieved pressure resulted in involution and atrophy of the glandular tissue, similar to that which occurs when a woman does not breastfeed. After this localized weaning, the tenderness in her axilla resolved. The woman's primary breasts were unaffected by these events.

The woman in **Fig. 186** has a milk pore located on the milk line. That is, she has an *ectopic duct* with no accessory breast or nipple tissue. When she experiences a milk ejection (a let-down), a drop of milk appears on the surface of her skin.

Areolar Skin Glands

Fig. 187 shows milk drops oozing from areola glands. The location suggests milk production in 2 of the shallow ductal systems of a *Montgomery gland.*

The human areola is endowed with skin glands that enlarge during pregnancy and lactation. (See also **Fig. 176**.) Areolar skin glands include eccrine glands, sebaceous glands, and small protuberances called Montgomery glands. Greasy secretions from these areolar skin glands may protect the skin from the corrosive action of the infant's saliva. The scent of the secretions from these structures appears to act as an attractive, potent signal to the infant, inducing nipple-seeking and sucking behavior (Doucet 2012).

Schaal (2006) and Doucet (2012) observed individual variation in the number and distribution of areolar skin glands. In Doucet's sample of 121 women, the majority had between 1 and 20 areolar glands on each areola. Infants of mothers with a higher number of areolar skin glands showed evidence of a lesser weight loss between birth and Day 3. They concluded that maternal endowment of areolar skin glands positively contributed to infants' breastfeeding performance, early growth, and the mother's lactation onset.

(**Fig. 170** shows a mother with a white spot on her nipple. Notice the lack of areolar glands. Interestingly, this mother's milk did not come in until day 6 with her first baby.)

Fig. 188 shows a breast in profile with a supernumerary nipple positioned slightly above the *mammary fold* (where the breast meets the rib cage). Some supernumerary nipples have a pronounced appearance, as in **Figs. 189**, and **190**, but they generally have only a rudimentary underlying ductal and glandular structure. Small drops of milk may be visible whenever milk ejection occurs, but such tissue typically does not produce copious amounts of milk. Mothers can be reassured that accessory breast and nipple tissue will not interfere with breastfeeding. Occasionally, this tissue develops mastitis and requires medical treatment.

Figs. 189 and **190** show well-developed accessory nipples (photos courtesy of Susan Gehrman). When this woman was born, the doctor told her mother, "Don't let anyone perform any cosmetic surgery until after she is fully developed, and then think twice if she is going to breastfeed." The woman's family has a history of accessory nipples, most of which are smaller and resemble moles. The brother of the woman in **Figs. 189** and **190** has an accessory nipple, as do an uncle and a female second cousin. Renal

anomalies also run in the family. The woman pictured, however, has no history of renal problems.

At age 19, the young woman pictured in **Figs. 189** and **190** delivered her first child, whom she breastfed for 16 months. Her extra nipples leaked milk at every feeding, and breast tissue was easily palpable below both nipples. She had to place cloths over her extra nipples during feedings to catch the leaking milk. In all other respects, lactation was uneventful. At age 22 she consulted a surgeon to discuss removing the accessory nipples. After the consultation, she opted to delay cosmetic surgery until after she completed her family.

Underdeveloped Breast Tissue

The young woman pictured in **Fig. 191** has underdeveloped breasts. When there is absent breast tissue, this is referred to as *amazia*. (*Amastia*, a similar term, is often used interchangeably, although it is medically different and specifically refers to an absence of breast, nipple, and areolar tissue.) This woman's medical history included infertility. Unable to conceive, she adopted 2 children, and attempted to induce lactation with both. She never made more than a few drops of milk, but was able to coax her infants to the breast using both a feeding tube device and a nipple shield. In this way, she enjoyed the experience of breastfeeding. The LC may encounter women whose lack of breast development motivates them to seek surgical implants. Their reduced capacity to lactate relates to the underdevelopment of the breasts, not specifically to the implants. It is vital that LCs ask women *why* they sought augmentation in order to solicit information about abnormal breast development.

Figs. 192 and **193** picture women with insufficient breast tissue that affected their ability to produce normal volumes of milk for their infants. Both women supplemented with infant formula to ensure infant growth.

Fig. 193 shows a woman with underdeveloped breasts. She was able to produce about 8 ounces (227 grams) daily for each of her 2 daughters. She breastfed her first daughter and offered supplements of formula by bottle. She breastfed her second daughter using a supplementer device.

Breast Variations

Vazirinejad (2009) investigated whether maternal breast variations such as flat or inverted nipples, large breasts, large nipples or other anomalies are barriers for weight gain in breastfeeding infants in the first week of life. In a prospective cohort study of 100 healthy term neonates, 50 mothers had "normal" breasts. The other 50 women had some type of breast variation. Newborns born to mothers in the normal breast group demonstrated significantly greater weight gain by Day 7. Health care professionals must enhance their assessment skills in order to identify women with breast variations. With appropriate, timely intervention, women can overcome problems that impact infant growth and contribute to early discontinuation of exclusive breastfeeding.

Breast development often occurs asymmetrically. Most women have one breast that is slightly larger than the other. Differences in milk output between the right and left breast are often observed, especially during simultaneous pumping (Engstrom 2007). In fact, comparisons of crematocrit and protein concentrations in milk taken from different ducts in the same breast indicate that different mammary lobes produce milk of varying composition (Murase 2009). The mechanism for these differences is probably related to local control mediated by feedback inhibition of lactation (FIL). If an individual lobe is poorly drained, for example, the retained milk triggers the same engorgement and subsequent downward regulation in that lobe that occurs in the entire breast during weaning.

Sometimes the LC observes marked breast asymmetry. One or both breasts have an unusual cone shape. This may not significantly impact lactation or it may be a marker of a physical problem that will inhibit full milk production.

Huggins (2000) prospectively studied 34 lactating women with abnormally appearing breasts to explore a possible relationship between breast *hypoplasia* (underdevelopment) and milk production. She found that "the majority of the women with some degree of hypoplasia and with an intramammary distance of 1.5 inches (approximately 4 cm) or more produced 50 percent or less of the milk necessary to sustain normal infant growth in the first week postpartum." Many of the women in the study reported no pregnancy-related breast growth or changes. While some of these women experienced gradual increases in milk volume after careful management to maximize their production, 61 percent of the women were unable to produce a full milk supply within the first month. Whenever physical markers such as hypoplastic breasts or a wide span between breasts are observed, it is prudent to monitor the infant's growth rate, and to provide extra assistance to the mother to encourage optimal milk production.

Good counseling skills are critical when a woman presents with abnormal breast markers, because they may not always predict difficulty with breastfeeding. The LC must avoid creating anxiety or a loss of confidence, as this in itself may create breastfeeding problems. However,

because the calibration of the milk supply occurs early in the process, women with unusual breasts deserve extra attention and extended follow-up to make sure they reach their full lactation potential.

Polycystic Ovary Syndrome

More than 40 years ago, a group of researchers (Balcar 1972) used soft tissue radiography of the breast to diagnose *polycystic ovarian syndrome* (PCOS), then called Stein-Leventhal Syndrome. The researchers found 80 percent agreement between abnormal ovarian findings and abnormal breast development, and commented that, "Decreases in [breast] gland parenchyma [even in large breasts] may serve to reveal a hormonal disorder…and may in such cases serve as an easy, simple screening test before a more complicated investigation."

Marasco (2000) proposed a connection between insufficient milk supply and PCOS. Full understanding of the complex metabolic relationships in this syndrome continues to evolve. Vanky (2008) observed that women with PCOS appear to have a reduced breastfeeding rate in the early postpartum, and hypothesized that gestational dehydroepiandorosterone-sulphate might negatively influence breastfeeding rates in women with the syndrome. Vanky (2012) reported that women with PCOS who experienced no changes in breast size seem to be more metabolically disturbed and less able to breastfeed.

In January, 2013, an independent panel held at the US National Institutes of Health reported that 5 million women in the US are affected by PCOS. Symptoms may include amenorrhea, infertility, hirsutism, hyperinsulinemia, ovarian cysts, persistent acne, obesity, elevated triglycerides, adult-onset diabetes, and possible pathological interference with breast growth. This pathological interference may affect all 3 phases of lactogenesis. Even subtle changes in a woman's hormonal balance appear to influence breast development, and may create a risk of insufficient milk supply that puts infants at risk for failure to thrive. Factors associated with better glucose tolerance predict earlier onset of lactation (Nommsen-Rivers 2012). Women with PCOS at significantly higher risk for depression (Hollinrake 2007). The expert panel proposed renaming the syndrome, although no decision on a name change was made. The panel also recommended clarifying the diagnostic criteria (Lewis 2013.)

Metformin therapy decreases hyperandrogenism and hyperinsulinemia in women with PCOS, reducing some of the symptoms noted above (Kolodziejczyk 2000). Metformin is compatible with breastfeeding (Hale 2012); however, Vanky (2012) found metformin had no impact upon breastfeeding and did not overcome the effect on lactation of having no breast growth during pregnancy.

Gestational Ovarian Theca Lutein Cysts

Failure to lactate following delivery is an abnormal event, and an endocrinology referral is appropriate (Hoover 2002, Betzold 2004). *Gestational ovarian theca lutein cysts* are brought on by pregnancy and emit androgens, specifically testosterone, in levels that may temporarily suppress lactation. Levels of suppressive testosterone lessen over a period of 3 to 4 weeks as the cycts resolve. Women are encouraged to continue stimulating their breasts with a breast pump or a baby at the breast with a supplementer in hopes that their milk supply gradually will increase.

Both Hoover (2002) and Betzold (2004) followed women whose initially high testosterone levels prevented lactation. As their testosterone levels declined, most of the women produced milk to satisfy 100 percent of their infants' caloric needs. It therefore seems reasonable to encourage maintenance of breast stimulation for at least 4 weeks in order to optimize the likelihood of developing a full milk supply. One case report describes a mother with a gestational ovarian theca lutein cyst whose milk supply suddenly appeared on day 31 postpartum. She had been stimulating her breasts with a pump since the delivery of the baby, during which time she had only been pumping small quantities of milk (Betzold 2004).

Insufficient Glandular Tissue

Women with insufficient glandular tissue (Neifert 1985) may not experience breast changes during pregnancy and do not report an engorgement phase postpartum. Palpation reveals only patchy areas of glandular tissue in an otherwise flaccid breast. In spite of good management, these women may be unable to produce an adequate milk supply. The occurence of insufficient glandular development of the breasts is unknown. It is assumed to be a rare condition.

Increasingly, concern is being expressed that exposure to environmental toxins and endocrine-disrupting chemicals are influencing female breast development (Diamanti-Kandarakist 2009). Agricultural chemicals, plastics that leak chemicals into food and water, and animal feed additives have been documented to affect body size and breast development in both rural and urban populations of girls (Bandera 2011).

Precocious puberty, with early breast development, has been observed in girls with cumulative exposure to environ-

mental chemicals, especially estrogens. While the breasts of some of the chemically-exposed girls studied seem to contain more *adipose* (fat) tissue, their glandular tissue was often poorly developed or, in some cases, absent (Guillette 2006). Additional studies are required to determine whether chemical exposure exerts wide-spread effects on human female breast development and disrupts lactation.

Other factors may influence breast development, including a connection between insufficient glandular tissue and thyroid disease. Pringle (1988) found abnormal sexual maturation secondary to primary hypothyroidism. The girls studied had abnormal breast development, and absent pubertal growth acceleration. Sharma (2006) reported the development of ovarian cysts in girls with long-standing primary hypothyroidism. Restoration of *euthyroid state* (a balanced state with regard to thyroid levels) was associated with resolution of the ovarian cycts. Such findings suggest a need to exclude hypothryoridism in young girls with ovarian cysts. Given the association between ovarian cysts and abnormal breast development, early treatment of hypothyroidism would perhaps protect optimal breast development and prevent potential lactation deficiency.

In **Fig. 194** the breasts have a tubular ("coke-bottle") shape, and were flaccid for a woman 3 weeks postpartum. Referred by her pediatrician, this mother sought help from an LC because her infant was failing to thrive. Test weights and use of a feeding supplementer during the next week determined that her milk supply was stable at about half of what the infant required. The mother decided to supplement with formula by bottle and continued to breastfeed for several months. Once supplementation began, the baby gained well. The mother, who initially blamed herself, was relieved to know that her baby's poor growth resulted from a physical condition over which she had no control.

Fig. 195 shows another woman with unusually shaped breasts. Her first baby did not gain well, but her second baby gained normally with exclusive breastfeeding. Glandular tissue of the breast increases with each pregnancy, and there is evidence that lactation itself causes additional maturation of the glandular tissue (Cox 1999). Perhaps this explains why this mother's second lactation was more successful. Her story serves as a reminder to encourage women to breastfeed to whatever level they can achieve. The effort may positively influence future lactations.

The phenomenon of more successful lactation with subsequent births may also be partially explained by the fact that women often enjoy increased confidence and typically find better social support the second time around. Ingram

(2001) followed 22 women who had trouble breastfeeding a first child, and documented significantly more milk production during their second locations.

Since some problems during a woman's first lactation may be related to poor management, lack of confidence, or some other secondary issue, it is wise to give good support and additional encouragement to women who have experienced breastfeeding difficulties in the past. Ingram concluded that, "Health professionals should encourage women to breastfeed all their children, whatever their experience with their first child."

The woman in **Fig. 196**, who has marked breast asymmetry, sought assistance from an LC when her third child was gaining poorly. Neither of her older children had gained weight well while exclusively breastfeeding. The woman followed all the recommendations that would normally result in improved production without noticeable effect. The LC therefore suspected lactation failure owing to insufficient glandular development.

The nipples and areolae of the woman in **Fig. 197** are located in the forward cone of hypoplastic, tubular breasts. This mother experienced low milk supply problems with her first child. The weight of her second child, a 3 week-old baby boy, stalled at 5 oz. (142 g) below birth weight. The LC obtained pre- and post-feed weights on a sensitive electronic scale. An hour of continuous breastfeeding augmented with breast massage produced only 1.8 oz. (53 g) of intake. Visual markers are suggestive of abnormal breast development. The lack of breast changes during pregnancy and the first week postpartum, and the confirmation of low intake by test weights suggest insufficient glandular tissue as a probable cause for the baby's failure to thrive.

After communicating with the physician, the LC began interventions to optimize milk production, and advised supplementation to support the baby's growth. The obstetrician wrote a prescription for 30 mg daily of domperidone. The pediatrician agreed that the infant required temporary use of supplemental formula. Because the baby's suck was too weak initially to make effective use of a feeding tube device, the mother used a bottle to deliver supplemental formula.

Within 4 days, the baby regained birth weight and was sucking strongly enough to begin using a feeding tube at breast, which was the mother's preference. The mother felt that her breasts were fuller and firmer as a result of stimulation from the galactagogue and the extra stimulation provided by post-feed pumping. Her production met the majority of her child's growth needs, and she continued to use formula as necessary. The obstetrician contin-

ued to prescribe domperidone for the first 4 months postpartum because the mother noticed an immediate decrease in production whenever she stopped using the drug.

Based on minimal research, domperidone likely has a galactagogue effect (Donovan 2012), although no research currently guides length of administration. The drug poses minimal risks to the nursing infant, but doses higher than 30 mg daily, preexisting cardiac problems, and interactions with common drugs increase maternal risk. Fluconazole, erythromycin, clarithromycin, and even grapefruit juice increase serum domperidone concentrations and add to the risk of cardiac arrhythmia (Anderson 2013). Larger, better designed studies are required to identify the maternal factors that determine response to galactagogues, identify optimal dosages, and establish clear guidelines for usage. European Union (EU) drug regulators have called for a full review of domperidone to examine whether cardiac-related risks outweigh the benefits of this medication (Lowes 2013.).

Breast Augmentation

Millions of women have undergone breast augmentation. The United States Food and Drug Administration (FDA) publishes online information designed to help women make informed choices about breast implants. Information is regularly updated as new studies on outcomes become available. The FDA website provides a useful overview for the lactation consultant as well as the consumer. Topics covered include different types of implants with complication rates listed by brand names and manufacturers. Specific risks and benefits of different implant insertion sites are also discussed. To access, go to www.fda.gov and use the search words "breast implants."

The FDA (2011) recommends that patients who have or are considering breast implants should be aware that they are associated with significant local complications including: breast pain, hardening, wrinkling, asymmetry, scarring, capsular rupture, and infection. Breast implants are not lifetime devices. Their average life-span is approximately 10 years. The longer they remain in place, the more likely complications occur, making removal necessary.

The most recent policy statement from the AAP (2001) does not identify implants as a contraindication for breastfeeding infants. The FDA considers breast implants to have "a reasonable assurance of safety," although implants may complicate visualization by mammography and may interfere with the detection of breast cancer (FDA 2011). Women are advised to report problems with implants to their medical providers as soon as they develop. Magnetic resonance imaging (MRI) can be used to identify implant rupture.

Women's reasons for obtaining implants are varied, and after childbirth many women express regret or embarrassment about their prior decision to seek cosmetic breast surgery. The LC must consider the psychological state of the mother. Unless the woman is experiencing specific problems related to the implants, the best counseling approach is to reflect her feelings in a supportive manner.

Many women lactate fully after augmentation mammoplasty, and lactation consultants should certainly encourage breastfeeding in this population. The FDA data reports that approximately 2 percent of patients reported lactation difficulties following augmentation (2011). These data do not describe details about the nature of the difficulty, but effects of the surgery may impair full milk production in some women. Certainly, mothers with a history of any previous breast surgery need close follow-up. Follow-up of the infant is also important to make sure growth proceeds normally (Hill 2004).

It is crucial to ask women who have had cosmetic surgery about their reasons for seeking augmentation as well as asking about their post-operative recovery. Occasionally, the LC will identify a woman who reports that she failed to develop normal glandular tissue during adolescence. While rare, *amazia* (lack of breast tissue, such as seen in **Fig. 191**) may occur unilaterally or bilaterally, and sometimes results from congential chest wall underdevelopment It may also be iatrogenic, as in women who have been injured or burned (Davis 1996). Breast augmentation is used to improve the body image of women with amazia. Amazia constitutes a primary problem that prevents lactation and is unrelated to the direct effects of augmentation mammoplasty.

Augmentation Incision Location

Breast implants are inserted through incisions in 4 different locations:

- Under the arm pit (axilla)
- Under the breast
- Along the edge of the areola (periareolar)
- Through an umbilical incision

Because breast augmentation is performed for cosmetic or reconstructive reasons, minimizing the appearance of the scar is felt to be important. Some surgeons prefer to "hide" the incision scar at the edge of the areola. However, the location of the incision influences future lactation. The implications of locating the incision in this area may not be fully discussed with women of childbearing age. Even if a woman denies interest in lactation, the consequences

of selecting an areolar incision should be discussed prior to her breast surgery.

The Risks of Periareolar Incisions

Neifert (1990) prospectively investigated the effects of breast augmentation surgery on lactation outcome. While any previous breast surgery correlated significantly with a 3-fold increase in risk of lactation insufficiency, periareolar incisions were almost 5 times more likely to result in problems. Hurst (1996) also found a greater incidence of lactation insufficiency in augmented women compared with non-augmented women and specifically associated the periareolar approach as the most likely cause.

Periareolar insertion of the implant is more likely to sever ducts and affect the nerves that supply sensation to the nipple. Ultrasound studies of breast anatomy describe an average of 9 ductal openings on the nipple (Ramsay 2005). Since there are fewer patent ducts than previously believed, interruption of even a few ducts could seriously impact milk production.

Nipple innervation is complex and variable between women, making it surgically challenging to avoid interupting nerves and impacting nipple sensation (Schlenz 2000, Geddes 2007). Visualizing the breast as the face of a clock, the lateral cutaneous branch of the fourth intercostal nerve enters the left breast at 4 o'clock and the 8 o'clock position on the right. Rotating the placement of the surgical incision to avoid damage to this critical nerve may result in greater post-operative nipple sensation and may be an important way for the surgeon to protect the potential for full lactation (Schlenz 2000).

Fig. 198 shows a woman who has had breast implants that were inserted with a periareolar incision. She sought breast augmentation between her first and second births. The surgeon who performed the mammaplasty felt that lactation had stretched the woman's nipples in an unattractive manner, so he also "trimmed" her nipples for cosmetic effect. The woman's subsequent nipple sensation was poor. Her right nipple lacked sensation, and a large fissure had opened on the nipple face. The LC speculated that the mother could not sense it when the baby was poorly latched.

Although the woman in **Fig. 198** had experienced a normal lactation with her first child, her second infant failed to thrive. She was committed to the experience of breastfeeding and opted to use a supplemental feeding tube device to offer formula to the baby. Breastfeeding on her left side and pumping the right breast with a hospital-grade electric breast pump allowed the nipple fissure to heal. Her milk supply failed to respond to the efforts to improve production, suggesting that the capacity to lactate fully was negatively affected by the breast surgery.

The mother whose breast is pictured in **Fig. 199** also had implants inserted with a periareolar approach; however, the surgeon avoided bisection of the primary nerves to the nipple. The mother reported good nipple sensation. Observation of a spontaneous milk ejection (the nipple is dripping milk) is evidence of an intact neural pathway between the nipple and the brain, permitting the appropriate hormonal responses to sucking to occur. The mother in this case made enough milk to fully feed her own baby and to donate 200 ounces of her milk to a local milk bank.

Breast Implant Rupture

The mother pictured in **Fig. 200** is 8 months postpartum and has been breastfeeding her daughter. She experienced a rupture of a silicone implant, and her breast developed an abscess at the location of the leak. The scar tissue in the mammary fold has become fragile, red, and swollen. The woman's obstetrician advised her to immediately wean. The LC provided information about the option of *unilateral weaning* which would permit continued lactation on the unaffected breast.

After consultation with other specialists, the mother was instructed to pump and discard milk from the abscessed breast and was prescribed antibiotics for the infection. She slowly reduced the milk supply in the affected breast, which lessened the tension on the fragile scar tissue. The immediate crisis resolved, and the mother continued to breastfeed on her unaffected breast. She decided to have the implants removed from both breasts, but elected to postpone surgery until the baby weaned.

Breast Implants and The Risk of Mastitis

An uncommon complication of breast augmentation is bilaterally massive engorgement after pregnancy. The key risk factor appears to be development of infection in the post-operative period (following insertion of the implant). The resultant formation of scar tissue blocks the mammary ducts and impedes milk outflow (Acarturk 2005).

Hurst (1996) speculates that pressure exerted by the implant itself might occasionally be detrimental to milk production. Prolonged, increased intramammary pressure may cause atrophy of the alveolar cellular wall, thus diminishing secretion. In some women, implants may thus simulate the same effects caused by unrelieved engorgement. It is also possible that implants contribute to increased risk of mastitis if pressure from the implants interferes with drainage of milk. Theoretically, it is also possible that pressure from poorly drained milk ducts may induce a leak in an implant, causing both milk and the contents of the implant to leak into the interstitial space, triggering a heightened immune response. Pro-inflammatory cytokines present in milk are capable of provoking severe inflammatory response (mastitis). Silicone leakage might exacerbate the inflammatory response more than saline leaking from an implant (Fetherston 2001).

Breast Reduction

Large, heavy breasts may cause shoulder and spinal problems resulting in poor posture, neck and back pain, headaches, and poor body image. Women who seek surgical relief of these symptoms via *reduction mammaplasty* may not have specifically discussed lactation with their surgeons. Surgeons should proactively counsel young women fully on options that influence future breast function.

Before 1984, most reduction mammaplasty was done using a technique that essentially removed the nipple and re-centered it on the smaller breast. Modern surgical techniques (referred to as pedicle or central cone procedures) theoretically permit lactation (Marshall 1994). Skin and subcutaneous tissue are lifted off the breast except for a conical base that extends to the nipple-areolar complex, which remains intact (Hagerty 1989). Excess breast tissue is carefully sculpted away in an attempt to preserve nerve and ductal systems. Owing to the intermixture of adipose and glandular tissue (Geddes 2007) this is challenging. However, reports describe positive lactation outcomes for women following reduction mammaplasty using superior, inferior, and horizontal bipedicle techniques (Brzozowski 2000, Kakagia 2005, Cherchel 2007, Cruz 2007). It should be noted that positive outcomes are defined as breastfeeding for a period of 2 weeks. Longer follow-up is needed to fully describe outcomes, especially with regard to infant growth.

Anecdotal reports describe wide variations in lactation performance after breast reduction, from total impairment to full lactation (West 2001). Cruz (2007) observed that the lactation performance of women who had breast reduction surgery using various pedicle techniques was not significantly different from women with *macromastia* (large breasts) who did not seek breast reduction surgery. This suggests that extremely large breasts present challenges for some breastfeeding women. The human body is resilient, but it is difficult to predict how breasts will function after such invasive surgery. Mothers can be encouraged to breastfeed, but the LC monitor the infant's growth.

The woman pictured in **Fig. 201** had very large breasts. She lactated normally with her first 2 children. **Fig. 202** shows the same woman after breast reduction surgery. One pound (455 g) of tissue was removed from one breast and 1.5 pounds of tissue from the other. Following an unplanned pregnancy several years after the breast reduction, her infant daughter was readmitted to the hospital on Day 5 with dehydration and severe jaundice. While her milk "came in," the severed ducts in her breasts no longer drained to the nipple. Over the next week, she endured painful engorgement, and then abrupt involution.

Other Types of Breast Surgery

The woman whose breast is pictured in **Fig. 203** had a lumpectomy to treat breast cancer. A fine scar from a previous biopsy is visible at the periareolar margin and runs parallel to the lumpectomy scar. The bronze color of the breast results from radiation therapy. Irradiation of the breast generally results in diminished capacity to lactate, although some case reports describe partial lactation following treatment (Higgins 1994).

The 46 year-old woman pictured in **Fig. 204** recently weaned a 6 year-old child. A benign tumor was removed from her breast. The placement of the biopsy incision is located away from her areola to minimize the effect such surgery might have on future lactation. Note the rather deflated appearance of the breast tissue. This appearance is common immediately following weaning. As fat tissue regenerates to replace the atrophying glandular tissue, breast shape typically regains a more rounded contour, although perhaps not so readily in older women.

Counseling Guidelines Concerning Breast Surgery

- The LC should inquire, as part of her routine intake process, whether a woman has had previous breast trauma or surgery. The woman's reason for seeking surgery should be identified (i.e., whether surgery was initially sought to cosmetically correct underdeveloped breasts).
- Observe the location of scars. Periareolar scars at 4 o'clock on the woman's left breast and 8 o'clock on the woman's right breast are associated with increased risk of lactation insufficiency.
- Ask whether nipple sensitivity was surgically altered.
- Inform the mother how to assess normal feeding (breasts softer after feeding, listening for swallowing sounds. frequent infant stooling, normal infant weight gain).
- Confirm these impressions by test-weighing on an accurate scale and recommend once-a-week weight checks until lactation is well established.

- Perform hand expression and observe pumping to assess for sprays of milk as opposed to drips and for evidence of milk ejection reflex.
- Counsel about full or partial supplementation and the benefits of partial breastfeeding.
- Allow the mother to verbalize feelings, especially of disappointment. Validate her feeling of loss.
- Support her in other ways to find closeness with the infant, such as sling use, co-sleeping, co-bathing, etc.

Areolar Hair

The mother pictured in **Fig. 205** has hair growing around the edge of her areola. She was concerned about whether the hair would bother her breastfeeding baby, and wondered if she should pluck or shave it. The LC can reassure the mother that hair on the areola is common. Shaving the hairs may make them grow back stiffer or cause breaks in the skin, making it more vulnerable to infection. Because areolar and nipple tissue come in repeated contact with pathogens in the baby's mouth and from the mother's hands, keeping the nipple and areolar skin healthy and intact is important.

Unusual Nipple Configurations

Human nipples come in all sizes and shapes. Sometimes an unusual nipple configuration such as the one pictured in **Fig. 206** causes prenatal caregivers to become concerned about potential breastfeeding problems. The LC pointed out to this woman's midwife that while the nipple seemed too long in the vertical plane for a baby's mouth to encompass, breastfeeding in the cradle hold would position the mouth "sideways," providing plenty of room for the nipple to fit between the corners of the baby's mouth. This proved to be the case. Even though the baby was small, she had no trouble managing her mother's nipples as long as she was positioned carefully.

A similar positioning strategy would permit the woman with double nipples (**Fig. 207**) to fit both nipples comfortably into her baby's mouth. Note the milk dripping from both sections of the double nipple.

Pierced Nipples

Fig. 208 shows a pierced nipple. Perhaps the skill of the piercing artist is a factor that influences the effect of piercing on lactation. Possibly the size of the ring or stud is a determinant. Breastfeeding following nipple piercing does not appear to be uncommon, and in most cases appears uneventful. However, a small percentage of woman may be adversely affected. Garbin (2009) reports that 3 women seeking help at the lactation clinic at the University of Western Australia reported that their infants were unsettled after feeding from a breast with a pierced nipple. Ultrasound examination identified significant duct obstruction. Neither the infants nor breast pumping removed significant quantities of milk from the affected breasts. Decreased blood flow to the affected breasts was also observed. The authors conclude that nipple piercing can present complications for lactation. In the event of complications, unilateral breastfeeding can be suggested.

BWC worked with 2 women who breastfed after having worn nipple rings. One woman was followed for 3 months, during which time her infant grew well on exclusive breastfeeding. She had no difficulties with sore nipples or mastitis. The second mother had minor problems with her right nipple, which had been pierced twice. It became infected the first time it was pierced, and the ring had to be removed while it healed. The nipple appeared to have more scar tissue, and the baby preferred the other breast. However, her child grew well during the 4 weeks of follow-up.

Fig. 209 shows a nipple that formerly was pierced. The nipple did not experience full healing (granulation of tissue) after the ring was removed, and it clearly is leaking milk through the incision site in the nipple shaft. This photograph was taken when the baby was 9 months old. Leaking from the incision site did not cause problems for the mother or her baby.

Another woman who breastfed for 2 years reported nipple pain where she had previously worn a nipple ring. She assumed the pain was from scar tissue and nerve injury.

Inverted Nipples

Fig. 210 shows a nipple at rest. As was previously discussed in Ch. 7 and earlier in this chapter, nipple inversion is a variation that can cause breastfeeding difficulty. It can be challenging to identify nipple inversion by appearance only. Some nipples invert only when compressed. **Fig. 211** shows what occurred when the nipple in **Fig. 210** was manually compressed. This mother's infant was very fussy when put to the breast. Identification of the nipple inversion helped explain to the mother why her infant found it so difficult to latch. A nipple shield was employed as a temporary measure to bring the baby to the breast until the nipples became more protractile.

Identifying Other Unusual Presentations

The mother in **Fig. 212** required open heart surgery as an adolescent. Following the delivery of her first

child, she was distressed by a low milk supply and her infant's poor weight gain. In the absence of other factors to explain her situation, the LC speculated that the invasive surgery involving the chest wall interfered with her capacity to fully lactate. There are case reports of women with breast deformity caused by intensive care to treat pneumothorax when they were preterm infants.

In order to spare girls the psychological distress of abnormal breast development, and to protect their option to breastfeed, it is recommended that neonatologists place chest tubes away from the breast tissue in female infants. Skin incisions to drain pneumothorax can be alternatively positioned 4-5 cm inferior to the nipple, and chest drains inserted through the fifth or sixth intercostal space during neonatal treatment (Rainer 2003).

The young mother pictured in **Fig. 213** has just delivered her first child. She had been treated 9 years previously for a condition called *hidradenitis* (inflammation of a sweat gland). Some of her axillary lymph glands were surgically removed. BWC was concerned that the mother might experience difficulty with milk drainage owing to scar tissue in the tail of Spence. In the immediate postpartum period, the mother complained of a plugged duct on this breast, slightly below the location of the surgical scar. The LC suggested careful positioning, frequent breastfeeding to keep the breast soft, and use of cold compresses to reduce swelling. The plugged duct resolved, and the mother continued breastfeeding. There is a case report of a woman with postpartum axillary breast engorgement who was mistakenly diagnosed with hidradenitis (Silverberg 2003).

Fig. 214 shows a scar from thyroid surgery. Previous history of thyroid disease has been implicated in abnormal pubertal breast development, and is associated in animal studies with diminished lactation. Generally women in this situation are medically monitored and are prescribed replacement thyroid hormone. If they are euthyroid, lactation should be unaffected. However, the presence of scars should prompt the LC to discuss the mother's health history carefully for issues that may impact breastfeeding.

Fig. 215 shows a tattoo on the breast. Tattoos do not impact breastfeeding. Donor milk banks have rules excluding milk donations from women who have acquired tattoos from an unregulated site within 12 months of the time of donation (HMBANA 2008). Many states in the US now regulate tattoo and piercing establishments, requiring them to use single-use instruments, dye pots, etc. Tattoos from regulated sites do not restrict milk donation.

Figs. 216 and **217** show the swollen feet and ankles of 2 women, both of whom are several days postpartum. Both sought help from an LC because of low milk supply. Some LCs have observed that when women present with edema in their extremities, they often experience significant delays in lactogenesis stage II. Hall (2002) identified maternal hypertension as a risk factor for weaning in the first week postpartum. Hall does not elaborate on the mechanisms.

BWC observes that mothers in her practice with dramatic swelling in their limbs (with or without elevated blood pressure) notice increases in milk production in an inverse ratio with the decline in edema. As their feet and ankles return to normal size, their breasts fill with milk.

Nommsen-Rivers (2010) reported that postpartum edema was a significant factor in delayed onset of lactogenesis in a model that excluded obesity (body mass index). Clinicians should follow women with peripheral edema in their limbs carefully, as they are at increased risk for delayed lactogenesis.

The mother in **Fig. 216** was 7 days postpartum. Her breasts were flaccid, and her infant was still losing weight. She had been diagnosed shortly before delivery with *Pregnancy Induced Hypertension* (PIH). She experienced swelling in her hands and legs, and complained to the LC of headache. The LC advised her to report all of these symptoms to her obstetrician so that her blood pressure could be monitored.

The woman in **Fig. 217** also was experiencing severe edema, although she had no history of hypertension.

How can women with extreme peripheral edema be assisted? Increased dietary consumption of protein is said to assist diuresis, as does eating foods with diuretic qualities (such as cucumbers, watermelon) which seem to reduce edema and increase urination. Keeping the feet elevated may also reduce swelling. It would be interesting to see how administration of a single dose of an oral diuretic medication would affect this phenomenon. This issue deserves more attention, discussion, and systematic clinical investigation.

Acarturk S, Gencel E, Tuncer I. An uncommon complication of secondary augmentation mammoplasty: bilaterally massive engorgement of breasts after pregnancy attributable to postinfection and blockage of mammary ducts. *Aesthetic Plastic Surgery* 2005; 29(4):274-279.

Adler D, Rebner M, Pennes D. Accessory breast tissue in the axilla: mammographic appearance. *Radiology* 1987; 163(3):709-711.

American Academy of Pediatrics (AAP). The transfer of drugs and other chemicals into human milk. *Pediatrics* 2001; 108(3):776-789, p. 777.

Anderson PO. The galactogogue bandwagon. *Journal of Human Lactation* 2013; 29(1):7-10.

Balcar V, Silinova-Malkova E, Matys Z. Soft tissue radiography of the female breast and pelvic pneumoperitoneum in the Stein-Leventhal Syndrome. *Acta Radiologica Diagnosis* 1972; 12(3):353-362.

Bandera EV, Chandran U, Buckley B, et al. Urinary mycoestrogens, body size and breast development in New Jersey girls. *Science of the Total Environment* 2011; 409(24):5221-5227.

Betzold C, Hoover K, Snyder C. Delayed lactogenesis II: a comparison of four cases. *Journal of Midwifery & Women's Health* 2004; 49(2):132-137.

Brown SL, Pennello G, Berg WA, et al. Silicone gel breast implant rupture, extracapsular silicone, and health status in a population of women. *Journal of Rheumatology* 2001; 28(5):996-1003.

Brozozowski D, Niessen M, Evans HB, et al. Breastfeeding after inferior pedicle reduction mammaplasty. *Plastic Reconstructive Surgery* 2000; 105(2):530-534.

Cherchel A, Azzam C, DeMey A. Breastfeeding after vertical reduction mammaplasty using a superior pedicle. *Journal of Plastic Reconstructive Aesthetic Surgery* 2007; 60(5):465-470.

Cox D, Kent J, Casey R, et al. Breast growth and the urinary excretion of lactose during human pregnancy and early lactation: endocrine relationships. *Experimental Physiology* 1999; 84(2):421-434.

Cruz NI, Korchin L. Lactational performance after breast reduction with different pedicles. *Plastic Reconstructive Surgery* 2007; 120(1):35-40.

Davis A, Kulig J. Adolescent breast disorders. *Adolescent Health Update: A Clinical Guide for Pediatricians*. American Academy of Pediatrics, Section on Adolescent Health 1996; 9(1):1-8.

Diamanti-Kandarakis E, Bourguignon JP, Giudice LC, et al. Endocrine-disrupting chemicals: an Endocrine Society scientific statement. *Endocrine Review* 2009; 30(4):293-342.

Donovan TJ, Buchanan K. Medications for increasing milk supply in mothers expressing breastmilk for their preterm hospitalized infants. *Cochrane Database System Review* 2012; 3CD005544.

Doucet S, Soussignan R, Sagot P, et al. An overlooked aspect of the human breast: areolar glands in relation with breastfeeding pattern, neonatal weight gain, and the dynamics of lactation. *Early Human Development* 2012; 88(2):119-128.

Engstrom JL, Meier PP, Jegier B, et al. Comparison of milk output from the right and left breasts during simultaneous pumping in mothers of very low birthweight infants. *Breastfeeding Medicine* 2007; 2(2):83-91.

Fetherston C. Mastitis and implants. *Lactnet*, April 15, 2001.

Garbin CP, Deacon JP, Rowan MK, et al. Association of nipple piercing with abnormal milk production and breastfeeding. *Journal of the American Medical Association* 2009; 301(24):2550-2551.

Geddes DT. Gross Anatomy of the Human Breast, in *Hale & Hartmann's Textbook of Human Lactation*, Amarillo, TX: Hale Publishing, 2007; p. 27.

Grossl N. Supernumerary breast tissue: historical perspectives and clinical features. *Southern Medical Journal* 2000; 93(1):29-32.

Guillette EA, Conard C, Lares F, et al. Altered breast development in young girls from an agricultural environment. *Environmental Health Perspective* 2006; 114(3):471-475.

Hagerty R, Hagerty R. Reduction mammoplasty: central cone technique for maximal preservation of vascular and nerve supply. *Southern Medical Journal* 1989; 82(2):183-185.

Hale T. *Medications and Mothers' Milk 15th ed.* Amarillo, TX: Hale Publishing, 2012; pp. 744-745.

Hall R, Mercer A, Teasley S, et al. A breast-feeding assessment score to evaluate the risk for cessation of breast-feeding by 7 to 10 days of age. *Journal of Pediatrics* 2002; 141(5):659-64.

Higgins S, Huffy B. Pregnancy and lactation after breast-conserving therapy for early stage breast cancer. *Cancer* 1994; 73(8):2175-2180.

Hill PD, Wilhelm PSA, Aldag JC, et al. Breast augmentation and lactation outcome: a case report. *MCN American Journal of Maternal and Child Nursing* 2004; 29(4):238-242.

Hollinrake E, Abreu A, Maifeld M, et al. Increased risk of depressive disorders in women with polycystic ovary syndrome. *Fertility and Sterility* 2007; 87(6):1369-1376.

Hoover KL, Barbalinardo LH, Platia MP. Delayed lactogenesis II secondary to gestational ovarian theca lutein cysts in two normal singleton pregnancies. *Journal of Human Lactation* 2002; 18(3):264-268.

Huggins K, Petok E, Mireles O. Markers of lactation insufficiency: a study of 34 mothers, in K Auerbach, (ed). *Current Issues in Clinical Lactation* 2000, Sudbury, MA: Jones and Bartlett, 2000; pp. 25-35.

Human Milk Banking Association of North America (HMBANA). *Guidelines for Establishment and Operation of a Donor Human Milk Bank.* Ft Worth, TX: Human Milk Banking Association of North America, Inc, 2011.

Hurst N. Lactation after augmentation mammoplasty. *Obstetrics and Gynecology* 1996; 87(1):30-34.

Ingram J, Woolridge M, Greenwood R. Breastfeeding: it is worth trying with the second baby. *Lancet* 2001; 358(9286):986-87.

Kakagia D, Tripsiannis G, Tsoutsos D. Breastfeeding after reduction mammaplasty: a comparison of 3 techniques. *Annals of Plastic Surgery* 2005; 55(4):343-345.

Kolodziejczyk B, Duleba A, Spaczynski R, et al. Metformin therapy decreases hyperandrogenism and hyperinsulinemia in women with polycystic ovary syndrome. *Fertility and Sterility* 2000; 73(6):1149-1154.

Lawrence RA, Lawrence RM. *Breastfeeding: A Guide for the Medical Profession* (7th ed). Maryland Heights, MO: Elsevier Mosby, 2011; p. 44.

Lewis R. PCOS diagnostic criteria clarified: name must change. *Medscape Medical News,* Jan. 23, 2013.

Lowes R. Domperidone under scrutiny in Europe Due to cardiac risks. *Medscape Medical News* 2013; March 8, 2013. www.medscape.com.

Marasco L, Marmet C, Shell E. Polycystic ovary syndrome: a connection to insufficient milk supply? *Journal of Human Lactation* 2000; 16(2):143-148.

Marshall D, Callan P, Nicholson W. Breastfeeding after reduction mammoplasty. *British Journal of Plastic Surgery* 1994; 47(3):167-69.

Murase M, Mizuno K, Nishida Y, et al. Comparison of creamatocrit and protein concentration in each mammary lobe of the same breast: does the milk composition of each mammary lobe differ in the same breast? *Breastfeeding Medicine* 2009; 4(4):189-195.

Neifert M, Seacat J, Jobe W. Lactation failure due to insufficient glandular development of the breast. *Pediatrics* 1985; 76(5):823-827.

Neifert M, DeMarzo S, Seacat J, et al. The influence of breast surgery, breast appearance, and pregnancy induced breast changes on lactation sufficiency as measured by infant weight gain. *Birth* 1990; 17(1):31-38.

Nommsen-Rivers LA, Chantry CJ, Peerson JM, et al. Delayed onset of lactogenesis among first-time mothers is related to maternal obesity and factors associated with ineffective breastfeeding. *American Journal of Clinical Nutrition* 2010; 92(3):574-584.

Nommsen-Rivers LA, Dolan LM, Huang B. Timing of stage II lactogenesis is predicted by antenatal metabolic health in a cohort of primiparas. *Breastfeeding Medicine* 2012; 7(1):43-49.

Pringle P, Stanhope R, Hindmarsh P, et al. Abnormal pubertal development in primary hypothyroidism. *Clinical Endocrinology* 1988; 28(5):479-86.

Rainer C, Gardetto A, Fruhwirth M, et al. Breast deformity in adolescence as a result of pneumothorax drainage during neonatal intensive care. *Pediatrics* 2003; 111(1):80-85.

Ramsay D, Kent JC, Hartmann RA, et al. Anatomy of the lactating human breast redefined with ultrasound imaging. *Journal of Anatomy* 2005; 206(6): 525-534.

Schaal B, Doucet S, Sagot P, et al. Human breast areolae as scent organs: morphological data and possible involvement in maternal-neonatal coadaptation. *Developmental Psychobiology* 2006; 48(2):100-110.

Schlenz I, Kuzbari R, Holle J. The sensitivity of the nipple-areola complex: an anatomic study. *Plastic Reconstructive Surgery* 2000; 105(3):905-909.

Sharma Y, Bajpai A, Mittal S, et al. Ovarian cysts in young girls with hypothyroidism: follow-up and effect of treatment. *Journal of Pediatric Endocrinolog and Metabolism* 2006; 19(7):895-900.

Silverberg M, Rahman M. Axillary breast tissue mistaken for suppurative hidradenitis: an avoidable error. *Journal of Emergency Medicine* 2003; 25(1):51-55.

US FDA Center for Devices and Radiological Health. FDA Update on the silicone gel-filled breast implants. www.fda.gov. 2011. Accessed May 2013.

West D. *Defining Your Own Success: Breastfeeding After Breast Reduction Surgery.* Schaumburg, IL: La Leche League International, 2001.

Vanky E, Isaksen H, Moen MH, et al. Breastfeeding in polycystic ovary syndrome. *Acta Obstetrica Gynecologica Scandinavica* 2008; 87(5):531-535.

Vanky E, Nordskar JJ, Leithe H, et al. Breast size increment during pregnancy and breastfeeding in mothers with polycystic ovary syndrome: a follow-up study of a randomised controlled trial on metformin versus placebo. *BJOG International Journal of Obstetrics and Gynecology* 2012; 119(11):1403-1409.

Vazirinejad R, Darakhshan S, Esmaeili A, et al. The effect of maternal breast variation on neonatal weight gain in the first 7 days of life. *International Breastfeeding Journal* 2009; 4:13.

Anatomic Variability: An Important Issue in Assessment

Breasts, nipples, and babies come in all sizes and shapes. For the most part, breastfeeding accommodates normal anatomic variability. However, anatomic variations that occur at the extremes of the normal spectrum may be an under-appreciated issue in breastfeeding assessment and management (Vazirinejad 2009). Problems related to poor "fit" between mother and baby may create substantial barriers in the early days of breastfeeding, especially if the baby lacks strength, size, and stamina. Over time, babies grow. Mothers and babies learn how to compensate for anatomic variations in ways that make breastfeeding easier.

Half a century ago, Mavis Gunther (1955) observed: "If the physical shape of the nipple is the sign stimulus of instinctive activity in feeding, it should be possible from the mother's breast shape to predict the baby's feeding behavior." This provocative statement resulted from her observations that infants of mothers with flat or inverted nipples often were "apathetic" when put to breast. (See Ch. 7 and **Figs. 210-211** in Ch. 9.) Other variations, in addition to flat and inverted nipples, may challenge early breastfeeding. These issues are explored in this chapter.

Dyadic Assessment

Assessing an activity that involves 2 people (a dyad) necessitates looking at each individual and at how the partners interrelate. Infant weight, size, tone, maturation, oral anatomy, and physical condition all influence breastfeeding ability. These issues become more critical if there is something challenging about the maternal breast anatomy. For example, a robust term infant may be able to latch onto an engorged, non-elastic breast with a large diameter nipple. Mastering such challenges may prove daunting to a baby born at 37 weeks, to a tongue-tied infant, or to an infant recovering from injuries sustained during a traumatic delivery.

An experienced LC evaluates dyadic issues such as size and fit in the development of feeding intervention plans. Careful assessment also influences decisions about equipment and alternative feeding choices.

Breast Size

Women with large breasts may have body image issues. They may experience consequences of breast size that impact health, contribute to physical discomfort, and affect quality of life (Kerrigan 2001). Pregnancy itself causes additional breast growth. Breast tissue also grows during the postpartum if stimulated by sucking (Cox 1999).

Breast changes associated with pregnancy and lactation may increase the concerns of women with large breasts who want to breastfeed (Hoover 2008).

The mother pictured in **Fig. 218** has large breasts and cannot easily see her baby. She may find it difficult to comfortably position herself and the baby for breastfeeding, especially since her arms are short. The side-lying position frees the mother's hands. Since the bed supports the breast, it prevents the drag of the weight of the breast from tiring the baby. Another helpful position for women with large breasts is to support the breast on a table. (See **Fig. 100.**)

Areola Size

Areolar tissue is usually elastic and more darkly pigmented than the surrounding skin. Such pigmentation may serve as a visual target that helps the baby locate the nipple. Areolae vary in size, and the range of normal is wide. Areolar diameter tends to decrease with increasing age and to increase with increasing weight (Brown 1999). Ramsay (2005) measured 14 women and found a mean areola radius of 27.8 ± 5.5 mm and 25.6 ± 5.5 mm for the left and right breasts resepectively. A large areola placed far forward in the cone of a hypoplastic breast is described in the plastic surgery literature as a marker for abnormal breast development (Williams 1981). (Ch. 9 reviews areolar skin glands, and more fully describes abnormal breast development.)

Figs. **219**, **220**, and **221** demonstrate the wide variability in areolar size. The woman in **Fig. 219** has a large areolar circumference. However, her breast demonstrates a full and rounded contour in all 4 quadrants. There is no sign of breast hypoplasia or any tubular appearance. The size of her areola is unlikely to affect lactation. The challenge she may face will be how to interpret the misinformed advice to get "all of the areola into the baby's mouth." Clearly, this would be impossible.

The mother in **Fig. 220** has a small diameter nipple and a small diameter areola. She has recently weaned after breastfeeding her third child for 5 years. The upper quadrants of both of her breasts lack a rounded contour; however, (given her history of successful lactation) this is more likely attributable to recent weaning rather than to breast hypoplasia. The rather "deflated" look of her breast probably results from atrophy of glandular tissue — common after weaning. The shape of the breasts typically will alter as fat tissue in the breast regenerates, especially in younger women. Over time, this woman's breasts assumed a more rounded contour. Her areolar diameter remained about 23 mm, the size of a US or Canadian quarter, an Australian 1 dollar coin, or a 1 Euro coin.

Nipple Diameter

Areolar size is unlikely to impact breastfeeding except when areolar placement serves as a marker for abnormal breast development. However, some clinicians are becoming increasingly interested in the impact of nipple diameter on breastfeeding.

Along with breast and areolar size, nipple size increases during early to mid-pregnancy (Rohn 1989, Cox 1999). While areolar and breast growth are positively related to plasma human placental lactogen (hPL) concentrations, nipple growth appears to be related to prolactin concentrations. We have observed women with large nipple diameters during the first week postpartum, who, when seen weeks later, presented with more normal sized nipples. Engorgement of the nipple may occur simultaneously with engorgement of the breast. Tissue edema or high levels of prolactin in the early postpartum may influence nipple size.

The anatomy of the nipple has clinical relevance because various diagnostic techniques access the breast through the nipple ducts, and because surgeons offer nipple-preserving mastectomy. Studies of the nipple show a range of ducts between 19 to 28; however, not all ducts have an openings at the nipple surface. Some ducts appear to merge and share common duct openings (Rusby 2007).

Several researchers have measured the female nipple in order to begin to quantify the range of sizes. Zeimer (1993) described a wide range of sizes in a group of 20 normal breastfeeding women in the first 2 weeks. The average size nipple in her study measured 16 mm in diameter, slightly smaller than a US or Canadian dime, the Euro 1 cent coin, or the Australian 5 cent piece. In Zeimer's 1995 study of 50 women, the average nipple diameter was 15 mm.

Ramsay (2005) measured 14 lactating women and described a mean nipple diameter of 15.7 ± 1.8 mm for the left and 15.8 ± 2.4 mm for the right breast. For her Master's thesis, Stark (1994) used calipers and measured nipple diameter in a group of 59 normal breastfeeding women who ranged from 1 to 36 weeks postpartum. She grouped nipple size into categories.

Small: <12 mm at base (14 percent)
Average: 12-15 mm at base (62 percent)
Large: 16-23 mm at base (24 percent)
Extra-Large: >23 mm at base (0 percent)

In the previous list, the average size nipple diameter is approximately 15 mm. Stark compared her measurements to those of 86 women with breastfeeding problems who were seen for consultation at the Lactation Institute in Encino, California. She described the following size ranges and percentages in this group of mothers:

Small: <12 mm at base (8 percent)
Average: 12-15 mm at base (47 percent)
Large: 16-23 mm at base (38 percent)
Extra-Large: >23 mm at base (7 percent)

Stark observed that: "In both groups, the larger the nipple [diameter] the more likely it was for the woman to have [latch] problems."

Using an engineer's circle template, BWC measured the base nipple diameters of 34 breastfeeding clients. She noted that many of the mothers' nipples varied in size between their right and left nipples; thus, 68 nipples were plotted as separate data points. BWC's measurements describe the following nipple sizes and percentages:

Small: <12 mm at base (3 percent)
Medium: 12-15 mm at base (15 percent)
Large: 16-23 mm at base (70 percent)
Extra large: >23 mm at base (12 percent)

KH measured the nipples of 100 consecutive women who sought assistance for breastfeeding difficulties. Using a ruler, she measured the diameter of the nipple in millimeters. Reporting only the size of the larger nipple, KH found that the average nipple diameter in this group of clients was 17.5 mm; the average nipple length was 9.5 mm. Sizes and percentages in each categories were:

Small: <12 mm at base (14 percent)
Medium: 12-15 mm at base (17 percent)
Large: 16-23 mm at base (58 percent)
Extra large: >23 mm at base (11 percent)

While the sample sizes of the nipple measurement studies described here are small and the measuring tools differed, there is reasonable agreement on the ranges. Larger averages in nipple diameter were seen in women seeking help for breastfeeding problems.

Since women who consult a community-based LC are likely to have breastfeeding problems, it is possible that the data collected by Stark at the Lactation Institute, and by BWC and KH are skewed for women with larger than average nipples. A common observation from all these studies is that women with large nipples have more breastfeeding problems.

One report of 18 babies readmitted to the hospital for dehydration identified one mother with "giant" nipples (Caglar 2006). KH observed that among the mothers she assisted with low milk supplies in 2002, a high percentage had large nipples. Nipple size has seldom been mentioned or identified as an issue in studies of low milk supply or readmission for dehydration, but if nipple size complicates early feeding, it may well be a factor in poor early milk supply calibration. Clearly, the impact of nipple size on lactation requires additional research.

Measuring Tools

Half a century ago, Gunther (1955) observed that, "For the tissues to be accessible, the nipple must not be too large to enter past the baby's bite, and the tissues when drawn forward must be able to pass the gums." If the nipple diameter is too large, a small baby may experience difficulty latching on. Thus size information is pertinent.

It can be difficult to visualize relative sizes. Comparisons with common items may be useful when teaching. **Fig. 222** shows an engineer's circle template with a pencil eraser (top row), a small diameter nipple (second row) and 2 US coins (bottom row) that represent the sizes of nipple diameters referenced. Standardizing nipple measurement is a desireable research goal.

Electronic calipers provide consistent, reliable readings. Sanuki (2008) used micrometer calipers to measure the characteristics of 600 breasts of women in Japan to determine the diameter of the nipple and areolae, and to measure the height of the nipple. The women were not lactating. The researchers found that the mean diameter of the areola was 4.0 cm. The mean diameter of the nipple was 1.3 cm, and the mean height of the nipple was 0.9 cm; similar to the size information obtained by less precise nipple measurement tools.

Sucking Mechanics and Nipple Size

Ramsay (2004b) used ultrasound and intra-oral pressure transducers connected to a feeding tube device to study infant sucking. She observed that, "Negative pressure generated by the infant as the [posterior] tongue moved down resulted in opening of milk ducts in the nipple and milk flow from the breast." In order for maximal suction to be generated, the back of the baby's tongue must first rise as high as it can in order to be able to drop far enough to generate significant amounts of negative pressure.

If an infant (particularly a weak or tongue-tied infant) encounters a large diameter nipple, the size of the nipple may block the tongue from rising high enough, limiting the ability of the baby to generate sufficient suction to

remove milk. Validated refinements in ultrasound techniques can now provide objective measurements representative of tongue movement (McClellan 2010). Variations in nipple diameter, along with anomalies of the tongue, may thus explain some cases of inadequate breastfeeding.

Figs. 223, 224, and **225** show mothers who have large diameter nipples. The mother seen in **Fig. 223** was breastfeeding normally on Day 2 postpartum. On Day 3, she became engorged, and the baby was no longer able to latch. The hospital nurses remarked to KH that the mother's nipple also had become engorged. The photograph shows the size of the mother's engorged nipple, which is now comparable to the diameter of a US quarter. On Day 4, the engorgement resolved, the nipple returned to normal size, and the baby was once again able to breastfeed. This experience suggests that nipples become engorged, and demonstrates how an increase in nipple diameter may frustrate a breastfeeding baby's latch attempts. More research is needed to observe nipple enlargement in the early postpartum, to record how often it occurs, and to note how long it takes to resolve.

The mother in **Fig. 224** is breastfeeding her third and fourth children, a set of twins. Her nipple, in profile, is long, and as large around as a US quarter. Her large, long nipples have not posed problems for her children; all of them grew normally. Note how pliable the nipple tissue appears, even in the photograph. Perhaps the softness of the nipple tissue allowed the babies to easily compress the nipple against the hard palate, permitting room for the posterior tongue to lift and drop. Perhaps the twins had large enough mouths to easily accommodate nipples of this size.

The woman pictured in **Fig. 225** has an abraded nipple and *erythema* (reddening) of the nipple and areola indicative of mastitis. Note the yellow, crystalized exudate that is characteristic of *Staphylococcus aureus*. She suffered the same type of nipple damage after the births of each of her infant sons. Neither baby was able to latch comfortably to her nipple during the newborn period. Her nipple tissue appeared rigid, "meaty," and difficult to compress. Her nipple diameter proved challenging even though both her babies weighed more than 7 pounds (3200 g) at birth.

Because these babies were unable to accommodate the size of her nipples, they sucked in ways that were painful to their mother and caused nipple damage. By about 6 weeks postpartum, each of her babies had grown enough to accommodate their mother's nipples, permitting her to breastfeed each child for over 2 years, emphasizing the temporary nature of such "fit" problems. In such cases, the main challenge is to preserve breastfeeding during the time period when the babies cannot latch. Because direct breastfeeding will be delayed until these babies grow into the nipple size, the size of the pump flange must also be examined closely. If a woman with large nipples pumps with a standard size flange, she may feel pain and ducts may be compressed, inhibiting milk flow (Geddes 2007).

Long Nipples

Nipple length varies considerably and may also be an unexplored issue in breastfeeding management. A ruler or caliper can assess nipple length (**Fig. 226**). The human nipple elongates with suction pressure (Ramsay 2004a). Nipples can extend 2 to 3 times their resting length (Smith 1988).

The primiparous mother in **Fig. 227** has a long nipple (2 cm at rest). She has a large diameter nipple with a bulbous shape (20.6 mm at base and 22.3 mm at the tip). One of her 36 week-old twins is pictured on Day 6 in **Fig. 228**. This twin, who weighed 5 lb 2 oz (2337 g) at birth, lost over 9 percent of his birth weight and had an elevated bilirubin level. He had not stooled in 2 days. The baby is unable to pass the bulbous nipple tip between his gums. While he appears to be breastfeeding, he is actually sleeping with the nipple only halfway in his mouth. Test weights following a feeding revealed no milk intake. The other twin had also lost excessive weight and was similarly unable to latch. These preterm twins were released home from the hospital on Day 3 "exclusively breastfeeding" with no early follow-up planned. They were scheduled to see their pediatrician at 10 days postpartum. Thankfully, parental awareness and concern about lack of stooling prompted their worried mother to call an LC. In this case, the large size of the mother's nipples, infant prematurity, and small infant size should have identified a need for closer follow-up.

After observing the twins' inability to latch onto their mother's breasts, the LC evaluated the mother's pumping technique. The mother had rented a hospital-grade breast pump; however, her pump flange was a standard size and was not a good fit to accommodate either the diameter or the length of her nipples.

Implications of Long, Elastic Nipples

The twins' mother is shown pumping in **Fig. 229**. Note the full extension (4 cm) of her nipple. Neither twin could accommodate the length of this nipple without gagging. The full extension of her nipples filled the entire chamber of the shaft of the pump flanges, and appeared to affect the

suction created by the pump. Almost no milk issued forth during pumping. The LC (BWC) called a pump company engineer to discuss the effect on pumping when a nipple entirely fills the flange shaft.

The engineer explained that in order to create suction, some space must be present between the nipple and the walls and end of the flange chamber. Without space for air movement, insuffient pressure is exerted upon the surface area of the nipple and no milk is withdrawn. LCs should observe pumping for several minutes to identify how nipples fit the flange once they begin to elongate and swell. It is important to observe for pumping adequacy in cases when the infant is not able to directly breastfeed.

At the time of this case, there were no larger sized flanges available to adapt the kit the mother was using. She could not afford the expense of purchasing another pump kit with a larger flange size, nor did she feel she had the time or energy to try to hand express enough milk for 2 infants. Reluctantly, she weaned her twins to formula.

Fig. 230 pictures a nipple that is narrower at the base than at the tip. Note the shadow of this nipple, which emphasizes a not uncommon "doorknob" shape. The LC should also be aware of different terms to describe variants of nipple shape, such as conical or cylindrical.

Note the size of the nipple pictured in **Fig. 231**, which KH measured as 30 mm in diameter. Compare the size of this nipple to the size of the 2.5 week old twin who weighs 7 lbs 5 oz (3310 g). Both of this woman's twins were unable to breastfeed until they reached about 9 lbs (4075 g). LCs must be educated about how to counsel the mother with a fit problem. The infant's milk intake and the milk supply must be protected in such cases until the infant grows.

BWC has taken oral measurements of 98 infants ranging from 35 gestational weeks of age to 3 months. BWC allowed babies to draw her finger into their mouths until it reached a depth that triggered sucking, a spot near the juncture of the hard and soft palates. BWC made an ink mark on her finger where lip closure occurred (**Fig. 232**), and measured this length with a ruler. The ranges extended from 1.9 cm to 3.2 cm (**Fig. 233**). Shallower "oral reaches" were associated with smaller infants, and longer reaches with larger babies. Infant size (weight), rather than age or head circumference, seemed to be the key predictor of longer oral "reach." The availability of ultrasound to see these sucking mechanics will enhance our understanding.

Perhaps when small babies with a short oral reach encounter a long maternal nipple, repeated triggering of the gag reflex occurs, contributing to development of feeding aversion. Further, a short reach may cause babies to grasp only the shaft of the nipple, creating nipple pain. Thus, having a short oral length may elevate lactation risk.

Since oral reach seems most related to the infant's size, mothers can be reassured that growth will often resolve the problem. It is useful to point to the dental literature, which describes rapid forward growth of the mandible in the first few months after birth. This growth alters the size of the baby's mouth so that it will eventually accommodate the mother's nipple. Both BWC and KH have worked with many infants who initially were not able to breastfeed owing to fit problems, and who ultimately breastfed well once they grew larger.

It is unnecessary to measure all mothers and infants. However, some mothers will benefit from the explanation that a fit problem is complicating lactation.

Implications of Size Variability on Equipment Choice

Several manufacturers of clinical grade breast pumps provide equipment that accommodates variations in nipple size. The LC must ensure that women who are using pumps have correctly fitting flanges.

Fig. 234 illustrates the difference between the openings in the Medela 24 mm and Personal Fit™ 30 mm flanges. Other Personal Fit™ flanges measure 27 mm and 36 mm. A 40 mm glass flange is also available.

Fig. 235 shows Ameda Custom Breast Flanges. The Standard Ameda flange size is 25 mm. The Custom Breast Flange with the inset is 28.5 mm and 30.5 mm without the inset. Specialty sizes also include 32.5 and 36 mm flanges.

Figs. 236 and **237** demonstrate the consequences of pumping with a pump flange that is too small. The mother in **Fig. 236** was given a standard size pump kit in the hospital. Observe how the nipple is wedged tightly into the flange opening, creating a strangulation effect that inhibits milk outflow. The woman's breasts remained full and lumpy following pumping, and her pumped volumes were low for a woman 6 days postpartum. At the time of the LC's home visit, the nipples were increasingly sore. In **Fig. 237**, note the cracks that have opened at the base of the nipples, resulting from friction trauma caused by the poorly fitted flanges. The infant was ill and unable to breastfeed, so poor flange fit jeopardized the milk supply, the infant's growth, and increased the risk of mastitis. These are unacceptable consequences of incomplete evaluation. The mother in **Fig. 238**, delivered her second term infant at home. She suffered substantial blood loss following

delivery of an unexpected second placenta. Methergine was administered to control her bleeding. The woman had relatively flat nipples with a large base diameter (approximately 24 mm). She experienced low milk production with her first child. Because the new baby was sleepy and could not latch well to the mother's large, flat nipples, and owing to past milk supply problems, the midwife suggested pumping to help bring in the milk. After 24 hours of pumping, both nipples were swollen and abraded. The LC was consulted on Day 4, and began to systematically address all the red flags for increased lactation risk. She informed the parents that milk production might remain low until the mother recovered from the metabolic stress of excessive blood loss and the exposure to methergine.

Frustrated by hunger and the large nipples, the baby of the mother seen in **Fig. 238** began rejecting the breast. Effective pumping would prove critical to this case. The LC provided larger pump flanges and wrote down careful pumping instructions. The mother reported greater comfort during pumping with the larger flanges, and thus was able to tolerate increased pumping frequency. At a follow-up visit 2.5 weeks postpartum, the mother's milk supply was still inadequate for the baby's needs. The LC speculated that the woman needed more recovery time from her blood loss. Also, given her history of previous milk supply problems, the LC was concerned that this mother might have a primary milk production insufficiency.

Both BWC and KH contend that more research is needed to investigate the variable responses of the human nipple to pumping. The authors have observed that nipples frequently appear to swell during pumping. Pre- and post-pumping measurements taken with a circle template reveal that nipple size can increase 3 to 4 mm. **Figs. 239** and **240** graphically demonstrate this phenomenon. The mother's pre-pumping nipple size is 20.64 mm. After pumping, her nipple size swells to 23.81 mm. Using coin comparisons, her nipples enlarged from the size of a US nickel to the size of a US quarter. Thus, if a mother has nipples that are 20 mm in diameter or larger, she should use a larger size pump flange if she needs to pump her breasts.

Meier (2004) also examined flange fit in a group of women exclusively pumping for preterm infants, and observed that most mothers required larger flanges. She comments: "...about half of the 35 mothers who served as subjects in the research initially required either the 27 or 30 mm (Medela) shield in order to achieve optimal, pain-free nipple and areolar movement during milk expression. As lactation progressed, 77 percent or slightly over three-quarters of the mothers eventually found they needed these larger shields."

Fig. 241 shows the 40 mm Medela blown glass flange. While expensive, the glass flange provides another option when mothers have unusually large nipples that exceed even the capacity of the 36 mm plastic flanges. KH provided a 40 mm flange for a hospital LC whose patient had an extra large nipple that was not accommodated by using the plastic flanges stocked in the hospital. The hospital LC watched the mother pump with the glass flange and observed milk spraying from a duct opening located on the areola. The mother commented that a firm area of her breast softened and became comfortable. Had it not been for the wider opening of this large flange, that section of the woman's breast would not have been drained.

Fig. 242 pictures a woman with PCOS. (See Ch. 9 for a review of PCOS.) This woman has a wide span between her breasts, conical, hypoplastic breast shape, and extremely large diameter nipples. She is shown pumping with a large plastic flange in Fig. 243. Her nipples fit tightly even in the larger flange. She is a good candidate for the 36 mm plastic or the 40 mm glass flange.

Both authors have been asked how to determine the appropriate flange size. There needs to be space around the base of the nipple, and we have found that the woman herself is the best judge of which size fits.

Routine lubrication of the nipples or the pump flange is unnecessary and should be suggested only if the mother complains of discomfort. Fig. 244 shows a woman lubricating her nipples with olive oil prior to pumping. In addition to its lubricating properties, olive oil contains oleocanthal, a natural anti-inflammatory compound that has a chemical profile similar to that of ibuprofen (Beauchamp 2005). Edible oils are safe for the baby.

Fig. 245 demonstrates the consequences of a poor flange fit. Note the abrasions on the nipple face caused by using a 24 mm flange on a nipple with a resting diameter of 29 mm. Note the periareolar scars from previous breast reduction surgery.

Variability in Pacifiers and Teats

Pacifiers, nipple shields, and bottle teats come in a variety of sizes (Fig. 246). Some sizes and shapes may be more or less useful in meeting a specific therapeutic goal. For example, NNS may exercise a baby's weak tongue by giving the baby opportunities to move the tongue and jaw at times other than feedings.

Bottle teats come in various sizes and shapes (Fig. 247), factors that influence milk flow rate and infant sucking (Matthew 1990). Additionally, teats are made of dif-

ferent materials, some of which may expose the infant to chemical ingestion. It is important to chose the most effective size bottle teat or nipple shield when using them therapeutically so as not to provoke the gag reflex with a long teat, or overwhelm the infant with a too-fast flow. A wide-based teat may stress an infant with weak ability to form a seal. Moving from a narrow teat to a wider base teat may assist in transitioning bottle-feeding babies to the breast.

Beauchamp GK, Keast RS, Morel D, et al. Phytochemistry: ibuprofen-like activity in extra-virgin olive oil. *Nature* 2005; 437(7055):45-46.

Brown T, Ringrose C, Hyland R, et al. A method of assessing female-breast morphometry and its clinical application. *British Journal of Plastic Surgery* 1999; 52(5):355-359.

Caglar MK, Ozer I, Altugan FS. Risk factors for excessive weight loss and hypernatremia in exclusively breastfed infants. *Brazilian Journal of Medical and Biological Research* 2006; 39(4):539-544.

Cox D, Kent J, Casey T, et al. Breast growth and the urinary excretion of lactose during human pregnancy and early lactation: endocrine relationships. *Experimental Physiology* 1999; 84(2):421-434.

Geddes DT. Gross Anatomy of the Human Breast, in *Hale & Hartmann's Textbook of Human Lactation*. Amarillo, TX: Hale Publishing, 2007; p. 29.

Gunther M. Instinct and the nursing couple. *Lancet* March 15, 1955; 576-578.

Hoover KL. Maternal obesity: problems of breastfeeding with large breasts. *Women's Health Report*: a dietetic practice group of the American Dietetic Association 2008; 6:10.

Kerrigan C, Collins E, Striplin D, et al. The health burden of breast hypertrophy. *Plastic Reconstructive Surgery* 2001; 108(6):1591-1599.

Matthew OP. Determinants of milk flow through nipple units. Role of hole size and nipple thickness. *American Journal of Diseases of Children* 1990; 144(2):222-224.

McClellan HL, Sakalidis VS, Hepworth AR, et al. Validation of nipple diameter and tongue movement measurements with B-mode ultrasound during breastfeeding. *Ultrasound in Medicine and Biology* 2010; 36(11):1797-1807.

Meier P, Motyhowski J, Zuleger J. Chosing a correctly-fitted breastshield for milk expression. *Medela Messenger* 2004; 21(1):8-9.

Ramsay D, Langton D, Gollow I. Ultrasound imaging of the effect of frenulotomy on breastfeeding infants with ankyloglossia. Abstract of the proceedings of the 12th International Conference of the International Society for Research in Human Milk and Lactation, Sept. 10-14, 2004a; Queen's College, Cambridge, UK.

Ramsay D, Mitoulas L, Kent J, et al. Ultrasound imaging of the sucking mechanics of the breastfeeding infant. Abstract of the proceedings of the 12th International Conference of the International Society for Research in Human Milk and Lactation: Sept. 10-14, 2004b; Queen's College, Cambridge, UK.

Ramsay D, Kent J, Hartmann R, et al. Anatomy of the lactating human breast redefined with ultrasound imaging. *Journal of Anatomy* 2005; 206(6); 525-534.

Rohn R. Nipple (papilla) development in girls: III. the effect of pregnancy. *Journal of Adolescent Health Care* 1989; 19(1):39-40.

Rusby JE, Brachtel EF, Michaelson JS. Breast duct anatomy in the human nipple: 3-dimensional patterns and clinical implications. *Breast Cancer Research and Treatment* 2007; 106(2):171-179.

Sanuki J, Fukuma E, Uchida Y. Morphologic study of nipple-areola complex in 600 breasts. *Aesthetic Plastic Surgery* 2009; 33(3):295-297.

Smith W, Erenberg A, Nowak A. Imaging evaluation of the human nipple during breastfeeding. *American Journal of Diseases of Children* 1988; 142(1):76-78.

Stark Y. Human Nipples: Function and Anatomical Variations in Relationship to Breastfeeding. Master's Thesis. Pasadena, CA: Pacific Oaks College, 1994.

Williams G, Hoffmann S. Mammoplasty for tubular breasts. *Aesthetic Plastic Surgery* 1981; 5(1):51-56.

Vazirinejad R, Darakhshan S, Esmaeili A, et al. The effect of breast variations on neonatal weight gain in the first 7 days of life. *International Breastfeeding Journal* 2009; 4:13.

Ziemer M, Pigeon J. Skin changes and pain in the nipple during the 1st week of lactation. *Journal of Obstetric, Gynecologic, and Neonatal Nursing* 1993; 22(3):247-256.

Zeimer M, Cooper D, Pigeon J. Evaluation of a dressing to reduce nipple pain and improve nipple skin condition in breastfeeding women. *Nursing Research* 1995; 44(6):347-351.

Engorgement, Oversupply, and Mastitis

Fullness of both breasts appears to be a normal event in the first several weeks postpartum. Newton (1951) suggested that failure of the breasts to manifest some sign of fullness during this time is a marker for risk of lactation difficulty. However, at the other end of the spectrum, intense, unrelieved engorgement is a marker for inflammatory conditions of varying severity. Regular breast emptying is the first line of defense against inflammatory breast disorders, and failure to remove milk has consequences in terms of breast health and maintenance of milk production. Down-regulation of milk supply occurs when a protein called feedback inhibitor of lactation (FIL) accumulates in the breast and interferes with calibration of the milk supply (Daly 1996). FIL provides localized control of milk production within each individual breast and within individual lobes of the breast (Murase 2009). Prolonged, unrelieved engorgement may result in diminished milk production that may prove impossible to reverse.

Engorgement

There is no standardized tool to evaluate breast engorgement. Although experienced LCs have observed that some women become more engorged with subsequent lactations, the effect of parity and engorgement has not been studied. More time breastfeeding in the first 48 hours has been associated with less engorgement (Moon 1989), but lack of research on engorgement hampers both prevention and treatment strategies (ABM 2009).

Several theories explain the phenomenon of breast engorgement. The delivery of the placenta alters the maternal hormonal milieu, triggering the onset of copious milk production, typically by 72 hours postpartum. The breasts react to this hormone change with temporary lymphatic edema indicated as swelling. Because of the swelling, some babies experience difficulty latching onto the distended nipple and areolar tissue. Pathologic engorgement may result when the non-latching baby cannot assist the mother in draining colostrum and milk.

Newton (1951) theorized that retained milk causes the alveoli to distend. This distention presses against the surrounding milk ducts, prevents the outflow of milk, and creates inflammatory swelling.

Fetherston (2001) describes one aspect of the inflammatory process that occurs during engorgement or periods of milk stasis. Whenever milk flow is blocked, normally tight seals between cells in the ducts become leaky. Protein components from milk and blood begin to seep into the space between these cells. Leaked substances, particularly *pro-inflammatory cytokines* in the milk, provoke a host defense reaction, causing localized changes such as breast reddening and pain, and systemic responses, such as fever and body aches. These symptoms may occur with or without actual infection of the breast. Inflammatory symptoms are associated with decreased milk production in cattle, and low milk supply is often observed in mothers who suffer from any form of mastitis. Thus, milk stasis and inflammation may initiate a chain of events that ultimately culminates in poor lactation outcome.

It is important for the LC to understand the relationship between prolonged engorgement and down regulation of milk supply owing to the mechanism of FIL. Some women may be more sensitive to inhibitory factors, explaining why one mother may easily recover full production after early inhibition, and why another does not. Removing milk from the breast helps reduce engorgement and swelling. Milk production is endangered when postpartum engorgement is inappropriately or ineffectively managed.

Patterns of Breast Engorgement in the First 2 Weeks Postpartum

Moon (1989) identified variables that closely correlated with breast engorgement:

- delayed initiation of breastfeeding
- infrequent feeds
- time-limited feeds
- delayed onset of copious milk production
- supplementary feeds (usually without replacement pumping)

In an important study, Hill (1994) and Humenick (1994) observed 4 distinct patterns of postpartum breast engorgement:

- Some mothers have *one* experience of very firm, tender breasts followed by a decline in symptoms.
- Some mothers have *multiple peaks* of engorgement before symptoms decline.
- Some mothers have *intense engorgement that persists* for 2 weeks or longer.
- Some mothers experience only *slight breast changes*.

Hill and Humenick thus concluded that the experience of engorgement is not the same for each mother. Not only

did 4 distinct patterns emerge, but their research identified variations in the time to peak engorgement as well.
Some mothers became engorged as early as Day 2. Others
reached peak levels between Days 9 and 14. During the
first 2 weeks, some women only experienced firmness with
slight tenderness for one day and others had 9 days of very
firm, very tender breast engorgement. The LC should avoid
describing only one pattern of engorgement. Mothers who
experience a variant pattern may otherwise worry.

Breastfeeding Outcome and Patterns of Early Engorgement

Hill and Humenick assert that there is some predictive value in assessing a woman's pattern of postpartum breast engorgement. Women with profound and
persistent engorgement appeared to be at greater risk
for problems related to milk oversupply. Similarly,
women who reported only low levels of engorgement
were more likely to report low milk supply concerns.
The former were more uncomfortable and discouraged about their experience of breastfeeding. The latter
reported the highest percentage of early weaning owing
to real or perceived insufficient milk supply.

Hill (1994) also observed that previous breastfeeding
appeared to be a more critical variable than was parity
in predicting engorgement. "...second time breastfeeding mothers appeared to experience breast engorgement sooner after delivery and at higher levels than did
first time breastfeeding mothers, regardless of delivery
method." Further, "Growth of the mammary glands during lactation may not be a rare phenomenon" (Cox 1999).
Previous lactation may stimulate (along with pregnancy-
related growth) the amount of functional glandular tissue
present, increasing the likelihood of higher levels of early
milk production with each lactation.

Pathologic Engorgement

The mother in **Fig. 248** is 3 days postpartum. She
is experiencing pathologic breast engorgement that
appears to be obstructing milk removal. Her breasts
are so swollen that the baby cannot latch. Note the taut
appearance of the areolar tissue. When a balloon is
over-inflated, it is necessary to let off some of the air
pressure before enough of the balloon tissue is available to be drawn up to tie a knot. Similarly, some of
the swelling in a pathologically engorged breast must
be reduced before the baby can draw in enough of the
breast tissue for a good latch.

Very engorged mothers used to be cautioned against
expressing milk from their breasts owing to concerns

that milk production would then be overstimulated and
engorgement prolonged. While avoiding overstimula-
tion by pumping is important, some LCs have observed
that one thorough softening of the breasts can sometimes resolve extreme engorgement (van Veldhuizen-Stass
2007). Other women must continue to occasionally use
hand expression or breast pumping to relieve engorgement
during this phase of lactation.

Fig. 249 shows a woman on Day 8 postpartum. The LC
explained to the woman that her breast fullness might continue for another week. The mother was advised to briefly
apply warm packs to her nipples prior to latching the baby,
and to hand express or pump just enough to soften the
breasts to help the baby more easily draw in the nipples.
Cold compresses helped relieve pain in between feedings.

The woman in **Fig. 250** is engorged on Day 6 postpartum.
She has large, dimpled nipples and her infant is unable
to latch onto her breasts. A hospital-grade electric breast
pump and hand expresssion helped soften her engorged
breasts. Careful assessment of nipple diameter is always
important when a mother uses a pump to manage engorgement. A poorly-sized pump flange restricts the ability of
the pump to adequately drain the breast.

Treatment of Engorgement

A Cochrane Review (Mangesi 2010) compared interventions to relieve engorgement including acupuncture
(2 studies), cabbage leaves (2 studies), cold gel packs
(1 study), pharmacological treatments such as oxytocin
spray (2 studies), and ultrasound (1 study). In most
of the studies, women tended to have improvements
in pain over time whether or not they received active
treatment. Most of the interventions failed to produce
statistically significant evidence of resolution of the
symptoms of engorgement. One study on acupuncture
showed evidence that, compared to women receiving routine care, engorgement symptoms improved in
the days following acupuncture treatment. However,
owing to the size of the study, it lacked the statistical
power to detect differences in outcomes such as progression to mastitis or abscess. A study examining the
use of cold packs suggested that cold does not cause
harm and may improve symptoms. Again, owing to
problems with study design, the results were difficult
to interpret. The Cochrane Review concluded that
more research is needed to assess the effectiveness of
various treatments.

Some researchers have suggested exploration of the use of
non-steroidal anti-inflammatory drugs, such as ibuprofen,
in the management of engorgement (Berens 2007).

Considering that virtually every breastfeeding woman will experience some degree of breast engorgement, it is puzzling why the phenomenon has received so little focused research.

Breast Massage

In Russia, breastfeeding mothers are routinely advised to use massage to relieve engorgement and plugged ducts (Witt 2012). In the US, massage therapists trained in a technique called manual lymphatic drainage may assist mothers experiencing severe breast engorgement. Gentle massage along the lymph drainage pathways improves lymph flow. Reduced lymphatic congestion may lessen swelling and improve milk flow. BWC has referred several clients to a manual lymphatic drainage therapist when nothing else seemed to relieve their pathologic engorgement. Three women who sought manual lymphatic drainage massage all reported improvement of symptoms, including reduced discomfort and better subsequent milk yields during breast pumping. Gentle massage is not likely to do harm, and, along with measures such as cold cabbage leaf compresses, can be suggested as safe self-care measures for mothers (Lawrence 2011).

Reverse Pressure Softening/Areolar Massage

Postpartum women commonly retain fluids and often experience generalized peripheral edema that affects their hands and feet. Such edema causes distention of the nipple and areola as well, and may collapse ducts, reducing milk outflow. Miller (2004) and Cotterman (2004) described similar techniques that Cotterman named Reverse Pressure Softening (RPS). Both techniques appear to temporarily shift nipple and areolar edema, permitting better milk outflow.

The LC or mother places her fingers or thumbs at the base of the nipple and presses into the breast tissue, holding for 1 minute. If effective, nipple elasticity improves, which assists the infant in drawing in more tissue. Because pumping may pull excess interstitial fluid toward the nipple and areola, shifting edema away from the areola with RPS also may help the mother pump more effectively.

Fig. 251 (courtesy of Colette Acker, BS, IBCLC) shows a mother performing reverse pressure softening.

BWC encountered a mother with extreme engorgement who was unable to remove any milk from her right breast. She instructed the mother to take her prescribed dose of ibuprofen, and to wait 15 minutes for the anti-inflammatory and pain relief aspects of the medication to take effect. At this point, BWC performed RPS. Afterward, the mother

was able to pump 18 ml of milk from her previously impacted breast. The milk flow stopped after several minutes of pumping, and it became necessary to repeat the technique, which facilitated removal of another 10 ml of milk.

A nipple shield was then used to help the baby latch to the somewhat softened breast. The baby's sucking stimulated a milk ejection (observed on the other breast). Test weights confirmed infant intake of 12 ml of milk with the nipple shield in place. After the baby stopped feeding, the mother pumped another 15 ml.

Removing a total of 55 ml of milk from her breast significantly helped relieve this woman's pain. The mother was advised to repeat the process at 2 hour intervals, and to continue taking ibuprofen as prescribed in her post-discharge orders.

By the next day, the mother was able to pump 90 ml from her previously impacted breast. The baby was latching more consistently with the shield. As the breasts softened over the next few days, the baby was able to latch without using the shield.

The Risks of Inadequate Management of Engorgement

The risks of inadequate management of prolonged engorgement are illustrated in **Fig. 252**. The mother has unusually flaccid breasts for Day 12 postpartum. Hand expression and pumping produce only occasional drops of milk, and test weights confirm that the infant is not transferring milk. The baby has not regained his birth weight. The woman described an intensely painful engorgement phase characterized by full, tight breasts. Believing that it would make her engorgement worse, she did not remove milk from her breasts. Although she put the baby to breast frequently, he was unable to latch well to her tight breast tissue, and mostly slept at the breast. Because milk was not being regularly removed, down-regulation of her supply occurred. The situation on Day 12 mimics that of a woman who never initiated lactation; whose milk supply has been allowed to dry up. The woman never regained a full milk supply in spite of an aggressive regimen of pumping and the use of a galactagogue.

Peau d'orange

Figs. 253 and **254** show 2 women with *peau d'orange* (orange peel skin). This appearance of the skin may occur during severe engorgement or mastitis and is an important symptom of inflammatory breast cancer. The marks on the breast made by the seams of a bra in **Fig. 253** also reveal high levels of edema.

Milk Oversupply

Some mothers appear to make more milk than others, creating as many potential lactation difficulties as undersupply (Wilson-Clay 2006). A singleton baby, while thriving, may become overwhelmed by excessive milk volume. The baby may choke, pull away, feed frequently, act colicky, and have explosive, watery bowel movements. The mother may become confused by the negative feedback from her baby and may conclude that the baby is hungry or is allergic to something in her diet. Some mothers go to extraordinary lengths to avoid certain foods in an effort to resolve the baby's behavior. The baby's aversive behaviors may escalate to the level of a nursing strike.

Livingstone (1996) described milk oversupply as *maternal and infant hyperlactation syndrome,* and characterized it by a rate of milk production of > 60ml per hour. It is important to appreciate the dyadic emphasis. The mother is at increased risk for developing milk stasis-related disorders such as plugged ducts, mastitis, and abscess. Owing to rapid milk flow rates and gulping, some infants may suffer from digestive disorders (and even respiratory problems if milk is chronically aspirated). The infant may present with some of the symptoms of gastroesophageal reflux disease (GERD). Both members, mother and baby, become deprived of opportunities for pleasureable feedings, thus affecting the interpersonal relationship.

Unless the mother is planning to return to work or school, the management plan should focus on decreasing the rate of milk synthesis. Skillful counseling is required because it is not always obvious to a mother that milk oversupply is the problem, especially if she has previously interpreted the baby's fussing as a sign of hunger. Consequently, it is difficult for some mothers to trust the LC's advice to reduce milk production. Taking test weights can greatly assist counseling in this situation. Test weights often reveal that the baby is, indeed, taking in large volumes of milk during very short breastfeeding episodes. Such information helps the mother see that her baby is complaining about too much, not too little, milk.

Management of Milk Oversupply

It is important to manage apparent milk oversupply carefully. Some women with prolonged engorgement phases may find that their milk supply will gradually normalize without the need for dramatic interventions. To initiate aggressive down-regulation strategies too early may jeopardize milk production in the longer term. Women with milk oversupply who plan to return to work or school may even wish to maintain some degree of overproduction. A plentiful milk supply may serve as a hedge to protect against reduction of milk supply owing to the stress and fatigue that many working mothers experience. As a comfort measure, these mothers can be advised to briefly hand express or pump to soften their breasts prior to breastfeeding, making it easier for the baby to latch. Brief expression also reduces milk spraying that contributes to gulping and possible infant digestive distress. Mothers can freeze their extra milk for later use or donate it to a milk bank.

Lawrence (2011) describes *hypergalactia* as excess milk production presenting as constant leaking of milk and the ability to easily express several ounces of milk after feeding. If the condition persists, mothers should be evaluated for *prolactinoma* (a pituitary tumor). Postpartum thyroiditis and hyperthyroidism have been associated with excess milk production. However, oversupply can be idiopathic and may not occur with subsequent pregnancies.

A Mechanical Method to Down-regulate Milk Supply

A mechanical method to reduce milk oversupply involves changing the pattern of breast usage. Instead of using both breasts at a feeding, the mother only uses one breast for a feeding period that extends over several hours. This is called *block feeding*. Block feeding should be employed carefully, and probably not during the engorgement phase unless carefully supervised. If initiated too early, before it becomes clear that oversupply is, indeed the problem, block feeding may lead to low calibration of milk supply.

Many women notice down-regulation of supply within a few days of initiating block feeding. Some women with dramatic oversupply must breastfeed from the same breast for as long as 3, 4, 5 or even 6 hours in order to sufficiently reduce their milk production. Excessive pressure in the unused breast can be partially relieved by hand expression or pumping, but the unused breast should not be emptied. Because of local feedback control mechanisms for lactation, the presence of residual milk retained in the breast triggers a gradual reduction in production. In time, the woman's body will make less milk.

In an adaptation of block feeding, van Veldhuizen-Staas (2007) suggests beginning the intervention by completely emptying both engorged breasts with a pump, and then breastfeeding the baby. The baby thus gets cream rich milk from both of the "emptied" breasts. The day is then divided into blocks of time, during which the baby feeds *ad lib*, but only from one breast during the block. The duration of the blocks may gradually be increased from 4, 6, 8, or even 12 hours. Some mothers will require only one thorough mechanical drainage of the breasts at the start; others may require occasional repetition to drain "milk lakes." However, mothers must avoid over-stimulation.

Mothers with oversupply need help interpreting the babies' behavior during the down-regulatory period. At the first feed in a block, the infant may spend only a few minutes at the breast gulping milk. The LC teaches the mother to view this as the first "course," not the entire meal. The LC reassures the mother not to expect the baby to stay on the breast too long. The baby is free to come back to the same breast several times over the course of the blocked time period to access the creamier hindmilk.

Consuming a more appropriate balance between foremilk and hindmilk tends to reduce the baby's watery, explosive stools. A thickening in the consistency of the baby's bowel movements may be the first sign that the milk supply is down-regulating. As the milk supply normalizes, feedings become calmer and more pleasant for baby and mother, and evening colic may diminish. Sometimes the baby will begin asking for both breasts at some feedings, although the LC counsels the mother to make sure that the baby significantly softens the first breast before switching sides.

Pharmacologic Management of Milk Oversupply

Medically supervised pharmacologic treatment may be required to manage milk oversupply that fails to respond to block feeding. Estrogen has been observed to reduce milk production in women (King 2007). Some physicians recommend a brief course of oral estrogen once daily for 4 to 7 days in order to regulate extreme oversupply when other methods have failed (Jain 2001, Lawrence 2011). The woman may experience an episode of bleeding afterward, interrupting lactatation amenorrhea and disrupting the contraceptive protection of breastfeeding. Women should be directed to employ contraceptive precautions once menstruation begins. Estrogen hormonal therapy is not advised for anyone with a clotting disorder, nor is it suitable for an immobilized person. It should be used with great care and probably not during the first 3 weeks postpartum (Jain 2001). BWC has worked with women for whom estrogen therapy was very effective.

Rapid Milk Ejection Reflex

The milk ejection reflex can be triggered by nipple stimulation or thoughts of the baby. Some women appear to have unusually forceful milk ejection reflexes. This phenomenon is sometimes seen in conjunction with (but may appear independently from) milk oversupply.

Note the milk squirting from the mother's nipple in **Fig. 255**. Rapidly ejecting milk may cause the baby to choke or pull off the breast, and gulping may contribute to symptoms of colic. Some babies exposed to constant rapid milk ejections appear quite distressed and anxious at feeding times. As in oversupply cases, the mother may misinterpret her baby's response. She may think the baby is fussing because there is not enough milk when actually the baby is complaining about being overwhelmed by the forceful milk spray.

Many women do not know that pressure on the nipple stops the milk ejection. The mother can use her hand or finger tip to put direct pressure on the nipple, and there are pads and devices that can be worn to control leaking between feedings. LCs should not minimize the concerns women express about milk leaking. Cooke (2003) studied significant predictors of weaning and identified milk leaking as an issue in women's decision to wean during the first 3 months.

Choosing a special breastfeeding position may help the baby to manage a forceful milk ejection. Some infants will cope better when breastfed in an upright position, as in **Fig. 103**, or in side-lying. Some mothers lie flat and place the baby prone (face down) as in **Fig. 256** or in a semi-prone position as in **Fig. 104**.

Mothers with forceful milk ejections may wish to manually stimulate a milk ejection prior to putting the baby to the breast. They can catch the forceful milk spray with a towel, wait a few moments, and then latch the baby. Occasionally, a nipple shield may be used briefly, at the start of the feed, when the milk ejection is most forceful. The shield acts as a mechanical barrier blocking the milk spray so that it does not choke the baby. When the force of the spray lessens, the mother removes the shield and the baby finishes breastfeeding without it. Employing a nipple shield is useful if the baby has been rejecting the breast in favor of a more consistent or controllable milk flow rate from a bottle.

Lactation Mastitis

Plugged ducts and mastitis represent worsening problems along the spectrum of milk stasis that initially starts with breast engorgement. When a mother suffers from inflammatory breast disorders, the LC works with the woman's health care providers to help her recover. Further, as the LC works to ease the symptoms, she tries to discover the factors that have contributed to the current crisis, and help the mother learn how to prevent recurrence.

The LC must also appreciate that some cases of mastitis can be stubborn to eradicate. Eglash (2007) describes a mother first seen at 5 weeks postpartum who experienced early cracked nipples and one episode of acute mastitis. The woman continued to complain of chronic deep breast pain, which resolved only after several months and numerous courses of different oral antibiotic medications.

Some women who experience chronic mastitis have difficulty obtaining adequate medical attention. Because breastfeeding continues to be viewed by some as a "lifestyle choice," mothers who complain of lingering breast pain often encounter pressure from family members and HCPs to wean instead of receiving help to resolve the problem. Women have told BWC that they were sure if their pain had been located in any other part of the body than the breast, it would have been taken more seriously.

Sadly, women are vulnerable to persuasion when others tell them that breastfeeding has become "inconvenient." In such cases, the LC may advocate for the baby's right to be breastfed and for the mother's right to a full medical assessment and adequate treatment. It may be necessary to help locate professional resources and references in order to assist the HCP in treating the mother, especially if the HCP appears unfamiliar with current guidelines for treatment. A useful source for physician information for treating lactation mastitis is the Academy of Breastfeeding Medicine's Protocol # 4 (ABM 2008) at their website: www.bfmed.org .

What is Mastitis?

Controversy exists over the definition of mastitis. Medical texts have tended to define mastitis narrowly as an infectious process of the breast. More recently, experts have begun to understand mastitis as a condition occuring along a spectrum ranging from non-infectious inflammation, to subclinical mastitis, and to infectious processes, including breast abscess. (Foxman 1994, Inch 1995, Michie 2003, Amir 2007).

Mastitis is a frequently cited reason noted in the research for early weaning (Fetherston 1998, Crepinsek 2012). Lactation mastitis is also a major cause of reduction in milk supply. Additionally, Michie (2003) commented that "...by altering the cellular composition of milk and local defenses within the breast itself, mastitis is a powerful risk factor promoting vertical transmission of infections." During mastitis, activated dendritic cells may be identified in the milk, which may more readily carry virus particles to the infant. This fact has obvious implications in the transmission of HIV, increasing the risk of vertical transmission from mother to infant via breastfeeding (Hansen 2004).

Fetherston (2006) describes increased breast permeability, reduced milk synthesis, and rising concentrations of immune components with increasing severity of breast and systemic symptoms. Such changes, while still not fully explained by current theories, appear to be temporary. Remarkably, human breasts appear to fully recover within about one week after resolution of the symptoms of mastitis. The same cannot be said about the effects of abscesses, which are more damaging.

Underrated organisms, such as *Staphylococcus epidermidis* (*S. epidermidis*) have been isolated from breast milk of women with infectious mastitis and are attracting scientific interest (Delgado 2009). *S. epidermidis* is an organism that has a resitance to a wide range of antibiotics and has a higher ability to form biofilms. Both drug resistance and formation of biofilms are reasons why mastitis is increasingly difficult to eradicate with current antibiotic treatments. *S. epidermidis* is emerging as a leading cause of chronic mastitis in both human and veterinary medicine (Arroyo 2010). Discoveries of new potentially virulent organisms involved in breast infection may explain chronic or recurrent mastitis and require more investigation.

Novel treatments for mastitis using lactobacilli isolated from human milk itself are being explored (Arroyo 2010). These probiotic therapies are based on the theory that in the healthy breast, much like the healthy gut, the microbiota community is in balance. In this model, mastitis occurs when certain bacterial species, mainly *staphylococci* and *streptococci* occur at higher than normal concentrations, resulting in inflammation that obstructs the ducts. Probiotic therapy using *Lactobacillus fermentum* is being investigated as an alternative treatment to antibiotic therapy (Arroyo 2010).

Incidence of Mastitis

Identifying the incidence of mastitis is challenging because available studies vary widely in their definitions, methodology, diagnosis, and duration. Most studies focus on the early weeks postpartum, the time when mastitis is most common.

In Foxman's (2002) prospective study, 9.5 percent of breastfeeding women reported mastitis during the first 12 weeks of lactation. Amir (2007) examined data from 2 studies and found rates of mastitis of 17 percent with most episodes occuring in the first 4 weeks postpartum. Amir concluded that improved management of nipple damage could potentially reduce the risk of developing mastitis.

Riordan (1990) and Fetherston (1998) found much higher incidence rates for mastitis in separate studies that looked at the incidence over longer time periods. Riordan speculated that because many women self-treat, the true incidence of mastitis may be under-reported and under-appreciated. Riordan (1990) retrospectively studied a group of women about their experience with mastitis over the full duration of lactation, rather than focusing only on the first few months postpartum. She found rates of mastitis as high as 33 percent. Some of the women in her study lactated for 60 months. While incidence of mastitis was highest during the early months of lactation, a third of the women recalled developing mastitis after 6 months. Nearly a fourth of them developed mastitis after 1 year.

The mothers in Riordan's study (1990) ranked the factors they perceived to increase the risk for developing mastitis:

- fatigue
- stress
- plugged (blocked) ducts
- changes in number of feedings
- engorgement/milk stasis
- an infection in another family member
- breast trauma

Fetherston's (1998) prospectively sought to identify predictive factors associated with occurrence of mastitis in a group of Australian women. She found a 27 percent rate of mastitis in the first 3 months postpartum and proposed a broader definition of lactation mastitis as an "inflammation of breast tissue...[that] affects different tissues and structures of the breast." Fetherston notes that symptoms vary among individuals, and whether infective or non-infective in origin, symptoms can be equally debilitating. Grouping risk factors into common themes, Fetherston's 1998 study identified 5 factors as most predictive of development of mastitis:

- blocked ducts
- stress
- latch difficulties
- tight, restrictive bras
- nipple pain during a feeding

Maternal stress is not noted as a predictive factor for development of mastitis in primiparous mothers, but was predictive in multiparous women (Fetherston 2001). Perhaps women with more children to care for feel more tired and stressed. Previous history of mastitis also appears to be a risk factor for recurrence. Perhaps mastitis creates internal breast changes or scar tissue formation that blocks the ducts in places (such as is noted in dairy cattle). It is also possible that anatomic anomalies contribute to increased risk of mastitis in some women. These include: ducts blocked by previous surgery, cysts, tumors, etc.

Foxman (2002) also identified mastitis risk factors similar to Fetherston's:

- previous mastitis history
- breast and nipple pain
- cracks in the nipple

Subclinical Mastitis

Subclinical mastitis is a condition well known in the dairy industry. While it may occur without obvious symptoms, milk production can be impaired in early lactation. Subclinical mastitis in women is well-documented. It is described as an "asymptomatic inflammation of mammary tissue" and has been associated with lactation failure, poor infant growth in early infancy, and increased risk of mother-to-child transmission of HIV (Aryeetey 2008). "Subclinical mastitis may not reduce breast milk intake in *established* lactation" (Aryeetey 2009).

Studies of HIV-infected mothers with subclinical and chronic low-grade mastitis have identified high concentrations of immunological factors and elevated sodium and potassium in the milk (Semba 1999, Kasonka 2006). These milk changes were associated with a higher HIV load in the milk and higher mother-to-child transmission of HIV.

If the mother is HIV-positive, the safety of the infant may be at risk if breastfeeding is resumed, even after subclinical mastitis is treated with antibiotics as the breast milk HIV load remains elevated (Nussenblatt 2006).

Arsenault (2010) described subclinical mastitis as "common" in HIV-infected women. A randomized, placebo-controlled, clinical trial reported that supplementation with multivitamins, and with Vitamin A, and beta carotene *increased* the risk of subclinical mastitis in this population.

Subclinical mastitis may be connected with milk stasis that triggers inflammatory host responses. Milk stasis may occur owing to a number of reasons, including poor feed frequency, ineffective infant feeding, and incomplete breast emptying. Whenever inflammatory breast changes occur, milk flow becomes further obstructed by swelling. The mother begins to feel aches and other flu-like symptoms. The chemical markers in her milk will be similar to those noted during pregnancy, the colostral phase, engorgement, and during weaning (Rand 2001).

Subclinical mastitis can be detected in women by an increase in a number of specific chemical markers. These chemical changes in the milk appear to reveal the presence of a true inflammatory process that may occur in the mammary glands without the classic, full-blown symptoms of mastitis, such as fever. Researchers have also identified chemical changes in the milk that initiate inflammatory stimuli in the gut of young infants. Such changes affect infant gut permeability, increasing the risk of infant susceptibility to infection (Hansen 2004).

The impact of improved postpartum health care, particularly management of maternal infection, on the prevalence of subclinical mastitis requires investigation. Clearly, more studies are needed to fully identify the true incidence of subclinical mastitis. HCPs must discover ways to assist mothers with subclinical mastitis, whose symptoms (mainly low milk supply and low grade breast pain) may be overlooked or dismissed.

Other conditions must be ruled out when evaluating and assessing a mother's report of breast pain. Episodic breast pain coincidental with lactation is also observed among women experiencing vasospasm of the nipple (Page 2006). The pain may radiate deep in the breast and may occur without obvious signs of infection. Identification of nipple blanching confirms this phenomonon. As has previously been discussed in Ch. 9, vasospasm is treated with palliative use of heat and, medically, with nifedipine therapy.

The Link Between Milk Oversupply and Risk of Mastitis

In her analysis of the mechanisms involved in mastitis, Fetherston (2001) observed that obstruction of milk flow works against the natural flushing mechanisms of the lactating breast. She further speculates that frequent breast drainage may ease intramammary pressure and reduce inflammatory symptoms.

The flushing mechanism of the breast may be hampered when the rate of milk production is too high and retained milk contributes to chronic breast engorgement (Amir 2000). Vogel (1999) also concluded that mastitis "may be a marker of an ample milk supply." Some mothers appear to produce more milk than one infant can comfortably consume. Milk oversupply needs time to down regulate, and perhaps some women are more prone to mastitis in the interim. Both BWC and KH have observed that mothers in their practices who have been copious milk producers tended to have more episodes of both plugged ducts and mastitis, and have often required assistance to diminish milk production.

The Link Between Cracked Nipples and Mastitis

There is a link between cracked nipples and mastitis (Fetherston 2001, Amir 2007). When nipples become

cracked in the hospital environment, nosocomial (hospital acquired) organisms can ascend into the breast and cause infections. Women may be particularly vulnerable if bacterial colonization of the breasts occurs via cracked nipples during the engorgement phase when milk stasis is common and the let down reflex is not well-conditioned. The protective flushing mechanism of the breasts may not be as functional as it will be when breastfeeding is more established.

Livingstone (1999) also observed a strong association between cracked, infected nipples and mastitis. After 5 to 7 days of treatment with topical mupiricin, 12 to 35 percent of the women with infected nipples who were not also being treated with systemic antibiotics developed mastitis.

Anatomic ultrasound studies lend support to Livingstone's hypothesis that pathogens introduced through nipple cracks can ascend ducts, causing infection of the breast. Ramsay (2004) observed that "...milk is not stored in the larger ducts close to the nipple but flows back into the smaller collecting ducts and ductules, a phenomenon we have observed as a reversal in flow of the echogenic fat globules within the duct." Thus, mothers with superficial nipple skin damage must be carefully managed in order to prevent infiltrating infection through the ductal openings.

Other Risk Factors for Lactation Mastitis

The literature on mastitis contains references to less common risk factors. When the lactation consultant assesses a mother, it is important to consider that occasionally these issues may be relevant:

- poor maternal health, especially a history of anemia (Minchin 1998)
- reliance upon an ineffective breast pump
- injury to the breast resulting from strenuous exercise or trauma (Fetherston 1997)
- structural abnormalities of the breast: duct anomalies, previous breast surgery, breast cancer, cysts, abscesses (Meguid 1995, Dahlbeck 1995, Olsen 1990)
- use of and/or poor cleaning of nipple shields (Fetherston 1998, Noble 1997)
- smoking (Furlong 1994)
- maternal IgA immunodeficiency (Fetherston 2001)

Treatment of Mastitis

When a mother experiences symptoms of mastitis, it is appropriate for the LC to advise the mother to notify her health care provider. Unless the LC is also her physician, midwife, or nurse practitioner, the LC should report to the mother's HCP. Her report should describe symptoms observed rather than presenting a diagnosis.

The role of bacterial pathogens in mastitis remains unclear (Kvist 2008). The Royal College of Midwives' (2002) recommendations regarding mastitis state: "...it might be appropriate to delay antibiotic therapy for 12-24 hours, whilst taking corrective measures [to reduce inflammation and promote thorough breast emptying]. If however, there was no improvement during this time, a broad-spectrum antibiotic would be necessary.... If it is not possible to provide close professional supervision and support for a mother with mastitis, prophylactic antibiotics will be needed from the outset."

Some HCPs will wish to see the mother; others may phone in a prescription for a drug such as dicloxacillin that is generally effective against *S. aureus*. The ABM's (2008) mastitis protocol (citing the WHO publication on mastitis) states that if there is no positive response to antibiotics within 2 days, if the mastitis recurs, if it is hospital-acquired mastisis, or if the mastitis is severe or unusual, breast milk cultures and sensitivity testing should be undertaken.

Once the HCP has been notified of the mother's symptoms, the LC endeavors to alleviate inflammatory symptoms. The HCP may suggest ibuprofen, and cold therapy may be employed as a mechanism of pain relief (if it is culturally acceptable). Flushing the breast (ideally by breastfeeding) is imperative. Mothers may need to use a hospital grade electric pump if breastfeeding is too painful. Gentle reverse pressure softening can be employed (if the mother can tolerate it) to help reduce edema around the nipple that may be hindering milk outflow.

Rest is critical to recovery and immune system health. Lawrence (2011) instructs women with mastitis to rest for 2 days if possible. They should be encouraged to take all medication as prescribed (including pain medication if indicated), to eat well, and to drink extra fluids. Breastfeeding should continue. Removing residual milk on the affected side with a pump after breastfeeding helps to keep the breast flushed and to resolve symptoms more quickly.

Mothers pumping for a medically fragile or preterm baby should be directed to discard the milk from the mastitic breast until their symptoms resolve (Neifert 1999, Behari 2004). Sometimes babies refuse to breastfeed from a mastitic breast owing to the salty taste resulting from high levels of sodium and chloride present in milk during mastitis (Newton 1997b). In cases of breast refusal, the mother breastfeeds on the unaffected side and pumps the affected side.

Nasal carriage of *Staphylococcus aureus* is a major risk factor for invasive *S. aureus* disease (Peacock 2003). Amir (2006) identified significantly more infants of mothers with mastitis as nasal carriers of *S. aureus*.

If the infant has been colonized in the hospital setting, mouth-to-nipple contact potentially reintroduces bacterial exposure with each breastfeeding. Staph infections may also appear as pustules in the infant's diaper area (Fortunov 2006). Because bacterial contamination of open nipple wounds contributes to the development of mastitis, nipple cleansing and maternal hand washing after diaper changes are important measures to prevent mastitis.

Wound specialists advise flushing open wounds with tap water or normal saline solution. BWC and KH encourage mothers with cracked nipples to rinse their nipples after feeding or pumping. Mothers are also encouraged to clean nipples once daily with mild soap and water. Topical antiseptics such as gentian violet (Saji 1995) or antibiotics may prevent or treat infection, but best practices for the effective care of cracked nipples are lacking.

Nipple cleansing and antiseptic measures should be considered as short-term first aid until nipples heal, especially in unhygienic environments. It is unnecessary to engage in special cleansing or topical treatments if nipple skin is intact. Over-cleansing may dry the skin or alter the scent of the nipple. Purified lanolin is a safe, beneficial lubricant. Mupirocin (Bactroban™) has antifungal and antibacterial properties (Hale 2012). It may be applied sparingly to cracked nipples and may be useful to treat superficial infection of nipple wounds.

Generally, worsening symptoms are thought to indicate the need for treatment with oral or IV antibiotics. However, a Cochrane Review states that, "While oral or IV antibiotic therapy is common, there is insufficient evidence to confirm or refute the effectiveness of antibiotic therapy in the treatment of lactational mastitis. There is an urgent need to conduct high-quality, double-blinded randomized, controlled trials to determine whether antibiotics should be used in this common postpartum condition (Jahanfar 2013).

If cracked nipples result from mechanical trauma, the LC must assess the positioning and latch, evaluate any "fit" issues, and assess the infant's oral anatomy and suck. Assessment and correction of problems help prevent recurrences of nipple trauma and reduce the risk that the breast will become reinfected.

Images of Mastitis

The left breast of the woman in **Fig. 257** is inflamed on Day 4 postpartum. She complained to the LC on the telephone that her breast felt painfully hot and swollen. When the LC visited, she observed erythema (redness) that extended from the nipple to the chest wall (from 4 o'clock to 12 o'clock). The mother's milk flow was blocked and breastfeeding was too painful for her to attempt. The mother reported headache and body aches but no fever; however, she had been taking acetaminophen, which may have masked febrile symptoms.

The mother in **Fig. 258** also was taking acetaminophen and was afebrile. Mastitis typically is unilateral, but bilateral mastitis can occur (**Figs. 258** and **259**). Bilateral pathological engorgement may present similarly, but *Streptococcus* infection should be ruled out when bilateral mastitis occurs.

Amir (1999) performed an audit of women treated for mastitis in an emergency room and found that almost 40 percent of the women were afebrile. Only 27 percent ran temperatures of 38.5°C (101°F) or higher. She also noted that some mothers were taking anti-pyretic medications that masked symptoms. Mastitic women without fever should be asked whether they have taken a medication that may be altering their symptoms. Based on this audit, Amir remarks, "...the evidence for the presence of a fever of 38.5°C in women with mastitis needs to be reexamined." Other practitioners have observed mastitis and even abscess without the symptom of fever. Some individuals may only develop fever late in the course of an infection. Therefore, breast pain must be considered as an important diagnostic indicator of mastitis.

Milk Cultures

Studies have examined the colony counts of bacteria in expressed milk as a way to definitively diagnose breast infection (Osterman 2000, Thomsen 1983). However, Fetherston points out that this technique, borrowed from bovine science, has limitations when trying to diagnose mastitis in humans. The human breast has a different structure from the udder, in which all lobes drain into a common reservoir. Love (2000) states that, in humans, it is more anatomically correct to think of "...not a breast but 6 to 9 ductal systems."

Because each of these ductal systems is separate from the others, researchers suspect that it may be possible to get confusing results when performing bacteriologic testing. Unless the milk is captured only from the infected ductal system, mixing of milk from other, healthy lobes may dilute the bacterial colonies obtained from infected lobes. Thus, a colony count may not provide accurate information. In practice, colony counts are seldom done owing to cost and the time it takes to get the culture results. However, milk cultures are useful, to identify the type of pathogens growing in the breast. Identification aids in selection of appropriate antibiotic therapy.

Some practitioners obtain cultures of the mother's milk or of the baby's nose and throat to identify pathogens (Wust 1995) to help in the selection of an antibiotic. These cultures are typically performed when a woman fails to respond to standard treatment with frontline antibiotics.

Candida

The role of *candida* in nipple and breast pain has yet to be fully elucidated. Prospective longitudinal studies are underway utilizing molecular techniques to test milk that are more sensitive than standard microbiological cultures (Amir 2013). The eventual results will help determine the role of fungal infection in postpartum mastitis, and will influence treatment.

Secondary *candida* infection may occur following antibiotic use or mothers may be exposed to fungal spores when their infants have thrush. Yeast spores can be washed off intact skin. Overgrowth of yeast on the nipple surface and subsequent tissue breakdown may be preventable by gentle rinsing of the nipples with clean water following each breastfeeding. The LC provides anticipatory guidance to assist women in identifying and obtaining treatment for topical fungal infections that may occur following the use of oral antibiotics or infection from an infant with thrush.

Both authors have encountered women with chronic nipple/breast pain who manifest an almost phobic fear of yeast infection. In some cases, these women avoid antibiotic therapy for mastitis owing to this fear. Some continue to self-treat for what they are convinced is fungal infection. They drastically modify their diets and incur exhausting extra laundry and housekeeping duties to treat for "yeast." Many are willing to repeat numerous courses of powerful systemic antifungal medications, in spite of experiencing only minor relief of symptoms. The LC must explore the possibility that they do not have a fungal infection.

Thomassen (1998) studied 3 groups of women: 20 with deep breast pain in one breast, 20 with superficial skin infection of the nipple, and 20 healthy women with respect to the growth of bacteria and fungi. *C. albicans* was found twice as often in the milk of women with superficial lesions compared to those with deep breast pain. Bacteria were more likely to be found on the nipple and in the milk of those complaining of deep breast pain. Women with persistent, chronic, unilateral deep breast pain should be evaluated for bacterial infection. If signs and symptoms of *candidiasis* of the nipple occur, topical antifungal medication can be prescribed by the HCP (see Ch. 8 for additional information).

Breast Abscess

We have emphasized that lactation mastitis occurs along a spectrum of severity. Failure to resolve symptoms successfully at any stage often results in progression toward more serious disease. Delayed or inadequate treatment of mastitis can result in the development of breast abscesses.

Breast abscesses are pus-filled cysts that develop as a complication of mastitis. A study from the United States puts the incidence of breast abscess as high as 11 percent (Foxman 2002). Incidence seems to vary significantly by country, and may be related to the quality of maternity services and the degree to which lactation management is skillfully provided. Amir (2004) cites an occurrence rate of breast abscess in Australia as approximately 3 percent. In a Swedish study, Kvist (2005) examined data for all singleton births from 1987 to 2000 and identified a rate of occurrence of breast abscess of 0.1 percent.

Abscesses are more common in primiparous women, in women older than 30, and in those who give birth post-term (Ulitzsch 2004, Kvist 2005). The risk of developing an abscess is increased if abrupt weaning occurs during inflammatory or infectious mastitis, if the wrong antibiotic therapy is chosen to treat a breast infection, if necessary antibiotic therapy is delayed, or if a woman fails to complete the full course of antibiotics.

Aspiration of Breast Abscesses

Abscesses constitute a medical emergency and require prompt medical treatment. Performing mammograms on women with mastitis is painful and breast changes caused by inflammation of the breast may result in increased radiographic density that can obscure focal lesions such as abscesses or galactoceles (Ulitzsch 2004). Ultrasound is a useful tool to identify cyst formation. If an abscess or galactocele is present, ultrasound can be used to define the area of the cyst and to guide the aspiration needle or catheter to the abscess for drainage (O'Hara 1996, Hayes 1991, Ulitzsch 2004).

Aspiration of material allows culture and sensitivity tests to determine the proper drug therapy to specifically treat the infection. Aspiration and irrigation of the abscess with sterile saline permits withdrawal of the purulent material from the cyst, allowing some abscesses to be treated without incision and drainage (Dixon 1988). For large abscesses (typically those in excess of 3 cm), catheter drains may be placed for several days, allowing for continuous drainage and irrigation (see **Fig. 265**). Such drains may prevent the need for surgical incision and speed healing (Karstrup 1993, Ulitzsch 2004).

Christensen (2005) studied the results of ultrasound-guided drainage of 151 patients who had puerperal (occuring after childbirth) and non-puerperal breast abcesses. Their abscesses were drained by needle or catheter under local anesthesia, and the women were treated with oral antibiotics. Of the women with puerperal abscesses, 97 percent recovered after the first round of ultrasound-guided drainage. Only one required subsequent surgical excision of the abscess cavity or of a fistula. This study supports the use of the aspiration technique as a less invasive treatment than traditional surgery, while providing a high rate of success.

Surgical Treatment of Breast Abscess

Recovery can be slow when incision and drainage are used to remove a cyst or abscess from a lactating breast. It is not unusual for the wound to take 4 to 6 weeks to heal. The incision must be kept open and draining so that the wound can fill in and granulate properly from the inside. If the external wound heals over too quickly, fistulas may form under the surface, leading to further complications. The open incision will leak milk during the time the internal healing is occurring. Leaking milk, while messy, may be beneficial, because milk contains human growth, anti-inflammatory, and immune factors that bathe the wound and may help prevent infection. However, the appearance of the open wound is alarming to women and their families. Leaking may be especially noticeable when the woman experiences a milk ejection. A clean disposable diaper held over the open incision works well to catch leaking milk and to wick the moisture away from the skin. Keeping the skin dry may help to prevent maceration and skin breakdown.

Types of Abscesses

Intramammary unilocular abscesses occur as a solitary locus of infected material deep in the tissue of the breast. Some 65 percent of abscesses are multilocular and have a high rate of recurrence (Olsen 1990).

Abscesses can occur close to the surface of the breast near the nipple (*subareolar abscesses*). These often "ripen" as a boil does, are easier to excise, and have a more favorable prognosis. The woman pictured in **Fig. 260** is 6 weeks postpartum. Seen from the side, the shape of a ripening abscess is apparent. Note the *induration* (pulling in) of the nipple. Induration of breast tissue is an important symptom of serious disease and should be reported to a physician.

The woman pictured in **Fig. 261** has an abscess that is ripening (coming to a head). She had been self-treating what she thought was a plugged duct for 3.5 weeks. Since she did not report a fever, the doctor's staff did not take her other symptoms seriously. Because of the risks associated with untreated breast disorders, unexplained breast masses that do not resolve within 3 days should always be examined by a HCP.

The mother pictured in **Fig. 262** developed a subareolar abscess in the 3 o'clock position on her right breast at 3 weeks postpartum. She had an oversupply problem and poorly managed engorgement. She began experiencing mastitis by the end of week 2, but delayed seeking medical treatment for her symptoms. She sought emergency room care with a walnut-sized breast mass that was identified as an abscess. It was incised and drained. The mother is shown at 1 month postpartum with an iodine wick that promotes drainage and prevents the surface of the wound from closing before internal healing is complete. The wound is leaking blood and milk. Normally, the mother wore a dressing over the wound, but the large dressing seemed to distract the baby during feedings. The mother learned to hold a small piece of sterile gauze over the wound while breastfeeding (**Fig. 263**).

This mother was advised by her doctor to pump the affected breast and to discard the milk; however, the pump flange was difficult to position so that it did not rub against the wound. Further, the mother was unable to soften her breast by pumping. She found that the baby's sucking brought more relief. While some mothers might be too distressed to breastfeed and would prefer to rely on the pump to keep the breast drained, this mother preferred to breastfeed. Because an ill or preterm infant might become sick if exposed to the high levels of pathogens in the milk of a mother with breast abscess, the infant should be medically monitored for illness. The infant did not experience any ill effects after breastfeeding from the mastitic breast.

Because of their location, periareolar abscesses create both breastfeeding and pumping challenges. From the standpoint of lactation, surgical incision should be placed as far as possible from the nipple in order to facilitate breastfeeding and pumping. Locating the incision radially, so that it runs along, rather than across the ducts, may be less likely to damage the ductal system.

Fig. 264 shows the same mother's breast at 7 weeks postpartum. The wound closed, and the mother continued to breastfeed uneventfully.

Case Study of MRSA-related Abscess Treated Initially with Percutaneous Drainage

A 36 year-old woman who is breastfeeding her first child is pictured in **Fig. 265**. She gave birth to a healthy male infant at 38 weeks. Both nipples became cracked in the hospital. Treatment with hydrogel dressings and lanolin failed to heal the nipples, and the cracks persisted for 7 weeks. The left breast produced 3 times as much milk as the right. Engorgement may have contributed to poor flushing. The pathogens that prevented nipple healing thus had ample opportunity to ascend into the interior of the breast.

At 4 weeks postpartum, the mother experienced plugged ducts in the left breast without the symptom of fever. Her physician phoned in a prescription for a 7-day course of cephalexin (500 mg twice a day). Owing to infant colic symptoms, the mother discontinued the medication on Day 5 of therapy. Symptoms recurred in the same breast 2 weeks later. Although the mother remained afebrile, she insisted on an evelatuion from her obstetrician. Her doctor prescribed dicloxacillin 250 mg 4 times a day for 10 days, which did not resolve her symptoms. The Academy of Breastfeeding Medicine Protocol on mastitis describes the dosage for dicloxacillin as being 500 mg 4 times a day (ABM 2008), so the second antibiotic dosage was inadequate. Incomplete, delayed, and inadequate antibiotic therapy is associated with increased risk of breast abscess. The mother was primiparous and older than 30, both issues identified in the literature as additional risk factors for breast abscess.

By Week 7 a red, swollen area developed at approximately 3 o'clock on the upper, outer quadrant of the left breast. A radiologist performed ultrasound investigation, which revealed a cluster of abscesses. As seen in the photo, a percutaneous drain was inserted to drain fluid from the abscess. Methicillin-resistant *Staphylococcus aureus* (MRSA) was isolated from material aspirated. The mother was immediately admitted to the hospital for incision and drainage of the abscess, along with intravenous vancomycin therapy. The mother requested emergency weaning advice, but the infant had difficulty tolerating formula. The mother opted to reverse the weaning and continued to lactate on the unaffected breast.

This case (Wilson-Clay 2008) demonstrates how serious infection can occur as the result of non-healing cracked nipples. The absence of fever resulted in treatment delays. Because persistent low-grade breast pain was the primary symptom, it failed to sufficiently alarm the HCP. This resulted in a failure to provide timely, appropriate care. The increasing prevalence of drug-resistant pathogens warrants timely adequate evaluation and treatment of soft tissue infection in postpartum women.

More than 14,000 pregnant or postpartum women in the US experience an invasive MRSA infection annually. The majority of these infections are mastitis and cost approximately $16.5 million dollars from the societal and payer perspectives (Beigi 2009).

Case Study of Multilocular Breast Abscesses in a Breastfeeding Mother

The 26 year-old primiparous woman in **Fig. 266** has 2 abscesses shown in the healing phase, following surgical incision. She visited her physician on Day 21 postpartum to report a pea-size lump in her right breast above the edge of her areola at 12 o'clock. She had no fever, but the area was tender. The doctor identified a plugged duct and recommended application of hot packs and more frequent breastfeeding. The mother had returned to graduate school at 2 weeks postpartum, and she was experiencing elevated levels of stress and fatigue as a result. She also had a copious milk supply with a prolonged engorgement phase. Her baby was unable to remove enough milk to prevent breast engorgement, and her busy school schedule interfered with adequate time for pumping.

By Friday of the same week, the mother phoned to report that the lump in her breast had grown to the size of a hen's egg. The woman still reported no febrile symptoms; however, mastitis can occur without fever (Amir 1999) and the mass was enlarging. BWC notified the obstetrician, and he immediately referred the woman to a surgeon. Using ultrasound, the surgeon located a subareolar abscess, and aspirated it for relief of pressure and to culture for drug sensitivity. When the mother asked about her lack of fever, the surgeon stated that approximately 25 percent of the women he treated for breast abscess were afebrile.

Fine needle aspiration did not resolve this mother's abscesses, nor did oral antibiotics. Incision and drainage were performed 2 days later. Multilocular abscesses were discovered. Drainage tubes removed purulent material. The mother pumped her breasts post-surgery to relieve engorgement, and decided to wean as a result of her emotional and physical trauma.

Slow Weaning on a Breast Pump

The LC devised a slow weaning plan to protect the healing breast from the stress of engorgement. The mother expressed milk with a breast pump, and gradually reduced the number of minutes for each pumping session and also slowly decreased the number of daily pumping sessions.

For example, on Day 1, the mother dropped one feeding. She pumped for 12 minutes at all the rest of her regular feeding times. The baby received bottles of pumped milk until it became necessary to use formula. The mother followed this schedule for several days until her breasts felt comfortable at the reduced level of milk production. She then reduced the duration of pumping at each session to 10 minutes, holding at this level for a few days until her milk production stabilized. Next, she dropped another scheduled pumping session. She continued in this manner, alternating between dropping minutes of pumping and dropping entire pumping sessions until milk production ceased. Whenever she became uncomfortable during the weaning process, she was instructed to use the pump briefly to relieve built up milk pressure. Because of her history of abscesses and milk overproduction issues, an extremely slow and careful weaning was necessary to protect her.

The LC recommended the mother hold her dressings in place using a sports bra. Wearing such a bra also helped to stabilize the mother's breast so that motion would not stress the healing incisions. The soft cotton-lycra bra material allowed the breasts to "breathe," while providing support.

Six months after treatment for the abscess, this mother returned to the breast surgeon when she discovered another mass in her breast. Ultrasound detected a galactocele, a sterile, milk-filled cyst. The surgeon reopened the upper incision and removed the cyst.

Subsequent Lactation Following Surgery for Breast Abscess

The mother pictured in **Fig. 266** became pregnant again when her older child was only 11 months old. Her surgically-affected breast appeared still to be healing, with reddened, keloid scar tissue that stretched and remained tender to the touch throughout her pregnancy. Her son was born at term, 20 months after the original abscesses were treated. The mother again experienced a copious milk supply. She was counseled to rest and to guard against excessive fatigue and engorgement.

Her nipples became cracked and she complained of a plugged duct in her right breast, although in a different location from the previous abscess sites. The breast surgeon was immediately consulted and placed the woman on prophylactic antibiotics. The mass in her breast persisted. She did not experience fever, but her right breast became increasingly tender, especially over the locations of the old scars. The surgeon detected another galactocele; however, he said that since it was not growing, no immediate action or any surgical intervention was required to excise it. Galactoceles are often left alone, provided they are not growing rapidly, are not painful, and do not impair lactation.

The mother in this case study experienced 4 episodes of mastitis over the next 6 months; 2 in each breast. When she introduced solid foods to the baby at 6 months, her copious milk oversupply began to resolve. Once production lessened, her baby was able to keep the breasts comfortably drained. She experienced no additional episodes of breast inflammation, and breast-fed her son until he was almost 2 years old.

When this woman's third child was born, the surgeon and the LC discussed her situation and suggested the use of prophylactic benadryl during the engorgement phase to see if the drying effect of this medication would help reduce the woman's milk supply and prevent mastitis. The mother was instructed to take the medication at bed-time because her baby slept 4 to 5 hours overnight, and her breasts often became painfully engorged by morn-ing. Oral benadryl appeared to be effective in slightly suppressing this woman's milk oversupply in the early weeks of lactation, and she avoided developing mastitis. However, benadryl causes maternal drowsiness, and is not ideal for new mothers.

Abscess Drainage Tubes

Fig. 267 shows drainage tubes being used to drain pus from an abscess in the breast of a woman who was breast-feeding twins. The mother had recently returned to a part-time job. Perhaps extra fatigue and incomplete breast emptying resulted in mastitis with subsequent abscess development. The woman initially had 3 drains, but one had fallen out at the time of the photograph.

Clumps in the Milk

In dairy herds, visible changes in the milk often signal the onset of mastitis. Clots or clumps of cellular debris (pus) in the milk alert the farmer to early stage illness in the animal (Milner 1996). Infected milk in cattle has been shown to contain higher amounts of free fatty acids, suggesting that it is susceptible to spontaneous and induced *lipolysis* (the breakdown of fat). Clumps in a woman's milk may indicate evidence of a similar mecha-nism in humans, or it might be the result of the activity of *coagulase*, a protein manufactured by *staphylococcus* microorganisms that produces *fibrin*, a substance that causes clotting.

Some women report that milk pumped during bouts of mastitis contains congealed globules of material. A mother with mastitis at 3 weeks postpartum has pumped milk from the affected breast and poured the milk through a tea strainer (**Fig. 268**). The clumping is clearly visible. If infection affects the chemical composition of milk, it may be more likely to coagulate (Newton 1997a). Women can be reassured that the clumps will go away. Mothers may breastfeed during mastitis (AAP 2012).

The American Academy of Pediatrics (2012) considers the presence of a breast abscess as a contraindication to breastfeeding, and advises mothers not to feed milk from a breast still draining pus owing to the number of pathogens the infant might consume. The mother with a healing abscess in **Fig. 263** is breastfeeding her baby. The pus has been drained, and she is taking antibiotics to protect against infection. The abscess is draining serous fluid, blood, and occasionally, milk. The ABM Protocol #4 supports this mother's actions; however, owing to concerns about emerging pathogens, such as MRSA, increased cau-tion is required in abscess cases. Behari (2004) reported that MRSA-infected breast milk contributes to increased morbidity and mortality in babies in special care nurseries, consequently, milk from a mastitic breast is usually dis-carded when the baby is medically fragile (Neifert 1999.) Milk from the non-affected breast is safe to feed to the baby.

Case Study of a Mother with Methicillin-resistant Staphylococcus Aureus

KH consulted with a G1 P1 mother at 4 weeks postpartum who requested a consultation for pain in her right breast.

On Sept. 3rd, 2 days before the initial LC visit, the wom-an's breast surgeon drained a cyst using needle aspiration at 9:00 AM. By mid-afternoon, the mother experienced sharp, shooting pains in that breast. The breast became engorged, and the baby refused it. By late afternoon, the mother began taking ibuprofen for pain. She used a pump to relieve the fullness, and observed blood-stained milk. In the middle of the night the woman began to feel ill. She experienced chills and fever of 103.5°F. She contacted her doctor and began treatment with dicloxacillin at about 5:00 AM. She noticed that her pumped milk had turned yellow.

Sept. 5. When the mother phoned the LC 2 days after the aspiration procedure, she was concerned about blisters that had begun to form on the face of her right nipple. She told the LC that her right breast remained full and firm. She could not get her baby to latch, and could no longer express any milk. She had been on antibiotics for 40 hours with only minimal improvement.

That evening, the LC made a home visit to evaluate the mother's situation. The mother's entire right breast was red and hot (**Fig. 269**), and her temperature was 102°F in spite of antibiotic therapy. The mother pumped for 2 hours and only obtained 2 ounces (57 g) from her right breast. The pumping had not succeeded in softening the area around the areola, although the breast was somewhat softened toward the chest wall. Milk dripped, rather than squirted, during pumping, suggesting that the flow was blocked. The milk was bright yellow (**Fig. 270**). The LC was concerned about the possibility of subareolar abscesses. She urged the mother to call the doctor immediately to report her symptoms.

Sept. 6. Because the next day was a holiday, the mother ignored the LC's advice and chose not to "bother" the doctor. She kept trying to soften the breast during the night, but was only able to extract an additional ounce (28 g) of milk from her right breast. The LC made a follow-up phone call in the morning. The mother's temperature was still elevated. When she learned that the mother had not reported her symptoms to the doctor, the LC explained that in her opinion, the mother's situation constituted an emergency. The mother agreed to phone the physician, who insisted she be immediately evaluated. After examining her, the doctor admitted the woman to the hospital and began antibiotic treatment with intravenous (IV) levofloxacin (Levaquin™). The baby was allowed to accompany her to the hospital.

Sept. 7. Ultrasound revealed no abscesses and suggested a diagnosis of cellulitis (mastitis of the interlobular connective tissue). The mother was now pumping orange milk (**Fig. 271**).

Sept. 9. After 3 days of IV antibiotics, the mother still had fever and her condition had not improved. The family was advised to discontinue feeding her milk to the baby due to concerns about prolonged infant exposure to levofloxacin.

Sept. 10. On Day 7 of the infection, cultures indicated that the breast infection was caused by methicillin-resistant *S. aureus*. IV vancomycin therapy was immediately begun. After this antibiotic therapy was initiated, the mother slowly began to improve.

Sept. 13. Within 3 days after beginning vancomycin therapy, the mother began breastfeeding again on the unaffected breast. The mother had maintained her milk supply through the crisis by pumping at 3 hour intervals. She was able to pump close to 24 ounces in 24 hours. This volume of milk is considered to constitute a full supply. The milk pumped from the affected breast had clumps of debris in it the size of large coins.

After her week-long hospitalization, the mother was discharged home still receiving IV vancomycin.

Sept. 15. The LC made a home visit to take photos. The breast looked more inflamed than it had appeared at the initial visit (**Fig. 272**). The mother was pumping red milk (**Fig. 273**). The area of the breast where infection had destroyed the connective tissue layer is evident in **Fig. 274**. Milk can be seen leaking though the broken skin at the site of the original needle aspiration. The mother used disposable diapers to absorb the leaking milk. **Fig. 275** shows a plug of congealed milk being pulled through a hole at the aspiration site on the breast. The woman's expressed milk still contained clots of congealed material (**Fig. 276**).

Oct. 5. Almost a month later, IV antibiotic therapy was terminated. The mother had been pumping and discarding milk from her mastitic breast during this time. For the next few weeks, the mother continued to pump her healing breast and fed the pumped milk to the baby by bottle.

Oct. 20. In **Fig. 277** the mother is shown feeding the baby from the unaffected breast. For 25 days from the night of the consultation, the baby received some formula supplements, but continued breastfeeding from the left breast. Over time, the milk supply increased in the left breast. Within one month the baby's milk needs were entirely satisfied by the healthy breast. The appearance of the mastitic breast was much improved, although milk can still be observed leaking from the wound in **Fig. 278**. Around this time, the baby resumed feeding from the affected breast with no ill effects observed.

Nov. 12. The mother saw the doctor for the last time. The broken skin on her right breast had healed and she was no longer leaking milk from the wound. A month later, the mother returned to full-time employment.

Fig. 279 shows the completely healed breast shortly before the baby's first birthday. The mother breastfed this child for 2.5 years, weaning midway through her next pregnancy.

Where did the woman acquire this virulent infection? MRSA may be acquired during the hospital stay via cracked nipples. Saiman (2003) described the cases of 8 postpartum women who developed skin and soft tissue infections with MRSA with a mean time after delivery of 23 days. The pathogen, in this case, may have entered the woman's breast at the time of the aspiration procedure. Her husband was a physician. It is also possible he may have unwittingly carried the infection home on his clothes or skin (Merlin 2009).

Follow-up is an important part of an LC's care plan. This case graphically illustrates the wisdom of close follow-up. Fortunately, KH recognized that this mother's condition was worsening. Her persistence was critical in assuring that the mother followed through in reporting her symptoms to a doctor. Sometimes the LC encounters situations that require immediate medical attention. In such cases, the LC should contact the HCP by phone for guidance. This case also documents the length of treatment sometimes required for full resolution of symptoms. Such experiences are traumatic for the whole family. The LC provides important emotional support to her client during this time. Sharing anonymous case details can often reassure families that this sort of thing has happened to other women and that the problem will eventually resolve.

Viral Mastitis

While the incidence of MRSA-related mastitis and breast abcess cases is increasing (Berens 2010), not every serious appearing inflamation of the breast and nipple is bacterial. The mother in **Fig. 280** was diagnosed with a viral herpes infection of the breast after weeks of self-treatment for *candida*. (Photo courtesy of Sue Cox RN, RM, IBCLC.)

Inflammatory Breast Conditions and Maternal Depression

Many women suffering from prolonged breast inflammation also appear to be struggling with some degree of depression. These mothers typically report feeling overwhelmed emotionally as well as physically. It may be that illness of any kind triggers some degree of depression; however, BWC routinely provides anticipatory guidance about managing transient symptoms of depression whenever mastitis occurs. This guidance may consist of simple reassurance that mood will lift as soon as recovery occurs. The mother must rest as much as she can, eat a nutritious diet, and seek temporary help with baby care and housework. The family's support should be enlisted. The LC should also discuss with her client and the family the importance of talking to a HCP if depression worsens.

A connection may exist between inflammation in the body and alterations in the brain that affect mood. Kendall-Tackett (2007) identifies inflammation as the key risk factor for depression. She explains that proinflammatory cytokine elevation is part of normal host defense; however, the chemical changes that result exert an effect upon the brain, including the increased release of *cortisol*, a stress hormone. Kendall-Tackett suggests that in order to prevent postpartum depression, care providers and families should reduce maternal stress and carefully treat inflammatory breast conditions to protect maternal mood.

Mastitis and the Baby-Friendly Hospital Initiative

A cross-sectional Brazilian study identified a lower prevalence of lactation mastitis in women who delivered in hospitals certified as Baby-Friendly (Vieira 2006). Consequently, the LC should advocate for policy implementations that facilitate more comprehensive care for postpartum women in order to ensure successful initation of lactation. Mastitis constitutes an important source of pain, physical and mental distress, and expense for women, their families, and national economies. Additionally, premature weaning resulting from mastitis puts infants at risk. More research is required to identify how to prevent mastitis. Optimal protocols for the management of inflammatory conditions of lactation need to be more widely disseminated among medical care providers. Lactation consultants need to be vigilant with follow-up to make sure problems resolve in a timely and expected manner. They should not fail to advocate for appropriate medical care for clients when necessary.

Academy of Breastfeeding Medicine (ABM) Protocol Committee. Protocol # 4: Mastitis. *Breastfeeding Medicine* 2008; 3(3):177-180. www.bfmed.org. Accessed March 2013.

Academy of Breastfeeding Medicine (ABM) Protocol Committee. Protocol # 20: Engorgement. *Breastfeeding Medicine* 2009; 4(2):111-113. www.bfmed.org. Accessed March 2013.

American Academy of Pediatrics (AAP). Committee on Infectious Diseases. 2012 Red Book: Report of the Committee on Infectious Diseases, 29th ed. Elk Grove Village, IL: American Academy of Pediatrics, 2012. p. 133.

Amir L. Mastitis: are we overprescribing antibiotics? *Current Therapeutics* April 2000; 24-28.

Amir LH, Donath SM, Garland SM, et al. Does *Candida* and/or *Staphylococcus* play a role in nipple and breast pain in lactation: A cohort study in Melbourne, Australia. *BMJ Open* 2013; 3: e002351.

Amir LH, Forster D, McLachlan H, et al. Incidence of breast abscess in lactating women: report from an Australian cohort. *BJOG: International Journal of Obstetrics and Gynaecology* 2004; 111(12):1378-1381.

Amir LH, Forster DA, Lumley J, et al. A descriptive study of mastitis in Australian breastfeeding women: incidence and determinants. *BMC Public Health* 2007; 7(147):62.

Amir L, Harris H, Andriske L. An audit of mastitis in the emergency department. *Journal of Human Lactation* 1999; 15(3):221-224.

Amir LH, Garland SM, Lumley J. A case-control study of mastitis: nasal carriage of *Staphylococcus aureus*. *BMC Family Practice* 2006; 7:57.

Arroyo R, Martin V, Maldonado A, et al. Treatment of infectious mastitis during lactation: antibiotics versus oral administration of lactobacilli isolated from breast milk. *Clinical Infectious Diseases* 2010; 50(12)1551-1558.

Arsenault JE, Aboud S, Manji KP, et al. Vitamin supplementation increases risk of subclinical mastitis in HIV-infected women. *Journal of Nutrition* 2010; 140(10):1788-1792.

Aryeetey RN, Marquis GS, Brakohiapa L, et al. Subclinical mastitis may not reduce breastmilk intake during established lactation. *Breastfeeding Medicine* 2009; 4(3):161-166.

Arveetey RN, Marquis GS, Timms L, et al. Subclinical mastitis is common among Ghanaian women lactating 3 to 4 months postpartum. *Journal of Human Lactation* 2008; 24(3):263-267.

Behari P, Englund J, Alcasid G, et al. Transmission of methicillin-resistant *Staphylococcus aureus* to preterm infants through breast milk. *Infection Control and Hospital Epidemiology* 2004; 25(9):778-780.

Beigi RH, Bunge K, Song Y, et al. Epidemiologic and economic effect of methicillin-resistant *Staphylococcus aureus* in obstetrics. *Obstetrics and Gynecology* 2009; 113(5):983-991.

Berens P. Management of Lactation in the Puerperium, in *Hale & Hartmann's Textbook of Human Lactation.* Amarillo, TX: Hale Publishing, 2007; p. 363.

Berens P Swaim L, Peterson B. Incidence of methicillin-resistant *Staphylococcus aureus* in postpartum breast abscess. *Breastfeeding Medicine* 2010; 5(3):113-115.

Christensen A, Al-Suliman N, Nielsen K, et al. Ultrasound-guided drainage of breast abscesses: results in 151 patients. *British Journal of Radiology* 2005; 78(927):186-188.

Cooke M, Sheehan A, Schmied V. A description of the relationship between breastfeeding experiences, breastfeeding satisfaction, and weaning in the first 3 months after birth. *Journal of Human Lactation* 2003; 19(2):145-156.

Cotterman KJ. Reverse pressure softening: a simple tool to prepare areola for easier latching during engorgement. *Journal of Human Lactation* 2004; 20(2):227-237.

Cox D, Kent J, Casey T, et al. Breast growth and the urinary excretion of lactose during human pregnancy and early lactation: endocrine relationships. *Experimental Physiology* 1999; 84(2):421-434.

Crekinsek MA, Crowe L, Michener K, et al. Interventions for preventing mastitis after childbirth. *Cochrane Database System Review* 2012; Oct. 17; 10:CD007239.

Dahlbeck S, Donnelly J, Theriault R. Differentiating inflammatory breast cancer from acute mastitis. *American Family Physician* 1995; 52(3):929-934.

Daly S, Kent J, Owens R, et al. Frequency and degree of milk removal and the short-term control of human milk synthesis. *Experimental Physiology* 1996; 81(5):861-875.

Delgado S, Arroyo R, Jimenez E, et al. *Staphylococcus epidermidis* strains isolated from breast milk of women suffering from infectious mastitis: potential virulence traits and resistance to antibiotics. *BMC Microbiology* 2009; 9:82. www.biomedcentral.com.

Dixon J. Repeated aspiration of breast abscess in lactating women. *British Medical Journal* 1988; 297(6662):1517-18.

Eglash A, Proctor R. A breastfeeding mother with chronic breast pain. *Breastfeeding Medicine* 2007; 2(2):99-104.

Fetherston C. Management of lactation mastitis in a Western Australian cohort. *Breastfeeding Review* 1997; 5(2):13-19.

Fetherston C. Risk factors for lactation mastitis. *Journal of Human Lactation* 1998; 14(2):101-109.

Fetherston C. Mastitis in lactating women: physiology or pathology? *Breastfeeding Review* 2001; 9(1):5-12.

Fetherston CM, Lai CT, Hartmann PE. Relationships between symptoms and changes in breast physiology during lactation mastitis. *Breastfeeding Medicine* 2006; 1(3):136-145.

Fortunov RM, Hulten KG, Hammerman WA, et al. Community-acquired *Staphylococcus aureus* infections in term and near-term previously healthy neonates. *Pediatrics* 2006; 118(3):874-881.

Foxman B, Schwartz K, Loman S. Breastfeeding practices and lactation mastitis. *Social Science Medicine* 1994; 38(5):755-761.

Foxman B, D'Arcy H, Gillespie B, et al. Lactation mastitis: occurrence and medical management among 946 breastfeeding women in the United States. *American Journal of Epidemiology* 2002; 155(2):103-114.

Furlong A, al-Nakib L, Knox W, et al. Periductal inflammation and cigarette smoke. *Journal of the American College of Surgeons* 1994; 179(4):417-420.

Hale T. *Medications and Mothers' Milk*, 15th ed. Amarillo, TX: Hale Publishing, 2012; pp. 805.

Hansen L. *Immunobiology of Human Milk.* Amarillo, Texas: Pharmasoft Publishing, 2004; pp. 196-203.

Hayes R, Michell M, Nunnerley HB. Acute inflammation of the breast— the role of breast ultrasound in diagnosis and management. *Clinical Radiology* 1991; 44(4):253-256.

Hill P, Humenick S. The occurrence of breast engorgement. *Journal of Human Lactation* 1994; 10(2):79-86.

Humenick S, Hill P. Breast engorgement: patterns and selected outcomes. *Journal of Human Lactation* 1994; 10(2):87-93.

Inch S, Fisher C. Mastitis: infection or inflammation? *The Practitioner* 1995; 239(1553):472-476.

Jain E. Personal correspondence, 2001.

Jananfar S, Ng CJ, Teng CL. Antibiotics for mastitis in breastfeeding women. *Cochrane Database System Review* 2013; 2:CD005458.

Karstrup S, Nolsoe C, Brabrand K, et al. Ultrasonically guided percutaneous drainage of breast abscesses. *Acta Radiologica* 1990; 31(2):157-159.

Karstrup S. Acute puerperal breast abscesses: US-guided drainage. *Radiology* 1993; 188(3):807-809.

Kasonka L, Makasa M, Marshall T, et al. Risk factors for subclinical mastitis among HIV-infected and uninfected women in Lusake, Zambia. *Paediatric Perinatology and Epidemiology* 2006; 20(5):379-391.

Kendall-Tackett K. A new paradigm for depression in new mothers: the central role of inflammation and how breastfeeding and anti-inflammatory treatments protect maternal mental health. *International Breastfeeding Journal* 2007; 2:6.

King J. Contraception and lactation. *Journal of Midwifery and Womens Health* 2007; 52(6):614-620.

Kvist LJ, Larsson BW, Hall-Lord ML, et al. the role of bacteria in lactational mastitis and some considerations of the use of antibiotic treatment. *International Breastfeeding Journal* 2008; 3:6.

Kvist LJ, Rydhstroem H. Factors related to breast abscess after delivery: a population-based study. *British Journal of Obstetrics and Gynecology* 2005; 112(8):1070-1074.

Lawrence RA, Lawrence RM. *Breastfeeding: A Guide for the Medical Profession*, 7th ed. Maryland Heights, MO: Elsevier Mosby, 2011; pp. 251-252, 564, 571-572.

Livingstone V. Too much of a good thing. Maternal and infant hyperlactation syndromes. *Canadian Family Physician* 1996; 42:89-99.

Livingstone V, Stinger LJ. The treatment of *Staphylococcus aureus* infected sore nipples: a randomized comparative study. *Journal of Human Lactation* 1999; 15(3):241-246.

Love S. *Dr. Susan Love's Breast Book*, 3rd ed. Cambridge, MA: Persues Publishing, 2000; p. 11.

Meguid M, Oler A, Numann P, et al. Pathogenesis-based treatment of recurring subareolar breast abscesses. *Surgery* 1995; 118(4):775-782.

Merlin MA, Wong ML, Pryor PW, et al. Prevalence of methicillin-resistant *Staphylococcus aureus* on the stethoscopes of emergency medical services providers. *Prehospital Emergency Care* 2009; 13(1):71-74.

Michie C, Lockie F, Lynn W. The challenge of mastitis. *Archives of Disease in Childhood* 2003; 88(9):818-821.

Miller V, Riordan J. Treating postpartum breast edema with areolar compression. *Journal of Human Lactation* 2004; 20(2):223-226.

Milner P, Page K, Walton A. Detection of clinical mastitis by changes in electrical conductivity of foremilk before visible changes in milk. *Journal of Dairy Science* 1996; 79(1):83-86.

Minchin M. *Breastfeeding Matters*, 4th ed. Victoria, Australia: Alma Press, 1998; p. 152.

Moon J, Humenick S. Breast engorgement: contributing variables and variables amenable to nursing intervention. *Journal of Obstetric, Gynecologic and Neonatal Nursing* 1989; 18(4):309-315.

Murase M, Mizuno K, Nishida Y, et al. Comparison of creamatocrit and protein concentration in each mammary lobe of the same breast: does the milk composition of each mammary lobe differ in the same breast? *Breastfeeding Medicine* 2009; 4(4):189-195.

Neifert M. Clinical aspects of lactation: promoting breastfeeding success, in CL Wagner, DM Purohit (eds). *Clinics in Perinatology: Clinical Aspects of Human Milk and Lactation.* 1999; 26(2):281-306.

Newton E. Personal communication; 1997a.

Newton E. Mastitis: Cause, Diagnosis, Treatment. Schaumburg, IL: La Leche League, Int., 1997b; p. 4.

Newton M, Newton N. Postpartum engorgement of the breast. *American Journal of Obstetrics & Gynecology* 1951; 61(3):664-667.

Noble R, Bovey A. Therapeutic teat use for babies who breastfeed poorly. *Breastfeeding Review* 1997; 5(2):37-42.

Nussenblatt V, Kumwenda N, Lema V, et al. Effect of antibiotic treatment of subclinical mastitis on human immunodeficiency virus type 1 RNA in human milk. *Journal of Tropical Pediatrics* 2006; 52(5):311-315.

O'Hara R, Dexter S, Fox J. Conservative management of infective mastitis and breast abscesses after ultrasonographic assessment. *British Journal of Surgery* 1996; 83(10):1413-1414.

Olsen CG, Gordon RE. Breast disorders in nursing mothers. *American Family Physician* 1990; 41(5):1509-1516.

Osterman K, Rahm U. Lactation mastitis: bacterial cultivation of breast milk, symptoms, treatment, and outcome. *Journal of Human Lactation* 2000; 16(4):297-302.

Page SM, McKenna DS. Vasospasm of the nipple presenting as painful lactation. *Obstetrics and Gynecology* 2006; 108(3 Pt 2):806-808.

Peacock SJ, Justice A, Griffiths D. Determinants of acquisition and carriage of *Staphylococcus aureus* in infancy. *Journal of Clinical Microbiology* 2003; 41(12):5718-5725.

Ramsay D, Kent J, Owens R, et al. Ultrasound imaging of milk ejection in the breast of lactating women. *Pediatrics* 2004; 113(2):361-367.

Rand S, Kolberg A. Neonatal hypernatremic dehydration secondary to lactation failure. *Journal of the American Board of Family Practics* 2001; 14(2):155-158.

Riordan JM, Nichols FH. A descriptive study of lactation mastitis in long-term breastfeeding women. *Journal of Human Lactation* 1990; 6(2):53-58.

Royal College of Midwives. *Successful Breastfeedin*g, 3rd ed, London: Churchill Livingstone, 2002; pp. 105-110.

Saiman L, O'Keefe M, Graham P, et al. Hospital transmission of community-acquired methicillin-resistant *Staphylococcus aureus* among postpartum women. *Clinical Infectious Diseases* 2003; 37(10):1313-1319.

Saji M, Taguchi S, Uchiyama K, et al. Efficacy of gentian violet in the eradication of methicillin-resistant *Staphylococcus aureus* from skin lesions. *Journal of Hospital Infection* 1995; 31(3):225-228.

Semba R, Newton K, Taha T, et al. Mastitis and immunological factors in breast milk of human imunodeficiency virus-infected women. *Journal of Human Lactatio*n 1999; 15(4):301-306.

Thomassen P, Johansson V, Wassberg C, et al. Breast-feeding, pain and infection. *Gynecologic and Obstetric Investigation* 1998; 46(2):73-74.

Thomsen A, Hansen K, Moller B. Leukocyte counts and microbiologic cultivation in the diagnosis of puerperal mastitis. *American Journal of Obstetrics and Gynecology* 1983; 146(8):938-941.

Ulitzsch D, Nyman M, Carlson R. Breast abscess in lactating women: US-guided treatment. *Radiology* 2004; 232(3):904-909.

van Veldhuizen-Staas C. Overabundant milk supply: an alternate way to intervene by full drainage and block feeding. *International Breastfeeding Journal* 2007; 2:11.

Vieira GO, Silva LR, Mendes CM, et al. Lactational mastitis and Baby-Friendly Hospital Initiative, Feira de Santana, Bahia, Brazil. Cad Suade Publica 2006; 22(6):1193-1200. (in Portuguese, abstract in English)

Vogel A, Hutchison L, Mitchell E. Mastitis in the first year postpartum. *Birth* 1999; 26(4):218-225.

Wilson-Clay B. Milk Oversupply. *Journal of Human Lactation* 2006; 22(2):218-220.

Wilson-Clay B. Case report of Methicillin-resistant *Staphylococcus aureus* (MRSA) mastitis with abscess formation in a breastfeeding woman. *Journal of Human Lactation* 2008; 25(3):326-329.

Witt A, Bolman M, Kondrashova T, et al. Incorporating Russian massage techniques in a US practice: A review of case studies (poster presentation abstract). *Breastfeeding Medicine* 2012; 7(S1):S12-S13.

Wust J, Rutsch M, Stocker S. *Streptococcus pneumoniaeas*: an agent of mastitis (letter). *European Journal of Clinical Microbiology and Infectious Diseases* 1995; 14(2):156-157.

Breast Cancer: Issues For Lactation

Epidemiological evidence suggesting that prolonged breast-feeding protects against breast cancer continues to accumulate (Chang-Claude 2000, Zheng 2000, Kim 2007, Shema 2007). Studies show a decreasing risk of breast cancer with increased number of months of breastfeeding. Additionally, preliminary data suggest that there are protective effects conferred by breastfeeding for mothers who are survivors of childhood cancers (Ogg 2011). The benefits consisted of reduced risk of metabolic syndrome, cardiovascular disease, and reduced risks of secondary tumors. Therefore, public health workers should continue to emphasize the risks of not breastfeeding for the mother, as well as the baby.

The top risk factors for breast cancer are a woman's age and having a first-degree relative with a history of breast cancer. Breastfeeding is thought to reduce the risk of breast cancer through 2 primary mechanisms: the reduction in lifetime ovulatory episodes, and differentiation of breast tissue. Full lactation delays a resumption of menstruation, sometimes for many months. Lactation amenorrhea is thus thought to be protective. Alpha-lactalbumin is a human milk component. Tumor cell death can be induced by HAMLET (a milk complex of oleic acid and alpha-lactalbumin). Healthy cells are not affected by the activity of HAMLET. It may be that this milk complex provides a defense for the tissues of the breast against the development of breast cancer (Franca-Botelho 2012).

Perhaps lactation also has a flushing effect on debris that accumulates in the breast ducts (Helewa 2002). The commonly yellow color of colostrum derives from the presence of carotenoid fat globules. Djuric (2005) studied nipple aspirate fluid taken from women who had never lactated and women who lactated only for short periods, compared to nipple fluid aspirated from women who lactated 6 months or more. Carotenoid and tocopherol levels were significantly higher in nipple aspirate fluid from women who lactated for 6 months or more. Carotenoids and tocopherols are thought to be protective against breast cancer. Carotenoids may dilute and help expel substances stored in the non-lactating gland such as DDT, PCB, and other environmental contaminants (Patton 1990).

At one point, it was thought that a woman's intake of dietary fat might increase her risk of developing breast cancer, and that increasing dietary fiber might reduce it. Studies do not support this theory (Rohan 1988, Willett 1992). However, exposure to breast milk in early childhood may decrease the risk of developing breast cancer later in life.

Freudenheim (1994) observed that *having been breastfed* is associated with a decrease in breast cancer. Martin (2005) performed a meta-analysis on a large cohort of cancer patients and identified a significantly reduced risk of premenopausal breast cancer in women who had been breastfed as infants.

A number of countries have noted increasing rates of breast cancer in their populations as rates of breastfeeding incidence and duration have fallen (Shema 2007, Kim 2007). Because having been breastfed as a child and breastfeeding each appear to be independently protective, the choice to breastfeed may be one of the few proactive measures that can be undertaken to lower a woman's lifetime risk of developing breast cancer. In fact, the evidence for a protective effect of breastfeeding is now sufficiently well-established to motivate changes in cancer prevention policy recommendations.

In 2002, the Collaborative Group on Hormonal Factors in Breast Cancer concluded that, "The longer women breastfeed the more they are protected against breast cancer. The lack of or the short lifetime duration of breastfeeding typical of women in developed countries makes a major contribution to the high incidence of breast cancer in these countries." Such statements have resulted in specific recommendations to women urging exclusive breastfeeding for 6 months, and the continuation of breastfeeding after the introduction of solids as a cancer prevention strategy (WCRF 2007).

The protective effect of breastfeeding does not alter the fact that it is still possible for an individual woman to develop breast cancer during pregnancy or lactation. Individuals who have been breastfed may still develop breast cancer. There is evidence that there is a transient increase in risk of breast cancer in the first 3 to 4 years after delivery of a singleton child (Helawa 2002). Following this transient period of increased risk, lifetime risk is lower than that of women who have never given birth.

Because breast cancer risk increases during pregnancy and remains elevated for some period of years afterward, cancer-associated proteins that are secreted into breast milk may provide a way to detect cancer in the lactating breast and to assess a woman's risk for future breast cancer (Arcaro 2012)

The incidence of breast cancer in young women has risen, and because many women now delay child-bearing, pregnancy following treatment for breast cancer is more common (Dow 1994). Owing to these demographic factors, the LC must be aware of the symptoms that require evaluation to rule out breast cancer.

Breast Cancer During Pregnancy and Lactation

Breast cancer is the second leading cause of cancer deaths among American women. The National Cancer Institute (at the National Institutes of Health) reports that 12.4 percent of women born in the US will develop breast cancer at some point in their lives (Howlander 2012). Of these, 25 percent develop tumors in their child-bearing years (Camune 2007). The incidence of breast cancers occuring in pregnant or lactating women is felt to be 2 to 3 per 1,000 (Steyskall 1996).

Unfortunately, diagnosis and treatment are often delayed in pregnant and lactating women. The reasons for this are complex and include lack of awareness, health care provider distraction, and psychological denial. According to researchers at M.D. Anderson Cancer Center in Houston, Texas, most women who visit a family physician with typical symptoms of inflamatory breast cancer (IBC) are diagnosed and treated for lactational mastitis (Kelly 2013).

While describing initial treatment for mastitis as reasonable, the IBC researchers remark that it is unreasonable to order a second or third round of antibiotics if the first round fails to produce improvement. Mammography and ultrasonography should be employed to determine if there is a mass that can be biopsied. While overdiagnosis is not desirable, the prognosis for survival with IBC is poor if treatment is delayed. As with other types of cancer, early identification provides the best chance of survival.

Prenatal care should include serial breast examinations, and women should continue monthly breast self-examinations during lactation. It is normal for lactating breasts to feel lumpy, and plugged ducts and mastitis are not unusual events. However, a discrete lump that is different from surrounding breast tissue may be a sign of breast cancer (Lind 2004). Breast exams increase the woman's familiarity with changes in her own breasts, alert her to masses that do not resolve with standard treatment, or that recur persistently in the same area of the breast. A physician should evaluate such masses.

Health care providers may be distracted by conditions such as pregnancy and lactation, dismissing or ignoring symptoms that would, in a non-lactating woman, trigger prompt evaluation. Misdiagnosis of carcinoma of the breast is the most frequent cause of malpractice litigation in the United States. The willingness to seek a second opinion has saved many lives.

Private practice lactation consultants may encounter situations where a woman presents with suspicious findings (Petok 1995). LCs must know the warning signs for breast cancer and refer women for prompt medical evaluation.

Red Flags and Warning Signs for Breast Cancer

The following warning signs require prompt referral to the woman's primary care provider:

- Skin color changes on the breast, red breast in the absence of fever (Dahlbeck 1995, Cristofanilli (2003)
- Skin texture changes, peau d'orange appearance, **Figs. 253** and **254**, edema, indurations, **Fig. 289**.
- Exaggerated hair follicle pits (**Fig. 253**) (Kelly 2013)
- Masses, especially fixed, irregular shaped lumps
- Copious, spontaneous, clear or bloody nipple discharge (typically unilateral)
- Mastitis that occurs repeatedly in the same area and does not resolve with conservative treatment (i.e., appropriate drugs and management)

Diagnostic Tests and Lactation

It is possible to perform diagnostic tests on pregnant and lactating women without weaning, although mammograms are more difficult to interpret, owing to the density of the pregnant and lactating breast. Ductal lavage is a technique to achieve non-invasive access to breast tissue. It involves duct cannulation and endoscopy. The duct is washed, and the flushed tissue is examined for breast cancer and precancerous changes (Love 1996). However, whether the ductal lavage technique is diagnostically useful during lactation is unknown.

Ultrasound (**Fig 281**) is a safe diagnostic technique that can be used during pregnancy and lactation. It is painless and useful in distinguishing between cystic (fluid-filled) and solid masses (Freund 2000, Lind 2004).

Galactoceles are a type of cyst that can form in the breast during lactation. The material aspirated from such a cyst is milk. Abscesses are another type of cystic lesion, and the aspirate will include purulent material (pus). Needle biopsy can be performed to examine cells aspirated from masses that have been identified by ultrasound. **Ch. 11** contains a full discussion of types of abscesses.

Tumors are solid (rather than cystic) masses. Many types of tumors (such as fibrocysts) are benign. A breast biopsy is the most definitive type of diagnostic measure used to identify the nature of a mass and to rule out cancer. Because it is a surgical procedure, it is also the most invasive diagnostic tool. While it is often necessary, biopsy poses a certain degree of risk to current or future lactation owing to incision and removal of tissue (Osuch 1998). Such risk, however, must be evaluated in terms of its potential for saving the mother's life.

Inflammatory Breast Cancer

Inflammatory breast cancer (IBC) is a particularly aggressive form of cancer with a high mortality rate. Although one of the rarer forms of breast cancer, it accounts for 1 to 5 percent of all breast cancer cases, but 10 percent of the breast cancer deaths (National Cancer Institute 2013). Early diagnosis is critical. However, diagnosis of inflammatory breast cancer may be delayed because it shares important symptoms with mastitis.

While a woman with inflammatory breast cancer typically experiences no fever, the breast becomes warm, red, heavy and edematous, often presenting with peau d'orange changes and exaggerated hair follicle pits. The area of redness is generally large, often covering the whole breast. The nipple appears flattened and indurated (retracted). The nipple may ooze fluid and nipple skin may become crusted (Dahlbeck 1995). Inflammatory breast cancer can be difficult to detect with mammography. Examination of malignant cells accessed by fine needle or excision biopsy confirms the diagnosis. Skin biopsy is indicated if there is no mass.

African American women have a higher incidence of inflammatory breast cancer (Cristofanilli 2003).

Breastfeeding after Treatment for Breast Cancer

Breastfeeding is discontinued during chemotherapy for breast cancer because the drugs used are toxic and may harm a breastfeeding baby.

Some women become infertile as the result of chemotherapy, which can cause *chemical menopause*. Other women succeed in becoming pregnant after cancer treatment and they can be encouraged to breastfeed. No survival disadvantage has been identified by subsequent pregnancy or lactation (Dow 1994, Kasum 2006, Camune 2007). There is no contraindication for breastfeeding after treatment for breast cancer (Danforth 1991). Lactation usually proceeds normally in the unaffected breast. In the treated breast, functional lactation is possible, but generally milk production is significantly diminished in the majority of patients (Moran 2005).

Breast conserving procedures such as lumpectomy rather than mastectomy are possible in many cases. However, radiation therapy and the damage to the structures of the breast caused by invasive surgery may render the breast incapable of lactation. Leal (2013) describes lactation following radiotherapy in at least 50 percent of patients but in reduced volume. Partial lactation has occurred in some cases, resulting in some ability to lactate on the treated breast (Higgins 1994).

David (1985) reports a case of a 36 year-old woman who had a "poorly differentiated infiltrating ductal carcinoma in the right tail of Spence area." The mass was excised and her nodes were unaffected. She received radiation therapy, and became pregnant a year later. Her treated breast did not enlarge as much as the untreated left breast during the pregnancy, but following the birth the treated breast did lactate. The milk was slightly thicker, and the breast produced about half the amount of milk that the left breast produced. Leal (2013) reports biochemical changes in irradiated breast milk.

BWC worked with a woman who breastfed unilaterally following treatment for breast cancer with lumpectomy. The lumpectomized breast became engorged following the birth of the baby. The mother observed spontaneous leaking. Because the woman elected not to stimulate that breast, it soon involuted. She breastfed her child uneventfully on the unaffected breast.

Lumpectomy

The 48 year-old woman shown in **Fig. 282** has a radial incision over the location of a lumpectomy. She had breastfed her children. A history of having breastfed does not justify complacency regarding the development of lumps in the breast, and the woman consulted with a surgeon who performed the lumpectomy. Interestingly, a faint scar from an earlier biopsy is visible, running exactly parallel to the lumpectomy scar, at the areolar edge. This earlier biopsy revealed a benign tumor. For a younger woman, with more childbearing years ahead of her, a radial rather than a circumferential incision might lessen the impact of such invasive surgery.

The same woman is pictured in **Fig. 283** during radiation therapy. Note the bronzed appearance of the skin. Approximately 90 percent of patients treated with radiation therapy will develop some degree of radiation-induced dermatitis (Harper 2004) that can produce significant discomfort and limit daily activity. Previously, soap and water washing of irradiated skin was discouraged due to concern that a drying effect of soap would exacerbate radiation dermatitis. When systematically evaluated, however, *moist desquamation* (shedding of skin) developed in 33 percent of those who did not wash the skin as compared with 14 percent of those who washed with soap and water. Roy (2001) hypothesized that washing may reduce moist desquamation by removing skin microbes that act as inflammatory stimuli at the basal layer of the skin. The study concluded that washing the skin does not increase skin toxicity.

Fig. 284 shows the scar from an axillary biopsy taken to see whether cancer has spread to the lymph nodes. The presence or absence of spread to the nodes defines the stage of the cancer. Staging is a way to conceptualize each case of breast cancer so that appropriate treatment can be selected. Stage 1 describes a tumor with no affected lymph nodes. Stage 2 is a small tumor with positive lymph nodes, or a larger tumor with positive or negative nodes, or a large tumor with negative nodes. Stage 3 is a large tumor with positive lymph nodes, or a tumor with "grave signs." Stage 4 is a tumor that has obvious metastasis (Love 2000).

The woman in **Fig. 285** was treated 8 years prior for breast cancer with lumpectomy, radiation therapy, and chemotherapy. Her left breast did not experience any changes during pregnancy or postpartum. She planned to breastfeed using her right breast. Note the size difference in her breasts from the increase in breast development during pregnancy.

Breastfeeding after Mastectomy

A 32 year-old woman is pictured in **Fig. 286**. She had 3 children at the time that she was diagnosed with breast cancer. Her affected breast was removed, and she was told that she would experience chemical menopause. She and her family were shocked when she became pregnant 4 years later. She described herself to the LC as having been "traumatized by my medical treatment." She had a home birth supported by a midwife, and 2 weeks later, requested to see the LC because of a cracked nipple on her remaining breast. Her baby was gaining well, and judging from the orientation of the wound, the main issue appeared to be a routine positioning and latch problem.

The mother was instructed to gently cleanse the wound in order to prevent nipple infection and mastitis and to pump the breast to give the nipple a chance to heal. The midwife presecribed topical mupirocin ointment to prevent infection. The baby was bottle-fed pumped milk for 5 days until the wound healed. An experienced breastfeeding mother who was determined to succeed, this woman was not worried about subsequent breast refusal. As expected, the baby easily transitioned back to breastfeeding.

The 28 year-old woman in **Fig. 287** is shown breastfeeding her 18 day-old third child following mastectomy for breast cancer. The woman's husband had discovered a lump in her left breast the previous summer. The mother was breastfeeding their 2 year-old son at the time. Because the mother was deaf, the father phoned BWC to describe the persistant mass in the breast. BWC recommended medical evaluation. A breast surgeon performed a needle biopsy and detected cancerous cells in the aspirate. The surgeon recommended immediate weaning and mastectomy to remove the breast and axillary lymph nodes.

BWC assisted with an emergency weaning and took photos of the process. In **Fig. 288** faint bruising appears over the location of the biopsy at 8 o'clock on the left breast. On Day 3 of the weaning (**Fig. 289**), engorgement has lessened to the extent that it is possible to perceive an induration on the underside of the breast where the tumor is located.

Chemotherapy and radiation treatment followed the mastectomy. During radiation treatment, the woman became pregnant, and her healthy daughter was born at term. Breastfeeding continued uneventfully for 5 months, during which time the baby grew normally, feeding only from one breast. Gradual weaning was begun at this point to allow the mother's physicians to perform diagnostic tests in response to elevated tumor markers in her blood. Sadly, 5 years after these photos were taken, the young mother died of breast cancer.

Biopsy to Rule Out Paget's Disease of the Nipple

The 32 year-old mother whose nipple is pictured in **Figs. 290-292** nursed her first child uneventfully for 15 months. After the birth of her second child, she developed an eruption on her left nipple that continued essentially unabated for 5 months. The LC observed an oozing, crusty left nipple on Day 7 postpartum. The right nipple was also cracked and irritated.

The LC adjusted the mother's positioning, and antibiotics were begun within 24 hours because the mother had developed febrile symptoms. After a week on antibiotics, the mother developed the symptoms of what she suspected was a yeast infection. At 6 weeks postpartum, after constant medical treatment, the nipples appeared to be healing. However, because the nipples were still slightly inflamed, the mother consulted the first of 4 dermatologists. The first dermatologist advised the mother to apply a hydrogel dressing after each feeding, which immediately worsened her symptoms, especially on the left nipple.

Over the next months, the mother consulted 3 other dermatologists and continued contact with her obstetrician and her LC. The mother was treated for yeast infection, staph infection, and contact irritant dermatitis. She was prescribed Diflucan, Loprox, Ketoconazole, Zithromax, Locoid ointment, Elocon cream and Vaseline. Cultures from her milk and the baby's mouth and nose all showed normal flora. For a period of 3 months, the mother exclusively pumped, feeding the baby by bottle. While her nipples improved during the time she pumped, they never healed completely and worsened as soon as she resumed any breastfeeding.

At 6 months, the left nipple again appeared erythematous and edematous. A fourth dermatologist advised a punch biopsy to rule out Paget's disease (a type of cancer of the nipple that resembles eczema and is also referrred to as *erosive adenomatosis*.) In **Fig. 290**, the dermatologist injects Lidocaine into the nipple to numb it. A numbing cream was applied previously to the nipple to reduce the sting of the injection.

In **Fig. 291** a small punch tool is used to remove a core of tissue (seen being removed in **Fig. 292**) that was sent to a lab for analysis. The sample indicated that there was no evidence of disease. In fact, there was no conclusive evidence even of a contact or irritant dermatitis. In short, nothing was discovered to explain this woman's chronic nipple irritation.

The dermatologist sutured the wound made by the biopsy. BWC expressed concern about the stitches, fearing they would interfere with breastfeeding. The mother phoned BWC several hours later to report that clots of blood had appeared in her pumped milk. Her breast was not draining well and felt engorged. In contrast to pumping, the baby was able to soften the breast, but the knot in the stiff sutures dug a deeper hole in her nipple each time the baby nursed. Additionally, her bra was rubbing on the sutures and this irritated the wound. The mother called the doctor who instructed her to remove the sutures. The doctor advised her to keep packing the hole in her nipple with mupirocin. However, within 24 hours, the mother's breast was bright red. She was diagnosed with mastitis and was treated with oral antibiotics. Once she began the oral antibiotics, healing proceeded uneventfully.

Several studies have discussed the development of atopic dermatitis, a chronic inflammatory skin disease, where colonization of skin with *Staphylococcus aureus* is known to produce toxins with superantigen activity. Perhaps sensitization occurred early in the course of this mother's situation. At the time of the biopsy, her results showed only a dilated vasculature, a very non-specific finding; however, the LC was uncertain whether tests for superantigen activity were performed.

Although the mother in this case stated that she had no food allergies, she consumed large amounts of dairy products, which she felt constituted the mainstay of her diet. BWC had advised a dairy elimination very early in the case, but the mother only abstained from dairy for about a week. During the biopsy, the LC and dermatologist discussed the possibility of a relationship between diet and the woman's sore nipples. After this discussion, the mother removed dairy products for several weeks and felt that it did make some difference. As time went on, the baby exhibited signs of atopic disease. He developed eczema and constipation around 6 months, and his mother had to remove dairy from his diet entirely by the time he reached toddlerhood.

Reaction from exposure to dairy protein in the mother's diet could have provoked salivary changes irritating to the nipple. It was interesting, however, that the nipple condition never totally resolved, even when the baby was not breastfeeding directly for long periods of time. The woman continued to breastfeed past the baby's second birthday. Her nipples, however, remained vulnerable, and breastfeeding was never comfortable for her. BWC stayed in contact with this woman, and 10 years later the woman reported no breast or nipple complications from her experience.

BWC is generally reluctant to advise dairy restriction; however, she observed another client whose sore nipples cleared up (after all other suggestions failed to bring results) when dairy protein was taken out of the woman's diet. Dairy elimination was trialed on the premise that a sensitive baby might experience salivary changes in reaction to exposure of the offending protein through the milk, and that these changes might irritate the nipple. A 3 week dairy elimination resulted in healed nipples. At the time, the supervising physician felt the improvement was merely coincidental; however, the mother was so relieved to have no more nipple pain that she remained on the dairy-free diet.

It became clear that her baby was allergic to dairy protein when, at age 5 months, the father gave the baby a taste of ice cream from a spoon. A drop of ice cream also spilled on the baby's cheek. The cheek was scalded where the ice cream touched it. Within an hour, the baby was taken to the emergency room with symptoms of anaphylactic shock. A similar event was described in an article about severely allergic children featured in the *New York Times* (Thernstrom 2013).

Extreme reactivity to minute quantities of allergen by skin contact is not unique. Another 5 cases are reported in the literature. One involved a 3 month-old male who later proved to have multiple food allergies. He developed localized skin irritation when his mother kissed him after eating cereal with milk (Tan 2001). In all 5 cases, reactions occurred while the children were being breastfed (exclusively in 4 and mixed feeding in one). A connection between food allergy and sore nipples deserves more investigation, and while it is important to rule out breast cancer (especially Paget's disease of the nipple), there may be alternate etiologies involved when nipples fail to heal.

Complex cases remind LCs that multiple causes exist for breast lumps and skin conditions of the nipples. Rarely are they cancer, but the LC has an ethical responsibility to not overlook suspicious symptoms that require further investigation by a qualified physician.

Arcaro KF, Browne EP, Qin W, et al. Differential expression of cancer-related proteins in paired breast milk samples from women with breast cancer. *Journal of Human Lactation* 2012; 28(4):543-546.

Camune B, Gabzdyl E. Breast-feeding after breast cancer in childbearing women. *Journal of Perinatal and Neonatal Nursing* 2007; 21(3):225-233.

Chang-Claude J, Eby N, Kiechle M, et al. Breastfeeding and breast cancer risk by age 50 among women in Germany. *Cancer Causes and Control* 2000; 11(8):687-695.

Cristofanilli M, Buzdar A, Hortobagyi G. Update on the management of inflammatory breast cancer. *The Oncologist* 2003; 8(2):141-148.

Collaborative Group on Hormonal Factors in Breast Cancer. Breast cancer and breastfeeding: collaborative re-analysis of individual data from 47 epidemiological studies in 30 countries, including 50302 women with breast cancer and 96973 women without the disease. *Lancet* 2002; 360(9328):187-195.

Dahlbeck S, Donnelly J, Theriault R. Differentiating inflammatory breast cancer from acute mastitis. *American Family Physician* 1995; 52(3):929-934.

Danforth D. How subsequent pregnancy affects outcome in women with prior breast cancer. *Oncology* 1991; 5(11):23-35.

David F. Lactation following primary radiation therapy for carcinoma of the breast. *International Journal of Radiation Oncology, Biology, Physics* 1985; 11(7):1425.

Djuric Z, Visscher DW, Heilbrun LK, et al. Influence of lactation history on breast nipple aspirate fluid yield and fluid composition. *Breast Journal* 2005; 11(2):92-99.

Dow KH, Harris JR, Roy C. Pregnancy after breast-conserving surgery and radiation therapy for breast cancer. *Journal of the National Cancer Institute Monogram* 1994; (16):131-137.

Franca-Botelho AC, Ferreira MC, Franca JL, et al. Breastfeeding and its relationship with reduction of breast cancer: a review. *Asian Pacific Journal of Cancer Prevention* 2012; 13(11):5327-5332.

Freudenheim J, Marshall J, Graham S, et al. Exposure to breastmilk in infancy and the risk of breast cancer. *Epidemiology* 1994; 5(3): 324-331.

Freund K. Rationale and technique of clinical breast examination. *Medscape Women's Health* 2000; 5(6): e2.

Harper J, Franklin L, Jenrette J, et al. Skin toxicity during breast irradiation: pathophysiology and management. *Southern Medical Journal* 2004; 97(10):989-993.

Helewa M, Levesque P, Provencher D, et al. Breast cancer, pregnancy, and breastfeeding. *Journal of Obstetrics and Gynaecology Canada* 2002; 24(2):164-180.

Higgins S, Huffy B. Pregnancy and lactation after breast-conserving therapy for early stage breast cancer. *Cancer* 1994; 73(8):2175-2180.

Howlander N, Noone AM, Krapcho M, et al. (eds). *SEER Cancer Statistics Review, 1975-2009 (Vintage 2009 Populations)*, National Cancer Institute. Bethesda, MD, 2012.

Kasum M. Breast cancer treatment - later pregnancy and survival. *European Journal of Gynaecological Oncology* 2006; 27(3): 225-229.

Kelly JC, Ueno NT. Inflammatory breast cancer: What you should know. *Medscape*. Feb. 1, 2013.

Kim Y, Choi JY, Lee KM, et al. Dose-dependent protective effect of breast-feeding against breast cancer among ever-lactated women in Korea. *European Journal of Cancer Prevention* 2007; 16(2):124-129.

Leal SC, Stuart SR, Carvalho H de A. Breast irradiation and lactation: a review. *Expert Review of Anticancer Therapy* 2013; 13(2):159-164.

Lind DS, Smith BL, Souba WW. 5 Breast Complaints. in Souba WW, Fink MP, Jurkovich GJ, et al. ACS Surgery Online. New York: WebMD Inc. 2004.

Love S. *Dr. Susan Love's Breast Book*. Cambridge, MA: Perseus Publishing, 2000; pp. 336-337.

Love S, Barsky S. Breast duct endoscopy to study stages of cancerous breast disease. *Lancet* 1996; 348(9033):997-999.

Martin RM, Middleton N, Gunnell D, et al. Breastfeeding and cancer: the Boyd Orr cohort and a sytematic reveiw with meta-analysis. *Journal of the National Cancer Institute* 2005; 97(19):1446-1457.

Moran MS, Colasanto JM, Haffty BG, et al. Effects of breast-conserving therapy on lactation after pregnancy. *Cancer Journal* 2005; 11(5):399-403.

National Cancer Institute Fact Sheet: *Inflammatory breast cancer*. 2013. www.cancer.gov. Accessed March 2013.

Ogg SW, Hudson MM, Randolph ME, et al. Protective effects of breast-feeding for mothers surviving childhood cancer. *Journal of Cancer Survivorship* 2011; DOI 10 1007

Osuch J, Bonham V, Morris L. Primary care guide to managing a breast mass step by step workup. Medscape/womens.health/1998/v03. n05/wh3.

Patton S, Canfield L, Huston G, et al. Carotenoids of human colostrum. *Lipids* 1990; 25(3):159-165.

Petok E. Breast cancer and breastfeeding: five cases. *Journal of Human Lactation* 1995; 11(3):205-209.

Rohan T, McMichael A, Baghurst P. A population-based case-control study of diet and breast cancer in Australia. *American Journal of Epidemiology* 1988; 128(3):478-489.

Roy I, Fortin A, Larochelle M. The impact of skin washing with water and soap during breast irradiation: a randomized study. *Radiotherapy & Oncology* 2001; 58(3):333-339.

Shema L, Ore L, Ben-Shachar M, et al. The association between breast-feeding and breast cancer occurrence among Israeli Jewish women: a case control study. *Journal of Cancer Research and Clinical Oncology* 2007; 133(8):539-546.

Steyskal R. Minimizing the risk of delayed diagnosis of breast cancer. Medscape/womens.health/1996/v0.n07/w65.

Tan B, Sher M, Good R, et al. Severe food allergies by skin contact. *Annals of Allergy, Asthma, & Immunology* 2001; 86(5):583-586.

Thernstrom M. The Allergy Buster: can a radical new treastment save children with severe food allergies? *New York Times Magazine* March 7, 2013. www.nytimes.com.

Willett W, Hunter D, Stampfer M, et al. Dietary fat and fiber in relation to risk of breast cancer. *Journal of the American Medical Association* 1992; 268(15):2037-2044.

World Cancer Research Fund (WCRF). Food, nutrition, physical activity, and the prevention of cancer: a global perspective. http://www. babyfriendly.org.uk/pdfs/World_Cancer_Research_Fund_2007-10.pdf. Accessed Feb. 2008.

Zheng R, Duan L, Liu Y, et al. Lactation reduces breast cancer risk in Shandong Province, China. *American Journal of Epidemiology* 2000; 152(12):1129-1135.

Twin, Triplet, and Tandem Breastfeeding

Slightly over 3 percent of infants born annually in the US are twin births. In the 1980s and 1990s, twin births occurring in the US and other developed countries increased as the result of drugs used to treat infertility. From 2000 to 2013, the twin rate stabilized in the US. The rate for triplet and higher order multiple births has also decreased in the last decade. The decline in higher order multiple births is seen as the result of practice guidelines issued by the American Society for Reproductive Medicine, and improvements in procedures that transfer fewer embryos per *in vitro* fertilization attempts (Martin 2012).

Birth rates have decreased in most segments of the US population since 2000, but rose in the 40 to 44 year-old group of women (Martin 2012). Presumably, many of these pregnancies resulted from fertility treatments. Consequently, multiple births in older first-time mothers in developed countries comprise a subset of mothers seeking lactation support. LCs assisting these mothers require skills in managing breastfeeding multiples and preterm infants. They must also be aware of health issues related to the older mother.

Many women who deliver multiples want to breastfeed, and the benefits of breastfeeding can be extremely important to them (Geraghty 2004). Generally health workers are supportive of this goal; however, encouragement must be realistic. Mothers should be informed that newborn twins are often inefficient feeders owing to small size, immaturity, etc. They may poorly stimulate the breasts, delaying the onset of copious lactation. During this delay, unacceptable levels of weight loss may occur if the infants are not spoon or cup fed colostrum. Weight monitoring is important. It is often necessary to augment breast stimulation on Days 1 and 2 to ensure that the milk comes in without long delays.

In Africa, the rate of *spontaneous twinning* (twin births that occur naturally) is the highest in the world (Steinman 2009). This may reflect a population's biologic attempt to protect its gene pool when environmental and economic conditions are stressful. Because poverty, violent conflicts, refugee situations, and natural disasters can affect populations anywhere, it is important for health workers to understand how to protect vulnerable infants with both high and low tech interventions. Electronic scales and electric breast pumps are efficient and effective, but hand expression, cup feeding, and skin-to-skin holding can also be employed to stabilize infants who are not initially able to breastfeed robustly. Health workers must be trained to support breastfeeding in any environment.

Increased Infant Risks Associated with Multiple Birth

Mothers struggling with the challenges of integrating 2 or more babies into the family often express feelings of concern about whether they will be able to give their babies as much maternal attention as a single child would receive. In fact, research suggests that this concern is valid, particularly in higher order multiples. Feldman (2005) reports that triplets scored lower than singletons and twins on developmental assessments at 6, 12, and 24 months. The smallest triplets showed decreased cognitive skills at 12 and 24 months compared to their siblings.

Greater medical risk at birth, multiple-birth status, limited access to exclusive parenting, and reduced infant social involvement in the first 2 years were each predictive of lower cognitive outcomes at 2 years of age. Mothers of multiples may find it reassuring to know that the interaction between mother and baby inherent in the activity of breastfeeding is a way to enhance infant stimulation and improve bonding and attachment.

Prematurity is a frequent complication of multiple births. Additionally, multiples tend to be small for gestational age (SGA). Morley (2004) identified improved cognitive outcomes of SGA infants in breastfed versus formula-fed babies. Given the higher risk of cognitive delay (especially in the smallest baby), breastfeeding is protective for multiples and their families. Fetal growth restriction, if followed by rapid weight gain owing to formula supplementation, increases the risk for adult diseases, including the metabolic syndrome. Human milk uniquely sustains normal growth without excessively increasing the infant's body fat mass or triggering insulin resistance (de Zegher 2013).

Sadly, research suggests that mothers of preterm multiples provide human milk less often than mothers of term singletons and term multiples. They are significantly at risk for providing milk for a shorter duration than other groups of mothers (Geraghty 2004, Yokoyama 2004).

Damato (2005) identified unique issues related to breastfeeding multiples that contributed to the early cessation of lactation. These included concerns about inadequate milk supply, the burden of milk expression, and general maternal fatigue. Issues relating to infant behavior included sleepiness, poor suck, disinterest in feeding, illness, or poor infant weight gain.

Depending on their size and condition, preterm babies often experience delays in going to the breast initially, and throughout the first days. Their behavioral cues are often indistinct, making it difficult for mothers to identify readiness to feed. This often results in too few daily feedings, especially if visitors are plentiful and interfere with the timing of feedings.

Many inexperienced mothers cannot accurately assess whether their newborn twins are feeding well. Hospital personnel, in an attempt to be supportive, often praise breastfeeding attempts that are not particularly successful from the standpoint of the babies actually transferring milk. Early weight loss in breastfeeding twins can thus be excessive, increasing the risk for elevated bilirubin and for dehydration when the twins are discharged from the hospital. Formula supplementation often begins at this point, especially if there has been deficient breast stimulation and the mother's milk supply is low.

New mothers of twins often do not know how much milk they should be producing or how much the babies should be drinking. (Ch. 5 reviews the normal, expected milk volumes for singleton babies.) Mothers of twins must be helped to understand that they need twice as much milk. Their breasts must be optimally stimulated, but small twins are often unable to accomplish this task. Hand expression or "insurance" pumping during the milk calibration phase can be crucial in establishing a milk supply that is sufficient for 2 babies. In a pilot study comparing 2 groups of mothers, Parker (2012) found that initiation of milk expression within 1 hour following birth increased milk volume and decreased the time to lactogenesis II in women who delivered low birth weight infants.

The transition to direct, exclusive breastfeeding is always easier if there is an ample milk supply and if the babies are not calorically deprived. Mothers who are using some form of milk expression to augment breast stimulation should be encouraged to feed the pumped milk to their babies immediately rather than freezing it for later use. Helping twins regain birth weight quickly will improve their breastfeeding abilities.

The LC should recommend frequent milk expression from both breasts. Morton (2009, 2012) described the best practices for improving early milk production of mothers of preterm infants using a combination of hand expression and double pumping with a hospital grade pump (See Ch. 14). The combination of techniques produced higher milk volumes and higher levels of fat-rich milk.

A Cochrane Review compared methods of milk expression (Becker 2008). Electric and pedal operated pumps obtained more milk than hand expression alone. The pedal pump is an important tool in populations without access to electricity. All mothers should be taught hand expression techniques for many reasons, for example if the power goes off. In the developing world, hand expression is a particularly critical skill for mothers to learn.

Increased Maternal Medical Risks Associated with Multiple Births

A large retrospective study comparing singleton with multiple-fetal pregnancies identified a higher incidence of maternal health complications in mothers of multiples (Walker 2004). These maternal risks included significant increases in cardiac morbidity, pre-eclampsia, gestational diabetes, postpartum hemorrhage, prolonged hospitalization, hysterectomy, and blood transfusion. Any of these conditions may delay the onset of lactogenesis II and thus negatively impact milk production. In addition, delivery at less than 28 weeks gestation may not allow for sufficient breast development during pregnancy to support full lactation (Geddes 2007).

McKenzie (2006) identified the need to understand and respect the fact that mothers pregnant with multiples require more resources during pregnancy than are often available to help them make informed infant feeding decisions. More breastfeeding education materials should be specifically adapted for mothers who are pregnant with multiples. Gromada (2010) published a 2-page resource for breastfeeding mothers of twins that may be freely photocopied for distribution (but not sold).

Mothers of multiples require extra support to successfully breastfeed or to preserve lactation with pumping. Lack of support from her partner and increased maternal anxiety when informed of a multiple pregnancy are factors that were significantly associated with the decision to bottle feed in a large study of Japanese mothers of multiples, compared to a control group of singleton mothers (Yokoyama 2004). Flidel-Rimon (2006) documented that mothers of multiples require the combined support of spouse, family, friends, and the medical team to make either full or partial breastfeeding possible. There is a case report of a woman who breastfed quadruplets with strong family support (Berlin 2007). The LC may need to counsel families to identify concrete ways the family can assist.

Postpartum care of mothers of multiples must include instructions on how to protect the option to breastfeed if the mother is ill or requires extended recovery time before being able to provide a robust milk supply. In the event that ill health or lack of breast development precludes a full or even a partial supply of own mother's milk, the LC may wish to provide information about donor human milk from an accredited milk bank.

Peer-to-peer milk sharing of unpasteurized human milk from unscreened donors is discouraged for medically fragile and preterm infants, owing to concern about the risk of transmission of viruses from human milk. The risks of artificial formula, especially in preterm populations, have created a renewed interest in human milk banking as a method of providing safe milk for hospitalized infants whose mothers cannot produce a full milk supply. (See Ch. 15.)

In the US and Canada, milk banks are regulated by the Human Milk Banking Association of North America (HMBANA), an organization comprised of representatives from member banks. Founded in 1985, it developed guidelines to establish donor requirements, donor screening protocols, pasteurization policies, and bacteriological quality control standards for dispensed milk. HMBANA guidelines are developed based on recommendations by the US Centers for Disease Control, the US Food and Drug Administration, and the American Association of Blood Banks for human donor tissues. The HMBANA guidelines can be viewed on-line at: www.hmbana.org.

Reducing Neonatal Necrotizing Enterocolitis in Preterm Populations

Necrotizing enterocolitis (NEC) is a devastating inflammatory condition that destroys the lining of the intestinal wall (Luig 2005). The causes of this painful disease are unclear, although 75 percent of cases occur in preterm infants. Research indicates that the use of human milk reduces the incidence of neonatal necrotizing enterocolitis (NEC) in populations of preterm infants (Lucas 1990, Kelley 2012, Lee 2012). This issue is meaningful to mothers of multiples, as many of these infants are preterm.

NEC accounts for a significant percentage of deaths in infants <1500 g. Many infants who develop NEC are treated surgically by removing affected sections of their bowels. With part of the intestine missing, the individual will have a life-long problem absorbing adequate nutrients from food intake.

Lucas (1990) reported that NEC was rare in those preterm infants receiving at least some human milk feeds. He observed that the incidence of NEC was 20 times more common in formula-fed infants. Dvorak (2003) reported that maternal milk is the major source of trophic peptides,

with significant healing effects on injured gastrointestinal mucosa.

Women who deliver preterm infants have higher concentrations of these peptides in their milk than are present in term milk or in formula. In the past, authorities were unclear whether donor human milk provided a protective effect similar to own mother's milk in the reduction of NEC. McGuire (2003) performed a meta-analysis of previous research and identified a significant association in reduction of relative risk of NEC in preterm infants fed donor human milk rather than formula. Evidence of improved neonatal outcomes in human milk-fed infants suggests an increased role of own mother's and donor human milk to reduce NEC and as a method to improve growth and development in preterm infants (Slusher 2003, Diehl-Jones 2004, Updegrove 2004, Maayan-Metzger 2012).

The LC has an obligation to share information with families about the prevention of disease in vulnerable babies. Such knowledge enables them to make informed decisions about how to advocate for their infants during hospitalization in the neonatal intensive care unit (NICU), or in emergency situations when clinical care may not be available.

Resources for Families of Multiples

Health care workers and mothers of multiples can find information, books, guidance about breast pumping, hand expression, and social support from organizations such as La Leche League International (LLLI), the Australian Breastfeeding Association (ABA), and Breastfeeding USA. (See the references for websites for these groups.) Community organizations such as Mothers of Multiples clubs and The Triplet Connection (which produces a newsletter) were founded to support the special needs of families with multiples. Many such organizations have local chapters in US cities. Internet searches can help parents locate additional resources in their communities.

The LC should review literature about breastfeeding multiples carefully before sharing it with parents. Inaccurate, unrealistic, or negative materials may undermine breastfeeding. Putting a mother in touch with a positive role model can be helpful. Some LCs maintain a phone or email list of willing former clients who are available to take phone calls from new mothers who have given birth to twins or higher order multiples. The LC may also be aware of other community resources that are available to help provide mothers of multiples with special types of assistance.

Simultaneous vs. Sequential Breastfeeding

Time management is important to the family adjusting to the birth of more than one baby. It makes sense to breastfeed twins simultaneously, although newborns often require more postural support than a new mother can manage with one hand. Small, immature, or weak infants require careful positioning at the breast in order to feed efficiently and to ensure adequate intake. Such increased positioning support may require both the mother's hands. In such cases, switching to sequential feeding (e.g., one baby at a time) may be an appropriate temporary strategy. Sequential feeding is often recommended if there is no helper available to assist the mother during latching.

The LC assesses, and, if necessary, assists the mother's positioning and latch technique. Special nursing pillows have been developed for simultaneous breastfeeding, but any firm pillow will work. A woman with multiples may find firm pillows helpful to assist with postural support for the babies. Babies require more physical support when young, but as they grow older they often become very creative in the feeding positions they devise.

The mother's family members require praise and encouragement for their contributions in caring for the new mother and her babies. The LC can provide valuable, specific information to these helpers; showing them how to assist with positioning, pillows, and equipment that make things easier for the mother and babies. The LC emphasizes the wisdom of resting and accepting help from the family, especially during the early postpartum weeks.

Breastfeeding Twins

Fig. 293 pictures *discordant twins*. The term refers to twins showing a marked disparity in size (greater than 10 percent difference in weight). Approximately 16 percent of twin gestations have discordance of at least 20 percent. The cause of the difference in weight is still unknown, but poor blood flow from the placenta may be implicated. Genetic or environmental factors may also be involved.

There have been published articles on the increased morbidity and mortality rates associated with discordant fetal growth, but there is scant information on how to manage these pregnancies optimally, and deliver them in a timely manner (Miller 2012).

LCs with clinical experience managing breastfeeding twins often observe that the larger twin is the stronger breastfeeder. There are some advantages to simultaneous

positioning in this situation, as the stronger of discordant twins may more effectively stimulate the milk release. However, the weaker, sleepier twin may require additional interventions (including supplementation with mother's own milk and more secure postural support than can be provided while simultaneously feeding).

Because of their small size and stamina issues, twins often require short, frequent feedings. Because of difficulties getting 2 babies well latched during the newborn phase, many mothers feed twins one baby at a time. The LC and pediatrician are well-advised to coordinate weekly weight checks to reassure families that twins are growing well. If parents are able to rent an electronic scale for home weighing, it can be a big time-saver when compared to the stress of taking twins to a clinic.

Once preterm twins reach 40 to 42 weeks or weigh approximately 7 lbs (3169 g), they typically become stronger feeders and need less help from their mother to achieve full feeds at the breast. At this point, or whenever they feel up to it, many mothers increase the frequency of simultaneous breastfeeding. Whenever mothers breastfed newborn twins simultaneously, they might be encouraged to switch each baby to the opposite breast midway through the feeding. This permits the larger, stronger twin to stimulate another let down. In some cases, it still may be necessary to pump after feeding to thoroughly drain the breasts and obtain hindmilk for supplementation.

Fig. 294 demonstrates the difficulty of positioning newborn, preterm twins for simultaneous breastfeeding. Neither twin pictured is latched well enough to feed effectively. The twin in the background appears to be falling asleep. The nose of the twin in the foreground is buried in the breast. A few seconds after this photo was taken, the twin with the blocked airway released the breast and began to cry. Repositioning (seen in **Fig. 295**) improved their milk intake. The LC used test weighing to verify the improvement.

In **Fig. 295**, the same mother is using a breastfeeding pillow to lift and support the babies so that her hands are free. However, pillows can often confuse positioning, especially in the newborn phase. Weaker or smaller babies may require far more active postural support to feed effectively without falling away from the breast. The LC may suggest that the mother rest her arms on the pillow for support, and use her hands and arms to support the babies. The mother may place her hands at the back of each baby's shoulders to stabilize their bodies and keep their chins pressed close to the breast. This position facilitates an open airway, and places the baby in an *en face* (face-to-face) gazing position with his mother.

Fig. 296 (courtesy of Els van der Wekken, RN, MS, IBCLC) shows a preterm Guinean twin feeding at the breast. The fraternal twins were born at 1600 g (3.5 lbs) and 1700 g (3.7 lbs) but their weight had fallen to 1000 (2.2 lbs) and 1100 g (2.4 lbs) by 1 week when the health worker came to their village and was invited to visit the twins (van der Wekken 2010). She observed the mother with the male twin in her arms trying to express milk into his mouth. The female twin was lying on the bed. Both babies were very cold, and the mother reported that neither baby could latch. Owing to unavailable prenatal care, the mother did not know their gestational age. The babies were placed briefly in the sun to warm them. Then, over the next few weeks, they were stabilized with intense kangaroo care and cup feeding of expressed milk.

At the time this photo was taken, after about a week of cup feeding, the baby boy pictured weighed 1250 g (2.7 lbs), and was able to latch and take 2 to 3 sucks. The mother was instructed to feed her twins every 2 hours and was given a small alarm clock to help her know when to hand express and cup feed. She was taught basic hygiene (hand washing and boiling of the cups). Both babies developed thrush and were treated with nystatin; their mother was treated with miconazole. The boy twin also required treatment for an eye infection. The twins were weighed weekly, and each gained only 50 g (1.75 oz) in the first 2 weeks. At the third weekly weight check, the twins finally began to exhibit more robust weight gains. By the fifth week, the boy twin pictured weighed 2000 g (4.4 lbs). With continued weekly supervision, the twins began to demonstrate improved breastfeeding behavior. Both twins weighed approximately 3000 g (6.6 lbs) at the third month check-up when they began their scheduled vaccinations.

Fig. 296 shows the twins' mother performing breast compression, which, according to the health worker, was a routine practice among the mothers she encountered in the villages that she served. It was her impression that the use of breast compression contributed to robust growth of healthy breastfed babies in Guinea. This observation is in line with published reports of higher fat content when breast compression is performed by mothers.

The 7 day-old twins (born near term) in **Figs. 297, 298, 299,** are being breastfed in various positions. The mother uses pillows under each elbow to support her arms (**Fig. 297**). The twin's legs come together in a "V" configuration, with support from the mother at their necks and hips to stabilize their bodies. It can be difficult to latch babies this way without help from a third person. Some mothers can accomplish simultaneous feeding by noticing which baby seems to need more assistance, and latching that baby first.

In **Fig. 299**, both of the twins are in a clutch or football hold. This mother's breasts are ideally shaped for breastfeeding twins because they are widely spaced. While widely spaced breasts can be a marker for PCOS, this mother has no history of that condition, and has ample milk to feed 2 babies. The wide span between her breasts and the angle of her nipple placement permits her to position the babies for simultaneous breastfeeding. Such a good "fit" between a mother and her twins is not always the case.

The 5 month-old twins in **Fig. 300** require far less physical support from their mother than they did as newborns. Here they are positioned on their knees, facing the breast. They use their hands to support the weight of the breast. Their mother leans slightly back, and stabilizes each baby with her arms. The twins have healing lesions on the backs of their heads. They are recovering from chicken pox.

In **Fig. 301**, 8 month-old twins are shown breastfeeding in a special sling. Older, stronger twins need little help from the mother in latching and staying on the breast, even if their mom is in motion.

Another view of the cradle-football combination hold is shown in **Fig. 302**. These 3 month-old twins have been exclusively breastfed and gaining well since birth. Their slender mother finds it challenging to obtain sufficient calories to maintain her own weight while breastfeeding.

The LC may discover that the mother of multiples needs dietary counseling. Caring for multiples is so time-consuming that meal preparation may be neglected. Breastfeeding mothers, especially mothers of multiples, may be protein deficient. This may manifest as an increased craving for sweets. Adding additional servings of protein to the daily diet provides a more stable source of energy, reducing the craving for sweets or carbohydrates. Strategies to help the mother obtain proper nutrition include:

- cooking and freezing meals during pregnancy
- organizing friends and family to bring meals during the first weeks postpartum
- using "rocking chair time" to mentally plan easy menus
- asking her partner to take over the responsibility of shopping and preparing meals
- having plenty of nutritious "finger foods" on hand such as fruit, carrots, yogurt, cheese, hard-boiled eggs, cold meats, etc.

Shopping lists may be drawn up with pre-planned menus in mind, and meals can be partially prepared during times when the infants are quiet or napping. The LC can remind mothers to keep a stash of non-perishable food in the house and in the car for nutritious snacking throughout the day.

Strategies to Increase Rest

The LC reminds the mother of multiples to take every opportunity to rest. Breastfeeding breaks can be relaxing for mother as well. A comfortable reclining chair, such as the one pictured in **Fig. 303**, became a useful tool for the mother of these 13 month-old twins. This mother put her feet up and relaxed at feeding times. Safe-sleep advocates warn new mothers not to fall asleep while breastfeeding newborn infants on couches or recliners owing to increased risk of suffocation on these surfaces.

Older Babies

The 13 month-old twins, pictured breastfeeding while standing up in **Fig. 304**, were just learning to walk. The typical bumps and bruises they sustained as toddlers created an ongoing need for reassurance from their mother. The easy and effective comfort provided from brief breastfeeding sessions helped this woman appreciate the advantages of *breast nurturing*.

Breastfeeding Triplets

Two 8 month-old triplets are pictured breastfeeding in **Fig. 305**. Higher order multiple births may or may not result in the need for supplementation. Some women who deliver triplets are able to exclusively, or near exclusively breastfeed. Baby A and Baby B are put to the breast. After they finish, Baby C breastfeeds from both breasts. At the next feed, the babies are rotated, so that Babies B and C each breastfeed from a full breast, and Baby A breastfeeds afterwards. An alternative plan for triplets involves breastfeeding 2 at each feeding, and offering the third baby (on a rotation basis) a bottle of banked human milk or formula.

Higher Order Multiples

The value of human milk for all infants is well established. Mothers of higher order multiples should be encouraged to pump their breasts and to provide as much milk as possible for their infants, who often will require treatment for prematurity related issues in special care nurseries. If the mother requires medical care and is unable to pump, donor human milk may be prescribed for temporary use until the mother recovers. When the infants are able to directly breastfeed, mothers should be encouraged to attempt whatever level of breastfeeding is achievable.

Tandem Breastfeeding

While most twins are identified during the pregnancy, sometimes their arrival is a surprise. The woman in **Fig. 306** did not know she was pregnant with twins. She is pictured breastfeeding her 2 year-old son, who breastfed mostly at nap time and bedtime. An older daughter, 4 years of age, still breastfed occasionally as well. The mother in this photograph continued to breastfeed her 2 older children for comfort as well as fully breastfeeding her twins.

In **Fig. 307**, a mother is pictured tandem breastfeeding a 4 year-old and a 16 month-old toddler.

In **Fig. 308**, a 4 year-old and a 19 month-old child are shown breastfeeding together. Some women choose tandem breastfeeding as a way to permit child-led weaning when births are closely spaced and to promote feelings of closeness (Hills-Bonczyk 1994). The experience can be enjoyable for the mother, who then benefits from the quiet moments that breastfeeding provides. She may also feel that tandem breastfeeding reduces sibling rivalry, providing the children moments of peaceful intimacy with each other. However, some mothers report that tandem breastfeeding contributes to emotional strain and a sense of feeling "touched out." Health workers or family members, sensing this, often pressure these mothers to wean. Such advice and weaning assistance may be appropriate; however, the mother may merely need more support and encouragement to continue breastfeeding.

The mother who is tandem breastfeeding generally has a robust milk supply, with ample milk for both children. The older child, responding to an increase in milk volume after the birth of the new baby, may temporarily increase breastfeeding, but typically returns to a pattern of less intense, less frequent breastfeeding over time. In some cases, however, it becomes important to ensure that the younger child gets sufficient nourishment for normal growth. Older children can obtain milk from the breast much faster than a newborn, and some mothers may need to ensure that the baby breastfeeds first.

BWC has seen 3 cases when infants have failed to thrive owing to older siblings, who, in feedings of surprisingly short duration, emptied the breast and jeopardized the newborn's milk intake. But if the mother has oversupply or a forceful milk ejection, the older child can drain off some of the milk pressure so that feeding is more comfortable for the infant. Mothers who are tandem breastfeeding soon work out the logistics of the activity (Flower 2003).

Fig. 309 shows a 2 year-old and her almost 5 year-old brother relaxing with their mother. Images such as this can be startling in a culture where breastfeeding the older child often becomes a closeted (hidden) activity. However, older breastfeeding children such as the 3 year-old child shown in **Fig. 310** are not uncommon, even in the US. Health care providers benefit from seeing visual images of what is a normal experience for many families (Dettwyler 1995, Sugarman 1995, AAP 1996, AAP 2012).

Legal Issues Related to Breastfeeding Past Infancy

Evidence associates the continuation of breastfeeding past the introduction of solids with reduced severity of infectious diseases and of food intolerances, and sensitization to gluten (AAP 2012), particularly in stressed environments (Prentice 1991). Many people in the US are unfamiliar with tandem and extended breastfeeding. Lactation consultants may receive requests for help from women accused of improper intimacy or sexual abuse of their children, solely because they are breastfeeding older children. The LC can provide written documentation from medical and anthropological sources and may provide expert testimony that toddler nursing and breastfeeding older children is normal behavior (Wilson-Clay 1990, Corbett 2001). The AAP policy statement on breastfeeding states that infants should be exclusively breastfed for 6 months "...followed by continued breastfeeding as complimentary foods are introduced, with continuation of breastfeeding for 1 year or longer as mutually desired by mother and infant" (AAP 2012).

Several books directed toward parents address breastfeeding past infancy: *How Weaning Happens* (Bengson 1999), *Mothering Your Nursing Toddler* (Bumgarner 2000), and *The Nursing Mother's Guide to Weaning* (Huggins 2007). *Breastfeeding: Biocultural Perspectives* (Stuart-Macadam, Dettwyler 1995) provides an anthropological view of weaning practices across mammalian species and human cultures.

American Academy of Pediatrics. Breastfeeding studies. *AAP News* 1996; 12(7):2.

American Academy of Pediatrics (AAP) Section on Breastfeeding. Breastfeeding and the use of human milk. *Pediatrics* 2012; 129(3): e827-e841.

Australian Breastfeeding Association: www.breastfeeding.asn.au

Becker GE, McCormick FM, Renfrew MJ. Methods of milk expression for lactating women. *Cochrane Database System Review* 2008; 8(4):CD006170.

Bengson D. *How Weaning Happens.* Schaumburg, IL: La Leche League International; 1999.

Berlin CM. "Exclusive" breastfeeding of quadruplets. *Breastfeeding Medicine* 2007; 2(2):125-126.

Breastfeeding USA. www.breastfeedingusa.org.

Bumgarner NJ. *Mothering Your Nursing Toddler.* Schaumburg, IL: La Leche League International, 2000.

Corbett S. The Breast Offense. *New York Times Magazine* May 6, 2001.

Damato EG, Dowling DA, Standing TS, et al. Explanation for cessation of breastfeeding in mothers of twins. *Journal of Human Lactation* 2005; 21(3):296-304.

Dettwyler K. A Time to Wean: The hominid blueprint for the natural age of weaning in modern human populations, in P Stuart-Macadam, K Dettwyler (ed). *Breastfeeding: Biocultural Perspectives.* New York: De Gruyter, 1995; pp. 65-66.

de Zegher F, Sebastiani G, Diaz M, et al. Breastfeeding vs formula feeding for infants born small for gestational age: divergent effects on fat mass and on circulating IGF-I and high-molecular-weight adiponectin in late infancy. *Journal of Clinical Endocrinology and Metabolism* 2013; 98(3):1242-1247.

Diehl-Jones W, Askin D. Nutritional modulation of neonatal outcomes. *AACN Clinical Issues* 2004; 15(1):83-96.

Dvorak B, Fituch C, Williams C, et al. Increased epidermal growth factor levels in human milk of mothers with extremely premature infants. *Pediatric Research* 2003; 54(1):15-19.

Feldman R, Eidelman A. Does a triplet birth pose a special risk for infant development? Assessing cognitive development in relation to intrauterine growth and mother-infant interaction across the first two years. *Pediatrics* 2005; 115(2):443-452.

Flidel-Rimon O, Shinwell ES. Breastfeeding twins and high multiples. *Archives of Diseases in Childhood Fetal and Neonatal Education* 2006; 91(5):F377-380.

Flower H. *Adventures in Tandem Nursing: Breastfeeding During Pregnancy and Beyond.* Shcumburg, IL: La Leche League International; 2003.

Geddes D. Gross anatomy of the lactating breast, in *Hale and Hartmann's Textbook of Human Lactation,* Amarillo, TX: Hale Publishing, 2007; p. 23.

Geraghty SR, Pinney SM, Sethuraman G, et al. Breast milk feeding rates of mothers of multiples compared to mothers of singletons. *Ambulatory Pediatrics* 2004; 4(3):226-231.

Gromada K. ILCA's Inside Track: Twins. *Journal of Human Lactation* 2010; 26(3):31-32.

Human Milk Banking Association of North America (HMBANA). www. hmbana.org. Accessed March 2013.

Hills-Bonczyk S, Tromiczsak K, Avery M, et al. Women's experiences with breastfeeding longer than 12 months. *Birth* 1994; 21(4):206-212.

Huggins K, Ziedrich L. *The Nursing Mother's Guide to Weaning.* Boston, MA: Harvard Common Press, 2007.

Kelley L. Increasing the consumption of breast milk in low-birth-weight infants: can it have an impact on necrotizing enterocolitis? *Advanced Neonatal Care* 2012; 12(5):267-272.

La Leche League International: www.lalecheleague.org

Lee HC, Kurtin PS, Wight NE, et al. A quality improvement project to increase breast milk use in very low birth weight infants. *Pediatrics* 2012; 130(6):e1679-1687.

Lucas A, Cole T. Breast milk and neonatal necrotizing enterocolitis. *Lancet* 1990; 336(8730):1519-1523.

Luig M, Lui K; NSW & ACT NICUS Group. Epidemiology of necrotizing enterocolitis - Part I: changing regional trends in extremely preterm infants over 14 years. *Journal of Paediatric Child Health* 2005; 41(4):169-173.

Martin JA, Hamilton BE, Ventura SJ, et al. Births: final data for 2010. *National Vital Statistics Report* 2012; 61(1):1-14. www.cdc.gov/nchs/. Search words: "birth data" Accessed March 2013.

Maayan-Metzger A, Avivi S, Schushan-Eisen I, et al. Human milk versus formula among preterm infants: short-term outcomes. *American Journal of Perinatology* 2012; 29(2):121-126.

McGuire W, Anthony M. Donor human milk versus formula for preventing necrotizing enterocolitis in preterm infants: systematic review. *Archives of Disease in Childhood Fetal Neonatal Education* 2003; 88(1):F11-F14.

McKenzie PJ. The seeking of baby-feeding information by Canadian women pregnant with twins. *Midwifery* 2006; 22(3):218-227.

Miller J, Chauhan SP, Abuhamad AZ. Discordant twins: diagnosis, evaluation and management. *American Journal of Obstetrics and Gynecology* 2012; 206(1):10-20.

Morley R, Fewtrell M, Abbott R, et al. Neurodevelopment in children born small for gestational age: a randomized trial of nutrient-enriched versus standard formula and comparison with a reference breastfed group. *Pediatrics* 2004; 113(3):515-521.

Morton J, Hall J, Wong RJ, et al. Combining hand techniques with electric pumping increases milk production in mothers of preterm infants. *Journal of Perinatology* 2009; 29(11):757-764.

Morton J, Wong RJ, Hall J, et al. Combining hand techniques with electric pumping increases the caloric content of milk in mothers of preterm infants. *Journal of Perinatology* 2012; 32(10):791-796.

Parker LA, Sullivan S, Krueger C, et al. Effect of early breast milk expression on milk volume and timing of lactogenesis stage II among mothers of very low birth weight infants: a pilot study. *Journal of Perinatology* 2012; 32(2): 205-209.

Prentice A. Breastfeeding and the older infant. *Acta Paediatrica Scandia/ Supplement* 1991; 374:78-88.

Slusher T, Hampton R, Bode-Thomas F, et al. Promoting the exclusive feeding of own mother's milk through the use of hindmilk and increased maternal milk volume for hospitalized, low birth weight infants (<1800 grams) in Nigeria: a feasibility study. *Journal of Human Lactation* 2003; 19(2):191-198.

Steinman G. Why the twinning rate is higher in Africa than elsewhere: an analysis of selected factors. *Journal of Reproductive Medicine* 2009; 54(10):609-613.

Sugarman M, Kendall-Tackett K. Weaning ages in a sample of American woman who practice extended breastfeeding. *Clinical Pediatrics* 1995; 34(12):642-647.

The Triplet Connection, www.tripletconnection.org. Accessed March 2013.

Updegrove K. Necrotizing enterocolitis: the evidence for the use of human milk in prevention and treatment. *Journal of Human Lactation* 2004; 20(3):335-339.

van der Wekken E. Personal communication 2010.

Walker M, Murphy K, Pan S, et al. Adverse maternal outcomes in multi-fetal pregnancies. *BJOG: An International Journal of Obstetrics & Gynaecology* 2004; 111(11):1294.

Wilson-Clay B. Extended breastfeeding as a legal issue: an annotated bibliography. *Journal of Human Lactation* 1990; 6(2):68-71.

Yokoyama Y, Ooki S. Breast-feeding and bottle-feeding of twins, triplets and higher order multiple births. *Nippon Koshu Eisei Azsshi* 2004; 51(11):969-974.

Alternative Feeding Methods

Breastfeeding is the biologically normal way to feed human infants. However, some babies are unable to breastfeed immediately, or their mothers need assistance improving their milk supply. During such situations, there are 3 basic rules: Feed the baby, Protect the milk supply, and Preserve breast focus. These interventions are often described as "triple feeding."

The baby must be fed so that growth and energy are protected. Breastfeeding cannot improve if the infant is hungry or weak. Many infants who initially appear to have sucking problems suck normally once they recover lost weight. Ideally, the baby receives the mother's own hand expressed or pumped milk whenever breastfeeding is interupted, but sometimes donor milk or formula may be required.

Utilizing evidence-based best practices, most healthy mothers can bring in a robust milk supply using a combination of hand expression and pumping. When possible, skin-to-skin contact with the baby maintains the baby's orientation to the breasts and provides opportunities for practice feedings.

Triple feeding is time-intensive and tiring for everyone. Written instructions and frequent follow-up during the intervention period are important for ensuring a good outcome. The extra effort is temporary in most cases, permitting eventual normal breastfeeding.

This chapter briefly reviews best practices for milk expression, types of electric breast pumps, and describes some of the alternate feeding methods that are available to deliver supplemental calories to infants. There is an absence of clear evidence demonstrating the superiority of one feeding method over another; however, some methods can be practiced at or near the breast, supporting the goal of protection of breast focus.

All alternative feeding methods appear to have differences that have not been fully evaluated, and there are risks and benefits of each method. Therefore, careful individual assessment and some degree of experimentation help determine the most suitable method for a specific baby. The primary consideration in selecting pumps and alternative feeding methods is to ensure the safety, efficiency, and effectiveness of the intervention. The feeding experience must be easily tolerated by the baby, and the logistics of "triple feeding" must be possible for the mother to accomplish. "The goal of any alternative feeding method is for restoration of full, direct breastfeeding whenever possible" (Wight 2001).

Legal and Ethical Concerns

It is important that practitioners understand the legal and ethical issues that arise whenever equipment is involved in a feeding care plan. Ethical principles require that equipment is selected because it serves a therapeutic purpose, is safe, and that profit motive is not placed before patient welfare. Legal principles (generally grouped under commercial code statutes) govern product liability. Consumers have the right to be informed about potentially negative outcomes of any intervention. Signed consent forms, careful case documentation, and malpractice insurance are all vital aspects of an IBCLC's practice (Hall 2002, Bornmann 2013, Brooks 2013).

The LC makes recommendations about pumping and feeding equipment that are based on available research, while being aware that research in this area is constantly evolving. The IBCLC should avoid making unsupported claims that various methods of alternative feeding are "most like breastfeeding."

Because of the specific and limited nature of product liability protection, manufacturers stipulate that they are not liable for any harm to the consumer if their product is used in a way other than what is described in the labeling and packaging instructions. This issue is relevant in various aspects of LC practice. For example, many LCs receive inquiries from women asking whether it is safe to borrow a used electric breast pump from a friend. If the pump was sold as a "single-user item," the LC potentially assumes legal risk in encouraging use of the equipment in a way that was not intended or warranted by the manufacturer.

Electric Breast Pumps

In the United States, the US Food and Drug Administration (FDA) oversees the safety and effectiveness of medical devices, including breast pumps. The FDA (2013) warns consumers to distinguish between multiple and single-user breast pumps and to avoid second-hand or used single-user pumps. Multiple-user pumps are typically rented rather than purchased. They are designed in various ways to prevent aspirated milk from coming in contact with the pump motor or other internal parts that cannot be cleaned and which are often hidden from view.

Detachable kits are sold with multiple-user pumps. The kit contains tubing, pump flanges, valves, and bottles. All of these parts can be sterilized, although tubing does not need to be washed unless it gets wet inside. Soap and water washing of external pump parts is generally adequate for healthy, term infants. Sterilization of pump parts is often required for medically fragile, hospitalized infants (D'Amico 2003). In the NICU, cleaned pump parts should be air dried on a clean towel, covered with a clean towel, and kept dry until the next use (Chiu 2012). (**Fig. 311.**) Dry pump parts can be stored in a large, clean plastic bag.

Dangerous organisms can grow on the outside of multiple-user hospital pumps. Hospitals should routinely disinfect the outside of breast pumps. There are case reports of both mold and pathogens such as *Serratia marcescens* growing inside of pump tubing (Faro 2011). (*Serratia marcescens* has a distinctive coloration; it turns contaminated surfaces and pumped milk bright pink.) Mothers should be instructed to replace moldy or discolored tubing.

Purchasable, single-user electric pumps have internal parts, including motors, that are difficult or impossible to sterilize. These pumps may become internally contaminated with aspirated milk particles and moisture, creating an environment in which pathogens can thrive (Blenkharn 1989). Without disassembling the pump, it is impossible to see that internal contamination has occurred. **Fig. 312** shows a single-user electric breast pump with black mold growing on a soft plastic diaphragm that is normally covered by a hard plastic plate containing an on/off switch and the pressure setting dials (Photo courtesy of Debi Wells, IBCLC).

Mothers should be instructed to follow the manufacturer's instructions on cleaning pumps and parts, and be informed about the potential risks of sharing non-sterilizable devices meant for single-use. They can be directed to the FDA website, where the search words: *single-user breast pump* provide more information.

Research indicates that mothers should select the highest *comfortable* pump pressure settings to enhance the milk flow rate and milk yield (Kent 2008). Because cold stress causes constriction of milk ducts within the nipple and inhibits milk ejection, using a warmed breast shield (pump flange) improves maternal comfort during pumping and appears to improve the efficiency of milk removal (Kent 2011).

Hospital-based LCs must be aware that long delays in initiating *effective* breast stimulation and milk expression put the mother at risk for low milk production. Parker (2012) conducted a randomized pilot study to establish the feasibility and effects of beginning milk expression within 1 hour of birth (compared to 1-6 hours of birth) in a population of women who had given birth to very low birth weight (VLBW) infants. The women in the early expression group produced significantly more milk and experienced earlier lactogenesis II. While it may be impossible for some mothers to begin pumping and hand expressing immediately following a traumatic delivery, the normal aftermath of birth includes immediate breast stimulation by the infant. These findings speak to the wisdom of imitating the biological norm as much as possible. The best available breast pump should be employed, utilizing technology designed to maximize milk production (Ramsay 2006, Slusher 2007)

Criteria for Selecting an Alternate Method of Infant Feeding

- It does not harm the infant.
- It is a good match for the infant's size, stamina, physical condition, and level of maturity.
- It is easy for the parents to manage.
- It involves equipment that the parents can obtain, afford, and clean.
- It is a suitable intervention for the length of time needed to remediate the feeding problem. Long-term interventions are the most stressful to maintain.
- It may help the baby learn to breastfeed.

Early Supplementation with Spoon Feeding

Sometimes a newborn needs only a brief period of supplementation, or a "jump start" of caloric energy, to rouse them sufficiently to latch to the breast. Using a spoon to feed hand-expressed or pumped colostrum is an excellent way to provide immediate calories to a non-breastfeeding newborn or to wake up a sleepy infant (Hoover 1998). The LC should instruct all mothers in the technique of hand expression (**Fig. 313**), which is cost free and ideal for obtaining a few swallows of milk for this kind of supplementation. Small bottles, called colostrum catchers, can be provided when available. (Pumping colostrum into a full-size bottle may give the mother the impression she is not making enough milk.)

About half a milliliter (ml) at a time seems to be a comfortable volume for a newborn to swallow (Lawrence 2011). Because a spoon holds only a small amount of fluid, parents may worry less about causing the baby to choke. In **Fig. 314** a baby is shown receiving approximately half a ml of expressed milk from a spoon.

Fig. 315 shows a sleepy, jaundiced 10 day-old infant who is not latching and still losing weight. The LC is demonstrating how to feed expressed milk with a spoon. In **Fig. 316** the same baby already appears more alert after only a few swallows. Note the baby's engaged affect. Once aroused, she was able to latch to the breast and her breastfeeding behavior improved.

Cup Feeding

Infant cup feeding implements have been used throughout the ages to supplement non-breastfeeding infants. Owing to cost issues and the increased risk of infant infection in settings where bottles and teats cannot be easily cleaned, there has been a resurgence of interest in cup feeding in the modern era (Fredeen 1948, Davis 1948). The current interest in cup feeding is also influenced by concerns about what is commonly called "nipple confusion" and a philosophical reluctance to expose infants to artificial teats.

A review of the literature on cup feeding identifies studies that suggest that cup fed infants are at lower risk for oxygen desaturation than are bottle-fed infants (Dowling 2002). Other studies (Freer 1999) describe physiological instability and oxygen desaturation of preterm infants during cup feeding. Dowling suggests that the better oxygenation noted in some of the cup feeding studies may be secondary to smaller intake volumes during cup feedings. While safer from the standpoint of oxygen desaturation, small intake volumes increase the risk of poor growth in cup fed populations.

Rocha (2002) observed similar weight gain in infants supplemented by cup or by bottle (Rocha 2002). However, Dowling (2002) reported that up to 48 percent of milk that was cup fed to one group of preterm infants was lost to spillage. This was not always apparent to their feeders, and was revealed only when careful test weights were performed on the infants and their bibs. Dowling recommends careful monitoring of intake and spillage in cup fed populations, especially preterm infants.

Some LCs have theorized that cup feeding leads to the acquisition of skills that facilitate breastfeeding. This idea is not supported by present available evidence. Dowling (2002) observed that cup feeding is a "closed mouth" activity and questioned whether lapping and sipping mimic or facilitate the development of oral behaviors required for breastfeeding. The activity of sucking, itself, provides state stabilizing benefits in addition to being the normal feeding method of infants. Therefore, depriving infants of the opportunity to suck during feeding may have negative consequences, including the development of oral aversions.

A Cochrane Review (Flint 2007) examined 4 randomized or quasi-randomized trials to determine the effects of cup feeding versus other forms of supplementation for newborns unable to breastfeed. Cup feeding conferred no significant benefit in maintaining breastfeeding and had the unintended consequence of significantly extending the length of infants' hospital stay. Cup fed infants remained hospitalized a mean of 10.1 additional days.

Another Cochrane Review (Collins 2008) described 4 trials that used a cup feeding strategy and 1 that used a tube feeding protocol to supplement non-breastfeeding preterm infants. There was a high degree of noncompliance in the largest cup feeding study. The reviewers perceived this as an indication of dissatisfaction with the method of cup feeding by both staff and parents. The reviewers concluded that cup feeding conferred no breastfeeding benefit and delayed hospital discharge.

The Cochrane Review findings do not mean that infants cannot be or never should be cup fed. Cups provide a hygiene benefit whenever a family's ability to procure and clean bottles is compromised. (See the case study of preterm African twins in Ch. 13.) Short-term cup feeding may also be useful in situations when only a few supplemental feeds will be required. Reducing the focus on bottles in such situations may provide a psychological benefit for the mother and help keep the focus on transitioning quickly to breastfeeding.

There is agreement in the cup feeding literature that technique is important (Howard 1999, Marinelli 2001). Thorley (1997) and Malhotra (1999) warn against "force feeding," citing concerns about the risk of aspiration.

During cup feeding, the infant's head and body should be stabilized as in **Fig. 317**. Lang (1994) suggests placing the rim of the cup level with the infant's lips and allowing the infant to sip or lap the milk rather than pouring milk into the mouth. Dowling (2002) cautions the feeder to observe the infant's respiration, allowing the baby to control the intake, pausing when necessary to allow the infant to reorganize respiration. Pacing the speed of the delivery of the fluid in this manner reduces the aspiration risk to the infant.

Cup feeding can be a difficult skill to learn from a text book. Some LCs practice the technique by taking turns cup feeding each other. Parents who want to cup feed should be observed while feeding the infant to make sure they are doing it safely. Return demonstration of the skill helps increase parental confidence.

Certain protective reflexes (for example, the cough) may be immature in some infants, placing them at heightened risk for silent aspiration (Wolf 1992). It is important to observe an infant's behavioral cues during feeding and to identify infant stress cues. Assessment of infant affect while feeding provides clues about whether the feeding method is well-tolerated. The term infant shown in **Fig. 317** manifests stable state behavior while cup feeding. Note the open eyes, calm facial expression, and absence of stress cues.

The infant in **Fig. 318** is being fed with a *paladai*, which is used on the Indian subcontinent to hold oil in religious ceremonies. The baby in **Fig. 318** drank 1 ounce (28 g) of expressed milk, but did not open his eyes or engage socially during the feeding. Malhotra (1999) documents less spillage with the paladai than with a cup, probably because the spout allows for greater directional control of the fluid. However, Malhotra also observed a tendency to pour milk from the paladai into the mouth of the baby, which increases the risk of aspiration. The infant pictured in **Fig. 318** may have become exhausted from the effort of swallowing rapidly. Note the infant's pursed lips which appear to block the insertion of the implement.

Finger Feeding

Finger feeding is another method of supplementation for the non-breastfeeding baby; however, there is no evidence to support claims that finger feeding is "more like breastfeeding." The belief that finger feeding facilitates breastfeeding has not been systematically evaluated. No research exists to guide practice with regard to finger feeding. However, some LCs report that finger feeding provides them with valuable information about how the baby is moving the tongue, thus facilitating a more sensitive assessment of nutritive sucking.

Because the adult finger is narrow, it is more similar to the diameter of a narrow base bottle teat than it is to the rounded contour of the human breast. Even more rigid than a bottle teat, the finger is inserted into (rather than shaped and drawn into) the mouth of the baby. Thus, finger feeding differs markedly from breastfeeding.

Technique is important during finger feeding. The feeder's hands should be clean and the nails clipped. Health care providers should be gloved or wear finger cots. Gentle massage around the lips may encourage the baby to open and willingly draw in the finger. The finger is inserted pad side up. Avoid inserting the finger too deeply into the baby's mouth. Inserting the finger beyond the hard/soft palate junction (past the mid-point of the tongue) will trigger a gag reflex; a noxious stimulus. Repeated triggering of noxious stimuli may create feeding aversion.

The feeder uses sensitivity and respect when inserting the finger into the mouth of the baby. If an infant has weak lip tone and cannot seal the lips around a wide base (such as a breast or a wide base bottle teat) the narrowness of the finger may make it easier for the baby to form a seal. Brief, light pressure on the tongue may help the infant form a central groove (Wolf 1992). Gentle stroking of the palate with the pad of the finger may stimulate the infant to keep sucking.

Finger feeding makes it possible to deliver larger volumes of fluid to the baby compared with spoon feeding. However, especially if done with a syringe, it can still be a slow method of feeding and may result in some infants (or parents) tiring before full feedings are achieved.

No safety data have been reported on the practice of finger feeding. While finger feeding is widely performed by LCs and frequently described in breastfeeding texts, only one research study on finger feeding has been published. Oddy (2003) examined breastfeeding rates in an Australian hospital before and after implementation of the Baby Friendly Hospital Initiative (BFHI). The study reports improved breastfeeding rates at discharge when staff discontinued use of artificial teats and began supplementing babies by finger feeding. However, the implementation of other aspects of BFHI rather than the specific intervention of finger feeding may explain the improved breastfeeding rates. Oddy did not investigate the respiratory stability of the infants during finger feeding or comment on safety issues.

Whether a curved-tip syringe or a feeding tube is inserted with the finger, feeders must be careful to avoid squirting liquids down the infant's throat. Anecdotal reports describe the practice in some hospitals of inserting a syringe filled with milk directly into the mouth of the infant without the finger. There is no advantage to inserting a narrow pointed device such as a syringe into the mouth of an infant. The resulting pursed mouth configuration does not facilitate breastfeeding, and there is increased risk of aspiration when milk is squirted directly into the mouth in this manner.

Fig. 319 shows the Monoject 412™ curved-tip syringe resting along the side of the mother's finger at the corner of the baby's mouth. Prior to inserting her finger, the mother gently stimulates the baby's lips. Finger feeding may provide the sensation of skin rather than plastic inside the baby's mouth, one possible additional advantage of the method. As the baby draws in the finger and begins sucking, the mother inserts the curved tip of the syringe, stabilizing it against her finger. The mother may allow the baby to suck for a few seconds before delivering the first bolus of milk. Briefly delaying the milk flow mimics the experience of sucking on the breast prior to milk ejection. Thus finger feeding becomes a behavior modification technique that may help the baby remain more patient waiting for the milk to let down while breastfeeding.

The mother in **Fig. 319** delivers a small bolus of about 1/2 ml of milk in response to the baby's sucking. (Half a ml is about half the width of the syringe's black gasket.) By pacing the delivery of milk in response to the baby's sucking, the mother rewards the baby for sucking effort. The LC helps teach parents to carefully observe their baby's ability to coordinate sucking, swallowing, and breathing. Notice how this mother has positioned the baby against her breast, skin-to-skin, as part of her effort to protect breast focus.

In **Fig. 320** a feeding tube has been inserted along the side of the feeder's thumb. If the aim of any alternative feeding method is to promote transition to the breast, the LC has to consider that finger feeding generally accustoms the baby to holding the mouth in a rather narrow position compared to the wide open jaw and flanged lip positions used when breastfeeding. The wider diameter of the thumb may be useful to accustom the baby to a wider mouth position. Notice, however, that this baby has a poor seal, as revealed by the milk leaking around the baby's lips. The baby also looks worried. Perhaps the narrower base provided by a finger would be a better option for this baby until lip tone improves.

Fig. 321 demonstrates a mother using a #5 French feeding tube attached to a Monoject 412™ curved-tip syringe. A Band-Aid™ has been taped to the mother's finger to help hold the tubing in place. When the baby naturally pauses, the mother stops the flow of milk. Once the baby begins sucking again, the mother delivers more milk. Swallowing too quickly may overwhelm some infants, causing vomiting. Parents should be encouraged to mimic the average feeding times of the breastfeeding infant, which range from 10 to 25 minutes (L'Esperance 1985).

Fig. 322 demonstrates an LC wearing a non-latex glove providing emergency supplementation to an infant. Gloves are not necessary when handling human milk, nor are they necessary for parents who are finger feeding. Gloves are required when the LC places a finger into the baby's mouth. Fungi and bacteria under the fingernails have been implicated in nosocomial infections (infections acquired in health care settings) (Parry 2001). The LC has an ethical obligation to protect the infant from exposure to pathogens that are not part of the baby's normal environment.

The preterm infant in **Fig. 322** was born at 36 gestational weeks, and presented at the lactation clinic with poor skin tone and turgor. The infant weighed 5 lbs 2 oz (2320 g) at birth. She was discharged from the hospital within 36 hours, before breastfeeding was established. On Day 6 postpartum, her mother became concerned that the baby was not stooling and brought her to the lactation clinic. The baby's weight on the LC's electonic scale was 4 lb 8 oz (2037 g). The baby had lost slightly more than 8 percent of her birth weight, appeared lethargic, and was showing signs of dehydration.

The LC contacted the pediatrician by phone. He directed her to provide immediate nutrition. The LC attempted to obtain expressed milk to feed the baby. Because the baby was sleepy and feeding poorly, the mother's breasts were understimulated and lactogenesis II had not yet occurred. Hand expression and breast pumping yielded only drops of milk. With the mother's permission and the doctor's approval, the baby was finger fed formula. The mother made arrangements to take the baby to the pediatrician for evaluation the same day.

Feeding Tube Devices

Feeding tube devices theoretically allow infants to be supplemented at the breast with pumped milk or formula. These devices were developed to permit adoptive mothers to feed at the breast, to facilitate relactation, and to induce lactation (Gribble 2004). They work well if the infant is strong enough to latch onto the breast, delivering a steady flow of milk to the infant who is capable of sucking normally. The skin-to-skin contact provided facilitates bonding and protects breast focus.

Another benefit of a feeding tube device is to deliver the scent and taste of human milk to preterm babies as an impetus to suck. Raimbault (2007) reported that exposure to mother's milk prior to early breastfeeding trials had a positive effect on sucking behavior and milk ingestion of preterm infants. It also resulted in shortened hospital stays.

Feeding tubes are less effective in stimulating the milk supply when the infant is too weak to suck normally in the first place. Many weak infants learn to suck the tube as if it were a straw and never actively latch onto the breast. The mother believes she is providing adequate breast stimulation and that this manner of sucking will calibrate a full milk supply. This is seldom the case. Many mothers lose their milk supplies owing to over reliance on these devices. When the weak, ill, or preterm infant feeds at breast with a feeding tube, the mother should be instructed to augment breast stimulation with a combination of hand expression and breast pumping, according to published best practices.

Weak infants may find feeding with a tube exhausting, and may fail to obtain adequate calories, thus prolonging their problems. In this situation, it is more beneficial to recommend pumping to protect the milk supply and to find another, more efficient, way to deliver calories to the baby. The use of a feeding tube device should be reconsidered if the infant takes an unacceptably long time (>30 minutes) to complete a feed, falls asleep while feeding, or fails to gain weight adequately while using the device. Tube feeding may be resumed when the infant stabilizes, and the focus shifts to transitioning the baby to fully breastfeeding.

Certain tricks can be used to manipulate feeding tube devices. The bottle can be elevated to create a greater gravity drop in order to increase the milk flow rate. Some mothers squeeze the feeding tube container to augment the milk flow rate. However, it is important to determine if a faster flow rate is well tolerated by the infant, especially if the infant has respiratory problems. There must be a sensitive balance between the feeder's need to complete feeds in a reasonable amount of time and the infant's experience.

Fig. 323 demonstrates a Monoject 412™ curved-tip syringe being used to supplement the baby at the breast in a way that mimics a feeding tube. This method may be appropriate for short-term use, and often assists in helping infants transfer to the breast after bottle, finger, or cup feeding. The mother latches the baby onto the breast and then stabilizes the curved tip of the periodontal syringe against her breast. She inserts the tip into the corner of the baby's mouth, and drips milk to entice the baby to suck.

An argument against feeding tubes in many environments is cost. **Fig. 324** shows a #5 French feeding tube inserted in a bottle of infant formula to create a homemade feeding supplementer that is taped to the mother's finger. Finger feeding in this manner requires the baby to actively suck the fluid rather than merely swallowing in response to the mother bolusing the milk. This activity may help strengthen the infant's suck. Once the infant becomes accustomed to the sensation of the feeding tube attached to the finger, it may be easier to transition the baby to a feeding tube worn at the breast.

Two commercially available feeding supplementers are the Medela™ Supplemental Nursing System (SNS)™ and the Lact-Aid™. Supplementers may be reimbursable under some US insurance plans because they are classified as medical equipment. Mothers report a range of opinions when discussing their experiences using feeding tube devices (Borucki 2005). However, the consensus among the women interviewed was that mothers seek alternatives when their infants are unable to breastfeed. The feeding tube device provides another choice.

Fig. 325 shows a woman breastfeeding her healthy, term, adopted baby with an SNS™ taped to her breast. The woman had lactated 15 years prior, and was inducing lactation for the new baby. Her baby easily adapted to the feeding tube device. At the peak of production the woman made approximately 6-10 ounces (170-283 ml) of milk daily. She and her son enjoyed the bonding benefits of breastfeeding. She continued to supplement him at the breast with only occasional bottles until he was 2 months old. She then returned to full time employment and discontinued using the feeding tube. She offered her breasts for comfort and supplemented with a bottle.

In **Fig. 326**, the LC has suggested using 2 tubes of an SNS™ at the same breast. Opening up both tubes simultaneously increases the milk flow rate and may assist the infant who has difficulty creating sufficient suction to obtain milk (idea attributed to Kittie Frantz). The infant in the photo was the third child born to her mother, and was 37 weeks gestational age at birth. The baby weighed 5 lb 10 oz (2551 g) at birth, and weighed only 5 lb 4 oz (2381 g) at 5 weeks. The LC observed a weak suck. The baby was unable to maintain continuous sucking bursts, took a long time to drain the SNS, and frequently lost suction. Using double tubes reduced the work of feeding and helped the baby complete feedings in a shorter period of time. Improved weight gain and increased energy strengthened the infant's feeding ability. However, in such situations, it should not be assumed that the breast is receiving sufficient stimulation to maintain full milk production. Pumping and hand expression will be necessary to protect the milk supply.

The infant pictured in **Fig. 327** is breastfeeding with a Lact-Aid™. Because this device features a soft plastic bag rather than a firm feeding bottle, some mothers feel that it is less obtrusive when worn under clothing and prefer it for discreet breastfeeding in public situations. The bag does not have to be worn around the neck and can be comfortably tucked between the mother and the baby. The feeding tube comes out of the top of the Lact-Aid™, requiring that the baby suck milk against the pull of gravity. This may assist in strengthening the suck more than the SNS™, which positions the tube at the bottom of the bottle, providing a gravity drop to augment milk flow. Some mothers may use both devices, or may progress from the SNS™ to the Lactaid™, depending upon the therapeutic plan.

In **Figs. 325-327**, all of the feeding tubes are shown positioned in the traditional manner. That is, the tubing is inserted under the upper lip and enters the baby's mouth centered along the palate. For some babies, particularly those with sensory defensiveness, the feel of the tube against the palate is a distraction. In **Fig. 328** the feeding tube is taped in a reverse position. That is, the tube will enter the mouth across the *lower* lip. **Fig. 329** shows a baby breastfeeding from a homemade feeding tube device with the tube positioned in contact with the tongue rather than the palate (idea credited to Peter Hartmann's team, Perth, Australia).

Nasogastric Tube Feeding

Research has demonstrated that breastfeeding is easier than bottle-feeding for preterm babies and that preterm babies can breastfeed before they can bottle-feed (Meier 1987, Meier 1988, Chen 2000). However, owing to the effect of maturation upon sucking, exclusive breastfeeding may not provide enough calories, and the baby may still need supplementation. Supplementation via nasogastric (NG) tube may be appropriate until the infant's sucking pattern matures.

Studies examining the use of NG feeding of preterm babies reveal that this type of feeding is an appropriate substitute for bottles when the mother is not present to breastfeed. NG tube supplemented infants also were more likely to be breastfeeding at 3 months and at 6 months vs bottle-fed babies (Stein 1990, Kliethermes 1999).

Some infants are unable to feed orally for extended periods of time Sucking in the absence of oral feeding stabilizes the rate of breathing and increases oxygenation (Dowling 2002). Therefore, pacifiers are often provided to infants during NG or gastric tube feeding. Preterm infants who sucked on pacifiers during NG feeds discontinued NG feeds earlier, had better weight gain, and were discharged from the hospital earlier (Measel 1979, Pinelli 2005).

Many breastfeeding advocates have negative views of pacifiers. However, the "highest level of evidence does not support an adverse effect of pacifier use on breastfeeding duration or exclusivity" (O'Connor 2009). Associations between shortened duration of breastfeedng reported in some observational studies probably reflect numerous complex issues related to breastfeeding difficulties, or intention to wean.

A randomized prospective study compared 4 feeding methods used to supplement 132 preterm infants ranging from 26 to 36 weeks of gestation at birth (Garpiel 2012). Preterm infants in this study fed with a NG tube and pacifier had significantly better breastfeeding ability at discharge than did infants fed with a cup, a bottle with a preterm nipple, or a Haberman infant feeder (Medela). Any cessation of breathing is referred to as *apnea*. Oxygen desaturation and *bradycardia* (slowing of the heart rate)

may result from apnea. The infants fed with nasogastric tube with pacifier had fewer episodes of apnea, bradycardia and oxygen desaturation than did the bottle feeding infants (Kelly 2006). More skin-to-skin episodes and more breastfeeding episodes also predicted better breastfeeding outcomes at discharge.

Sometimes an infant is so premature, ill, or weak, that oral feedings are impossible. **Fig. 330** shows a 3 month-old baby who is recovering from infant botulism. A symptom of infant botulism is sudden onset of sucking dysfunction and lack of stooling. The baby is recovering from the illness and is being fed by a nasogastric tube.

Infants who have had lengthy periods of NG or oral gastric tube feeding may have erosions of the tissue surrounding the tube. Adults who experience these procedures often complain of sore throats and irritated nasal passages, and infants may be equally uncomfortable following gavage feeding. They may develop anxiety owing to this pain. Sometimes this contributes to sensory defensiveness and aversive behavior surrounding feeding when the child begins oral feeds (Palmer 1998).

Bottle Feeding

Supplementation of breastfeeding infants with infant formula without a medical reason significantly reduced the duration of breastfeeding in both multiparas and primiparas in a Swedish study (Ekstrom 2003). Tender (2009) surveyed 150 low-income US breastfeeding mothers, and found no clear medical need for supplementation in 87 percent of the infants receiving bottles of infant formula in the hospital.

The Ten Steps of the Baby-Friendly Hospital Initiative wisely suggest giving newborns time to learn to breastfeed without interference or unnecessary interventions, especially bottle feeding (UNICEF 1991). However, research has yet to definitively describe best practices for supplementation (Cloherty 2005). In the event that an infant requires medically neccessary supplementation, Wight (2001) points out: "The main advantage of supplementing without a bottle is the nonverbal message to parents that the alternative method is temporary."

Ekstrom (2003) observed that if parents were aware that supplementation was medically necessary, it did not undermine confidence in breastfeeding. For infants who are unable to breastfeed and will require long-term supplementation, a method of feeding must be selected that is manageable for both the infant and the parents. It is unclear in such instances whether the use of bottles creates a major risk to eventual breastfeeding.

Some parents object to feeding tube devices because of expense, unfamiliarity, or difficulty of use. Others object to frequent milk spilling and the time consuming nature of spoon or cup feeding. Finger feeding is not a well known technique and some parents may prefer a more "normal" feeding method.

Physicians may object to some forms of alternative feeding on the grounds that there are few studies demonstrating the safety or developmental suitability of the various feeding methods (Dowling 2002). In such situations, bottles may constitute the most acceptable method of supplementation. In some situations, practitioners are beginning to reexamine the practice of bottle-feeding, adapting it to provide therapeutic advantages to the nonbreastfeeding infant.

As with other feeding methods, the LC has an obligation to learn how to make bottle-feeding a safe and pleasant experience for the baby, and to advocate for the use of human milk in the bottle. Additionally, with the goal of eventual breastfeeding in mind, the LC assists in using the bottle as a therapeutic intervention to transition the baby to breastfeeding.

When a baby is not breastfeeding well, it is wise to avoid planting negative suggestions about "nipple confusion." Many parents, hearing this term, become convinced that there is no point in trying to breastfeed after the baby has been exposed to bottles. It is important to reassure parents that breastfeeding problems can be complex, and that it is doubtful whether exposure to bottles prevents subsequent breastfeeding (Victoria 1997, Dowling 2001). Many babies who get early bottles learn to breastfeed once their problems resolve as long that the mother has a robust milk supply.

It is vital to assess each infant as an individual and to identify those for whom some aspect of bottle-feeding may be overwhelming. This includes infants with respiratory or swallowing problems. Many LCs find that observing infants during alternative feeding provides valuable clues into the nature of an infant's specific feeding problems. Stress cues (see Ch. 2 and 3) can be identified during bottle-feeding.

In **Fig. 331** a 6 week-old infant with failure to thrive (FTT) struggles with a flow rate from a bottle that is too fast for him to control. Note his furrowed brow and closed eyes.

The infant shown in **Figs. 332** and **333** was born with abnormally small nasal passages. (See **Fig. 37**.) This infant was unable to breastfeed or to bottle feed comfortably. When his mouth was filled, he was unable to draw in

enough air through his nostrils to sustain normal respiration. His typical bottle-feeding behavior is shown in **Fig. 332**. He gulped as much milk as he could while holding his breath. Then he fought to push the bottle away and panted in an attempt to reorganize his breathing. Such stressful feeding creates physiological and psychological distress for both the infant and the feeder. Slowing the feeding with pacing techniques (as is demonstrated in **Figs. 333** and **335**) assisted this baby.

External Pacing Techniques (Paced Feeding)

Infants who are at risk for apnea, bradycardia, and oxygen desaturation include those experiencing prematurity, illness, anatomic anomalies, or those with a history of respiratory problems. Infants with respiratory distress while feeding can be identified by behavioral cues. They will experience nasal flaring, stiffening of the extremities, or will begin spilling milk from the corners of their mouths. Their eyes may widen, they may grimace, or the skin around the baby's lips may turn blue. Some struggle to push away from the feeding device (**Figs. 331-332**). Others appear to fall asleep in an attempt to end the feeding as is the case with the 36 week gestational age twin in **Fig. 334**.

Special feeding techniques are recommended by Speech-Language Pathologists (SLPs) and Occupational Therapists (OTs) to help the infant who has difficulty maintaining respiratory stability during feeding (Wolf 1992, Alper 1996). Palmer (1998) described uncoordination of sucking and arrhythmic breathing in immature or compromised infants. She proposed systematic pacing of feeds to promote better infant organization of feeding in preterm infants. No matter the gestational age, when an infant is unable to appropriately self-regulate breathing with sucking and swallowing, the feeder must assume responsibility for ensuring the stability of the baby's respiratory status. This is called *external pacing*.

A perceived benefit of breastfeeding is that it allows the infant maximum control over his own food intake. A guiding principle of external pacing is that the feeder strives to partner with the infant, and attempts to return as much control as possible to the infant (Wilson-Clay 2005).

When employing external pacing techniques, the feeder closely observes and counts the number of sucks and swallows (Law-Morstatt 2003). If the baby does not take a spontaneous breath after 3 to 5 sucks, the feeder interrupts the delivery of fluids to impose a brief, few seconds long, pause for breathing. Parents and other care providers can be taught that the infant's motor and behavioral cues reliably signal the need for a brief pause to regain respiratory stability. Pacing techniques are adaptable to a variety of feeding methods, including cup and finger feeding.

Bottles lend themselves well to paced feeding techniques because they do not spill and are relatively easy for the feeder to control. The flow rate from bottle teats is dependent on the firmness of the teat material, the number and size of holes, the shape of the teat (Mathew 1990), and the elevation level of the bottle. A feeding specialist or LC can select teats based on suitability of size, shape, and flow rate by observing carefully to see what works best for the baby.

Once the mother learned how to use pacing techniques (**Fig. 333**) the infant with the small nostrils relaxed. He was able to enjoy bottle-feeding because he no longer had to struggle to breathe.

Pacing with a bottle can be done 2 ways. Some feeders prefer to withdraw the bottle and rest it lightly on the upper lip of the baby, waiting for a cue that the baby is ready to suck again. This method is seen in **Fig. 333**.

Some LCs observe that as the bottle is removed, some infants resist the withdrawal. They suck harder to hold onto the bottle, and may then swallow excessive amounts of milk as a consequence. Instead of directly withdrawing the bottle, the feeder should first drop the level of the bottle, letting the milk flow out of the teat and back into the bottle, leaving an empty teat in the baby's mouth. When the baby reorganizes and starts to suck again, the feeder tilts the bottle so that milk flows back into the teat.

As with cup feeding, it is important during bottle feeding to maintain fluid level with the infant's lips. Pouring milk into the baby's mouth is generally an unsafe practice. Undue concern over "air swallowing" has caused most parents and even some HCPs to elevate the bottle so that there is no air in the teat and it is almost entirely filled with milk (as is shown in **Fig 334**). The angle of elevation of the bottle puts an excessive gravity drop on the fluid and increases the rate of flow so that it often floods even normal, term infants. Milk spilling and choking result.

Simply holding the fluid horizontally in the bottle will slow the rate of milk transfer. This makes feeding more comfortable for the baby (**Fig. 335**) and makes it unnecessary to remove the teat from the baby's mouth. Parents can be reassured that air in the bottle teat will not cause dangerous amounts of air going into the baby's stomach. All infants swallow some air while feeding. Burping (winding) will bring up swallowed air. It is far more unpleasant and potentially dangerous for the baby to aspirate milk, which may occur when the flow rate is too fast.

Since the goal of the lactation consultant is to transition infants to breastfeeding as soon as possible, it is useful to teach parents to bottle feed in a breastfeeding position (**Fig. 336**). Peterson's book (2010) describes other ways to combine breast and bottle feeding.

Some feeding therapists contend that certain types of bottle teats can be useful to help transition poor feeders to the breast (Noble 1997, Kassing 2002). In their experience, BWC and KH find that an experimental approach is best. Some infants require a narrow-based teat owing to poor lip tone and inability to seal to a wide base. Some infants will gag if the teat is too long. Other infants seem not to respond if the teat is too short and insufficient proprioreceptive stimulation is provided along the tongue.

Some older breastfeeding babies refuse bottle feedings, for example when their mothers return to work. Perhaps this is because the breastfeeding child is used to prolonged eye contact with his or her mother. In situations when the baby refuses the bottle, it may be helpful to use a feeding position that does not force the baby into eye contact with the feeder (demonstrated in **Fig. 337**). As the baby adjusts to the new way of feeding and to new care givers, a more face-to-face position can be resumed.

Conclusion

Rationales for selecting one method of alternate feeding over another will vary, even among experienced lactation consultants. No method is guaranteed to work well every time, and it is possible for any method to result in a preference in the infant for continuing to be fed that way (Wilson-Clay 1996). In most cases, such preferences can be changed with gentle persistence, patience, and practice. However, there will always be infants who suffer from organically-based dysfunctional feeding problems; these infants may not be so easily transitioned to full or even partial breastfeeding (Neifert 1995).

The goal of therapy is not to strand patients in the middle of an intervention, but to resolve a problem and move forward to have a normal experience. Some families become psychologically dependant upon alternate feeding methods, perhaps because they have come to trust things they can see and measure. However, the time commitment of "triple feeding" serves to jeopardize maintenance of lactation (Buckley 2006). The LC uses counseling skills to help families see that the burden of pumping and feeding by alternate methods can be relieved as the infant is gradually transitioned to the breast. Such transitions often require outpatient follow-up or referral to a community-based LC to complete. No intervention should be prematurely abandoned just because the patient has been discharged. Adequate follow-up is routine in other areas of medicine, and should be regarded as such until the infant is successfully transitioned to breastfeeding.

Alper B, Manno C. Dysphagia in infants and children with oral-motor deficits: assessment and management. *Seminars in Speech and Language* 1996; 17(4):283-309.

Blenkharn JI. Infection risks from electrically operated breast pumps. *Journal of Hospital Infection* 1989; 13(1): 27-31.

Bornmann PG. A legal primer for lactation consultants. in R Mannel, P Martens, M Walker, *Core Curriculum for Lactation Consultants* 3rd ed. Burlington, MA: Jones and Bartlett. 2013; pp. 218-219, 221-222.

Borucki LC. Breastfeeding mothers' experiences using a supplemental feeding tube device: finding an alternative. *Journal of Human Lactation* 2005; 21(4):429-428.

Brooks L. *Legal and Ethical Issues for the IBCLC*. Burlington, MA: Jones & Bartlett Learning, 2013. pp. 24, 337,

Buckley KM, Charles GE. Benefits and challenges of transitioning preterm infants to at-breast feedings. *International Breastfeeding Journal* 2006; 1:13.

Chen CH, Wang TM, Chang HM, et al. The effect of breast and bottle feeding on oxygen saturation and body temperature in preterm infants. *Journal of Human Lactation* 2000; 16(1):21-27.

Chiu K. Clinical tips: caring for breast pump parts. *Journal of Clinical Lactation* 2012; 3(1):30-31.

Cloherty M, Alexander J, Holloway I, et al. The cup-versus-bottle debate: a theme from an ethnographic study of the supplementation of breastfed infants in hospital in the United Kingdom. *Journal of Human Lactation* 2005; 21(2):151-162.

Collins CT, Makrides M, Gillis J, et al. Avoidance of bottles during the establishment of breast feeds in preterm infants. *Cochrane Database System Review* 2008; 8(4): CD005252.

D'Amico CJ, DiNardo CA, Krystofiak S. Preventing contamination of breast pump kit attachments in the NICU. *Journal of Perinatal and Neonatal Nursing* 2003; 17(2):150-157.

Davis HV. Effects of cup, bottle and breastfeeding on oral activities of newborn infants. *Pediatrics* 1948; 2:549-558.

Dowling D, Meier P, DiDiore J, et al. Cup-feeding for preterm infants: mechanics and safety. *Journal of Human Lactation* 2002; 18(1):13-20.

Dowling D, Thanattherakul W. Nipple confusion, alternative feeding methods, and breast-feeding supplementation: state of the science. *Newborn and Infant Nursing Review* 2001; 1(4):217-223.

Ekstrom A, Widstrom AM, Nissen E: Duration of breastfeeding in Swedish primiparous and multiparous women. *Journal of Human Lactation* 2003; 19(2):172-178.

Faro J, Katz A, Berens P, et al. Premature termination of nursing secondary to *Serratia marcescens* breast pump contamination. *Obstetrics and Gynecology* 2011; 117(2):485-486.

Flint A, New K, Davies M. Cup feeding versus other forms of supplemental enteral feeding for newborn infants unable to fully breastfeed. *Cochrane Database System Review* 2007; (2):CD005092.

Fredeen RC. Cup feeding of newborn infants. *Pediatrics* 1948; 2:544-548.

Freer Y. A comparison of breast and cup feeding in preterm infants: effect on physiological parameters. *Journal of Neonatal Nursing* 1999; 5:16-21.

Garpiel SJ. Premature infant transition to effective breastfeeding: a comparison of four supplemental feeding methods. *Journal of Obstetric Gynecologic & Neonatal Nursing* 2012; 41:S143. doi:10.111/j/1552-6909.2012.01362_35.x

Gribble K. Adoptive breastfeeding beyond infancy. *Leaven*, Oct-Nov. 2004; pp. 99-104.

Hall JK. *Law & Ethics for Clinicians*. Vega, TX: Jackhal Books. 2002; pp. 179, 275-279.

Hoover K. Supplementation of the newborn by spoon in the first 24 hours. *Journal of Human Lactation* 1998; 14(3):245.

Howard C, de Blieck EA, ten Hoopen CB, et al. Physiologic stability of newborns during cup and bottle-feeding. *Pediatrics* (Supplement) 1999; 104(5):1204-1207.

Kassing D. Bottle-feeding as a tool to reinforce breastfeeding. *Journal of Human Lactation* 2002; 18(1):56-60.

Kelly BN, Huckabee ML, Jones RD, et al. Nutritive and non-nutritive swallowing apnea duration in term infants: implications for neural control mechanisms. *Respiratory Physiology & Neurobiology* 2006; 154(3):372-378.

Kent JC, Geddes DT, Hepworth AR, et al. Effect of warm breastshields on breast milk pumping. *Journal of Human Lactation* 2011; 27(4):331-338.

Kent JC, Mitoulas LR, Cregan MD, et al. Importance of vacuum for breastmilk expression. *Journal of Human Lactation* 2008; 3(1):11-19.

Kliethermes PA, Cross ML, Lanese MG, et al. Transitioning preterm infants with nasogastric tube supplementation: increased likelihood of breastfeeding. *Journal of Obstetric, Gynecologic, and Neonatal Nursing* 1999; 28(3):264-273.

Lang S, Lawrence CJ, Orme RL. Cup feeding: an alternative method of infant feeding. *Archives of Disease in Childhood* 1994; 71(4):365-369.

Law-Morstatt L, Judd D, Sndyer P, et al. Pacing as a treatment technique for transitional sucking patterns. *Journal of Perinatology* 2003; 23(6):483-488.

Lawrence RA, Lawrence RM. *Breastfeeding: A Guide for the Medical Profession* (7th ed). Maryland Heights, MO: Elsevier Mosby, 2011; p. 236.

L'Esperance C, Frantz K. Time limitation for early breastfeeding. *Journal of Obstetric, Gynecologic, and Neonatal Nursing* 1985; 14(2):114-118.

Malhotra N, Vishwimbaran L, Sundaram KR, et al. A controlled trial of alternative methods of oral feeding in neonates. *Early Human Development* 1999; 54(1):29-38.

Marinelli KA, Burke GS, Dodd VL. A comparison of the safety of cup feedings and bottlefeedings in premature infants whose mothers intend to breastfeed. *Journal of Perinatology* 2001; 21(6):350-355.

Mathew OP. Determinants of milk flow through nipple units: role of hole size and nipple thickness. *American Journal of Diseases of Children* 1990; 144(2):222-224.

Measel C, Anderson G. Non-nutritive sucking during tube feedings: effect on clinical course in premature infants. *Journal of Obstetrical, Gynecologic and Neonatal Nursing* 1979; 8(5):265-272.

Meier P. Bottle and breastfeeding: effects on transcutaneous oxygen pressure and temperature in preterm infants. *Nursing Research* 1988; 37(1):36-41.

Meier P, Anderson GC. Responses of small preterm infants to bottle and breastfeeding. *Maternal Child Nursing* 1987; 12(2):97-105.

Neifert M, Lawrence R, Seacat J. Nipple confusion: toward a formal definition. *Journal of Pediatrics* 1995; 126(6):125-129.

Noble R, Bovey A. Therapeutic teat use for babies who breastfeed poorly. *Breastfeeding Review* 1997; 5(2):37-42.

O'Connor NR, Tanabe KO, Siadaty MS, et al. Pacifiers and breastfeeding: a systematic review. *Archives of Pediatriac and Adolescent Medicine* 2009; 163(4):378-382.

Oddy W, Glenn K. Implementing the Baby Friendly Hospital Initiative: the role of finger feeding. *Breastfeeding Review* 2003; 11(1):5-9.

Palmer MM. Sensory-Based Oral Feeding Disorders, presentation, Fourth Annual Breastfeeding and the High Risk Neonate Conference, Albuquerque, NM: University of New Mexico, March 6, 1998.

Parker LA, Sullivan S, Krueger C, et al. Effect of early breast milk expression on milk volume and timing of lactogenesis stage II among mothers of very low birth weight infants: a pilot study. *Journal of Perinatology* 2012; 32(3):205-209.

Parry M, Grant B, Ykna M, et al. *Candida osteomyelitis* and diskitis after spinal surgery: an outbreak that implicates artificial nail use. *Clinical Infectious Diseases* 2001; 32(3):352-357.

Peterson A, Harmer M. *Balancing Breast & Bottle: Reaching Your Breastfeeding Goals.* Amarillo, TX: Hale Publishing, 2010. pp. 61-83.

Pinelli J, Symington A. Non-nutritive sucking for promoting physiologic stability and nutrition in preterm infants. *Cochrane Database System Review* 2005; (4): CD001071.

Raimbault C, Saliba E, Porter RH. The effect of the odour of mother's milk on breastfeeding behavior of premature neonates. *Acta Paediatrica* 2007; 96(3):368-371.

Ramsay DT, Mitoulas LR, Kent JC, et al. Milk flow rates can be used to identify and investigate milk ejection in women expressing breast milk using an electric breast pump. *Breastfeeding Medicine* 2006; 1(1):14-23.

Rocha N, Martinez F, Jorge S. Cup or bottle for preterm infants: effects on oxygen saturation, weight gain, and breastfeeding. *Journal of Human Lactation* 2002; 18(2):132-138.

Slusher T, Slusher IL, Biomdo M, et al. Electric breast pump use increases maternal milk volume in African nurseries. *Journal of Tropical Pediatrics* 2007; 53(2):125-130.

Stein MJ. Breastfeeding the premature newborn: a protocol without bottles. *Journal of Human Lactation* 1990; 6(4):167-170.

Tender JA, Janakiram J, Arce E, et al. Reasons for in-hospital formula supplementation of breastfed infants from low-income families. *Journal of Human Lactation* 2009; 25(1):11-17.

Thorley V. Cup-feeding: problems created by incorrect use. *Journal of Human Lactation* 1997; 13(1):54-55.

Victoria C, Behague D, Barros F, et al. Pacifier use and short breastfeeding duration: cause, consequence, or coincidence? *Pediatrics* 1997; 99(3):445-453.

UNICEF. Baby-Friendly Initiative 1991. http://www.unicef.org/programme/breastfeeding/baby.htm#10. Accessed June, 2013.

US Food and Drug Administration. Breast pumps: Don't be misled - Get the facts. www.fda.gov. Accessed June 2013.

Wight N. Management of common breastfeeding issues, in RJ Schanler, (ed). *The Pediatric Clinics of North America, Breastfeeding* 2001, Part II, The Management of Breastfeeding 2001; 48(2):321-344.

Wilson-Clay B. Clinical use of nipple shields. *Journal of Human Lactation* 1996; 12(4):279-285.

Wilson-Clay B. External pacing techniques: protecting respiratory stability during feeding. Independent Study Module, Amarillo, TX: Hale Publishing, 2005.

Wolf L, Glass R. *Feeding and Swallowing Disorders in Infancy.* Tucson, AZ: Therapy Skill Builders, 1992; pp. 108, 115-116.

Donor Human Milk Banking

Wet nursing describes the practice of a woman breast-feeding a baby other than her own. Historically, wet nurses were employed either by choice or necessity as the only reliable method to ensure an infant's survival if the infant's own mother did not breastfeed. Wet nursing was a well-established custom in many cultures. Historical records include laws, codes of conduct, and contracts pertaining to the practice. Many societies established standards governing the selection of a suitable wet nurse (Fildes 1986). History also documents that in many cultures, including the pre-Civil War US, wet nursing was a coerced activity, associated with slavery.

Wet nursing of infants persists into the modern era. Obed (2007) tracked the mortality rates of infants born to mothers who died in childbirth in Nigeria. According to local customs, orphaned infants are fed animal milk or wet-nursed by an aunt or grandmother. Only 31.3 percent of infants in the study who were orphaned at birth survived to age 5. Factors favoring survival included surrogate breastfeeding.

In many instances, infants receiving milk from another mother are not directly breastfed. Informal peer-to-peer milk sharing networks and institutional donor human milk banks provide milk, and infants are fed by an alternative method.

Epigenetics

Plant, animal, and human studies have demonstrated that transfer of genetic material can take place by means other than sexual reproduction. For example, genetic material is identifiable in and transmissible from human milk (Baumgartel 2013). An *epigenetic mechanism* is a biochemical alteration to DNA that does not change the sequence of a gene but influences the way the gene is expressed. These alterations are influenced by environmental factors, including toxic exposures, medications, diet, circadian patterns, gestational age at delivery, pumping method, and number of days since delivery.

The discovery of epigentic factors in milk has numerous potential implications. In a fascinating discussion, Ozkan, et al., describe the presence and activity of *exosome*s in human milk. Exosomes contain microRNA material. Both microRNA and stem cells present in human milk affect gene expression, and may affect or alter the child in ways that may be inheritable. In this way, environmental exposures in one generation potentially affect subsequent generations.

Human milk may one day serve as a source of genetic information obtainable in a non-invasive manner. Breast cancer risk factors may become more readily detectable by evaluating genes in milk. Milk composition varies greatly between women. Epigenetic studies may also be able to more fully explain variations in outcomes between breastfed infants. Perhaps it will become possible one day to correct for any deficiencies in an individual mother's milk by adding some amount of donor milk to the infant's diet. Transfer of microRNA from a healthy wet-nurse to a neonate through human milk could result in permanent correction of the clinical manifestions in genetic diseases (Irmak 2012). These issues are provocative, but largely unexplored.

Culture and religion affect perceptions of and rules about consuming milk from a woman other than a child's mother. In Islamic law, breastfeeding confers milk kinship. The Koran (Qur'an) explains that a child who has breastfed or received milk from a woman becomes her relative, and becomes a milk sibling to others who have shared the woman's milk (Ozkan 2012). Milk siblings cannot marry; the same incest prohibitions apply as between birth siblings.

It is curious that the concept of consanguinity conferred by milk sharing, expressed centuries ago, appears to have a basis in fact when viewed in light of information about epigenetics. "So, if infants are fed by the same mother regularly, they may share similar epigenotypes. If these epigenetic modifications can be heritable to the next generations, marriages between individuals breastfed by the same woman may result in the same consequences as consanguineous marriages" (Ozkan 2012).

Dry Nursing

Infant feeding vessels, often found in graves, provide anthropological evidence that infants were also *dry nursed* or *hand fed*; that is, fed a human milk substitute. Feeding implements have been made out of various materials. Some contain residues of animal milks and other substances that may be described as ritual beverages (Fildes 1995).

In the modern era, most infants not fully breastfed receive commercial infant formula. The recipes for making artificial baby milks have changed over time in an effort to more closely imitate human milk; however, milk is a living tissue, and formula cannot duplicate its cellular activity or its ability to respond to changing infant nutritional and immunological needs. Defective, contaminated formula, and high levels of potentially toxic metals in formula pose risks to infants, especially preterm or medically fragile infants (Navarro-Blasco 2003, Iversen 2004, Fattal-Valevski 2005, WHO 2008).

Peer-to-Peer Milk Sharing

Milk sharing between families has become commonplace in the internet era. Various websites and Facebook groups facilitate access to human milk, and describe the roles and responsibilities of donors and recipients. Safety issues are reviewed on these sites, including instructions for home pasteurization; however, there is no compliance monitoring or mechanism for reporting adverse health outcomes. Recipients must rely on donors being fully aware of their health status, their honesty in reporting use of medications, herbs, and recreational drugs, and their compliance with safe food handling principles throughout the milk collection and distribution process (Wilson-Clay 2013).

The US Food and Drug Administration (USFDA 2010) "...recommends against feeding your baby breast milk acquired directly from individuals or through the Internet... because the donor is unlikely to have been adequately screened for infectious disease or contamination risk... it is not likely that the human milk has been collected, processed, tested, or stored in a way that reduces possible safety risks to the baby."

Cohen (2010) reviewed blood screening tests of 1091 women seeking to donate their milk to the Mothers' Milk Bank of San Jose, California, a member of the Human Milk Bank Association of North America (HMBANA). The women had passed a preliminary health history screening similar to questionaires developed by blood banks to rule out donors with life-style risk factors. All believed themselves to be healthy. Blood testing revealed that 6 of the women had syphilis, 6 had HTLV, and 4 tested positive for HIV, diseases that are transmissible in unpasteurized human milk.

The first documented case of an infant acquiring HIV from a wet nurse has been reported in South Africa (Goedhais 2012). A 10 week-old baby contracted the disease after being breastfed by her aunt while her mother was at work. The infant's mother was HIV negative and continued to test negative. The infant was negative at birth. The aunt was unaware of her HIV positive status and that of her own HIV positive infant.

While the motivation of peer-to-peer donors is to do good, health workers have a relationship with clients/patients that includes an ethical obligation to first Do No Harm. Information about the risks of informal milk sharing must be provided to both donors and recipients.

It is impossible to set standards for milk donation that universally apply. In some countries, donor milk is not always pasteurized in order to preserve components of milk that are altered or destroyed when heated. In some countries where AIDS is pandemic, home sterilization of milk is common. In emergency situations where a baby may sicken or die unless wet-nursed, wet-nursing and raw milk sharing might well be the most ethical things to do. However, health professionals everywhere should mobilize to develop many more non-profit milk banks, and to develop better pasteurization techniques so that risks of milk sharing can be minimized.

The Importance of Human Donor Milk for Preterm Infants

The American Academy of Pediatrics recommends that all preterm infants receive mother's own milk, fresh or frozen, (fortified when appropriate). If mother's own milk is unavailable, pasteurized human donor milk should be used. The AAP states that "Quality control of pasteurized donor milk is important and should be monitored" (AAP 2012).

Evidence suggests that preterm and medically fragile infants benefit from exclusive human milk feedings (Oddy 2004, Shoji 2004, Ronnestad 2005). Yet, mothers of preterm infants may have difficulty initiating or maintaining milk supplies sufficient for their infant's needs. Additionally, small for gestational age infants, those with feeding intolerances, short gut syndrome, burns, renal failure, and other medical illnesses, benefit from exclusive human milk feeds (Hanson 2004).

Own mother's fresh milk best protects the infant. Because of a shorter duration pregnancy, some mothers of preterm infants may not experience full glandular development of their breasts. This may result in a functional inability to make a full milk supply. The stress of caring for a preterm or sick child also causes many mothers to struggle to maintain adequate milk supplies. Lactation strategies must be in place to help mothers maximize milk production. Adherence to best practices for establishing a full milk supply will ensure that more mothers are able to provide milk for their hospitalized infants. Screened, pasteurized, donor human milk provides a safe nutritional and therapeutic alternative to formula when a mother is unable to produce sufficient quantities of her own milk (Underwood 2013).

Neonatal Necrotizing Enterocolitis (NEC)

A Cochrane Review compared formula with donor human milk for feeding preterm or low birth weight infants (Quigley 2007). While formula produced a higher rate of short-term growth, it led to a higher rate of risk for the development of necrotizing enterocolitis. NEC is a devastating inflammatory condition that destroys the lining of the intestinal wall (Luig 2005). 75 percent of cases occur in preterm infants, and NEC accounts for a significant percentage of deaths in infants <1500 g. Many infants who develop NEC are treated surgically to remove affected sections of their bowels. These infants then develop short gut syndrome, which creates problems absorbing nutrients for the rest of their lives.

Lucas (1990) reported that NEC was rare in those preterm infants receiving at least some human milk feeds. He observed that the incidence of NEC was 20 times more common in formula-fed infants. Dvorak (2003) reported that maternal milk is the major source of trophic peptides with significant healing effects on injured gastrointestinal mucosa. Women who deliver preterm infants have higher concentrations of these peptides in their milk than are present in term milk or in formula (Chuang 2005). In the past, it was unclear whether donor human milk provided a protective effect similar to own mother's milk in the reduction of NEC. McGuire (2003) performed a meta-analysis of previous reseach and identified a significant association in reduction of relative risk of NEC in pre-term infants fed donor human milk rather than formula. Improved neonatal outcomes in human milk-fed infants suggest an increased role for own mother's (Stout 2008) and donor human milk to reduce NEC and to improve growth and development in preterm infants (Slusher 2003, Diehl-Jones 2004, Updegrove 2004).

History and Guidelines for Human Donor Milk Banking

Proponents of human milk banking have argued that receiving human milk is a human right of the infant (Arnold 2006). Lording (2006) observed that in spite of demonstrated cost-effectiveness, milk banking is "largely invisible from national breastfeeding policies." This observation prompted recommendations that human milk banking should become an integral component of national breastfeeding policies. Best practices for the operation of donor human milk banks are being developed on a country-by-country basis, and in association with milk banking organizations. These practices include

screening and processing criteria, traceability, and maintenance of records of all processing and storage conditions (Hartmann 2007, Landers 2013).

Although, as mentioned, some cultures impose prohibitions or restrictions on the use of both wet nursing and on the use of donor human milk, milk banking has been common in Western European countries, Scandanavia, South and Central America, and China since the early 1900s. However, the trend toward formula feeding, hospital budgetary crises, and the HIV/AIDS epidemic saw the closure of many North American milk banks (Jones 2003). Since the 1980s, there has been a resurgence of interest in donor human milk banking in the US, using screened donors and pasteurized milk. This renewed interest led to the formation in 1985 of the Human Milk Banking Association of North America (HMBANA).

As of 2013, HMBANA consists of representatives from 13 member banks. They develop guidelines establishing donor requirements, screening protocols, pasteurization policies, and bacteriological quality control requirements for dispensing donor milk. The HMBANA guidelines are similar to those developed for other human donor tissues by the US Centers for Disease Control, the US Food and Drug Administration, and the American Association of Blood Banks.

Ethical issues and policies regarding donors and recipients and the conduct of the milk banks are addressed by individual milk bank regulations and more broadly at the level of HMBANA. There currently is no regulation of donor milk banks by the US government; however, there is consensus among the existing milk banks to adhere to HMBANA standards. Policies can be viewed on the HMBANA website: www.hmbana.org.

Various models exist for milk banks, including at least one for-profit company. Some milk banks are associated with research institutions or universities. These institutions may provide milk samples to scientists studying topics relevant to human milk, including the best methods for processing, storing, labeling, and dispensing human milk (Geraghty 2005). Some milk banks are hospital-based, collecting and dispensing own mothers' milk to infants who are patients in their special care nurseries. While referred to as "milk banks," these do not meet the HMBANA definition of a milk bank because they do not provide donor milk. Other milk banks are free-standing, not-for-profit corporations funded through grants, program fees, and donations. While most prioritize the care of preterm and medically fragile infants, some milk banks provide milk for older children and even for adults who require nutritional support in special situations.

HMBANA milk banks do not sell milk; however, they do establish fees that are calculated to recover some of the costs of screening, processing, and distributing the milk. The costs of screening and processing (but not of distributing) donor milk is sometimes reimbursed by private US insurance companies or government programs such as Medicaid. The HMBANA milk banks advocate for increased private and public funding resources for donor human milk. HMBANA is committed to maintaining a non-profit approach to human donor milk banking, and to avoid creating a profit-driven "industry."

Donor Recruitment, Screening, and Exclusions

As demand for donor human milk increases, recruitment of adequate numbers of donor mothers has become an issue in some countries. To facilitate donor recruitment, several studies have examined the characteristics of human milk donors. Altruism and concern for the health of fragile infants have been identified as qualities of milk donors (Osbaldiston 2007, Azema 2003). Additional research has identified encouragement of a health professional as the primary reason for donation (Pimenteira 2008). Consequently, health care providers should initiate discusssions about milk donation with breastfeeding patients.

The first step in establishing the safety of donor human milk involves the careful screening of donors. HMBANA milk banks follow a specific protocol. A preliminary questionnaire is administered during a telephone interview. The interview elicits general information about travel history, health history, and screens for lifestyle risk factors. A more comprehensive written questionnaire is administered to prospective donors who progress beyond the phone interview stage.

Blood tests (paid for by the milk bank) screen for HIV-1, HIV-2, HTLV I & II, Hepatitis B and C, tuberculosis, and syphilis. Donors must be healthy and breastfeeding a healthy, well-growing child under 1 year of age. They must be non-smokers, not drink more than 2 alcoholic drinks daily, or use herbs or illegal drugs. A woman cannot donate if she or her partner is at risk for HIV, if she has obtained a tattoo in the past year, or received a blood transfusion or organ transplant in the past 6 months. Women from certain African countries are excluded as donors (see HMBANA website).

Women who lived in the United Kingdom for more than 3 months prior to 1996, or who lived in specific areas of Europe for more than 5 years between 1980-1996 are also excluded, owing to concerns about Creutzfeldt Jacob disease (the human form of *mad cow disease*).

Donors may use either progestin-only birth control pills or low dose (a maximum of 20mcg estrogen) estrogen/progesterone pills (Hale 2003). Women who have received Depo Provera injections and IUDs are also acceptable as donors. Synthroid (thyroid replacement hormone), insulin, and prenatal vitamins are also permitted. Donors may not be regular users of other medications, herbal supplements or mega-vitamins.

Mothers who wish to donate are asked to commit to donating a minimum amount of milk (generally 100-200 oz). The establishment of a minimum level of donation assures that the milk bank will not incur the expenses related to screening with no return benefit. Exceptions are made for bereaved mothers, from whom smaller amounts of milk are accepted. For some mothers, donating to a milk bank becomes an important part of the grieving process if their own babies have died (Tully 1999). These women find comfort in being able to provide life giving assistance to another baby.

The donor screening process seeks to ensure that the milk is safe and that no monetary incentive (or other issue) will deprive an infant of his own mother's milk. Of special interest to milk banks are donors who deliver prematurely and those who are on dairy-free diets. Milk from both special categories of donors is processed and stored separately. This milk is dispensed to preterm infants or to those who exhibit dairy protein intolerance. Preterm milk differs from term milk in a variety of ways (Ronayne de Ferrer 2000, Dvorak 2003, Bielicki 2004). Preterm milk has higher protein levels (for about 4 weeks after the birth) than term milk (Lemons 1982, Butte 1984).

Milk may be mixed with fortifiers to obtain the ideal mix of protein, minerals, and calories to help very small preterm babies grow. Most current milk fortifiers are bovine- and plant-based, and deprive the baby of the benefits of an exclusive human milk diet. Human-milk-based fortifiers have been developed by concentrating pasteurized donor milk and adding vitamins and minerals (Underwood 2013), and are available in the US and elsewhere (Czank 2010).

Collecting, Processing, and Storing Donor Milk

A screening program in a Chinese hospital tested the milk of mothers who were expressing breastmilk for their own hospitalized preterm infants. Unusually high rates of pathogens were discovered in their milk, including *enterococci* and *Staphylococcus aureus* (*S. aureus*). Researchers suspected that bacteriological contamination may have resulted from cultural traditions that prohibit bathing for one month after childbirth (Ng 2004).

This study suggests that anticipatory guidance on hygiene is an important part of the education provided to mothers who are expressing milk for their own or other babies.

Human milk is not sterile; it contains many types of bacteria. Pasteurized milk is dispensed as sterile. According to HMBANA guidelines, once a woman has been accepted as a donor, she receives written instructions relating to the hygienic collection of her milk. The mother temporarily stores milk in her own freezer until she accumulates enough to take a quantity of it to a collection site or directly to the milk bank. The raw, frozen milk is labeled, carefully logged, and stored in large freezers (**Fig. 338**).

Pasteurization of human donor milk is undertaken to protect fragile infants from viral and bacterial illness. While the pasteurization of own mother's milk has been shown to reduce fat absorption and growth in some preterm infants compared to unpasteurized own mother's milk (Andersson 2007), most donor milk is pasteurized, and many benefits remain after pasteurization.

Biologically active compounds such as oligosaccharides, for example, play an "emerging leading role" in protecting preterm infants (Bertino 2008). Holder pasteurization does not affect the concentration or pattern of oligosaccharides in human donor milk. New methods of high-temperature short-time pasteurization (HTST) are being studied. Research has concluded that HTST is effective in the elimination of "bacteria and certain important pathogenic viruses" (Terpstra 2007). As milk banks struggle to accommodate increasing demands, new technologies for pasteurizing donor milk are needed.

All milk banks discard milk that grows bacteria following pasteurization. Because it is expensive to pasteurize milk, some milk banks test raw milk before pasteurization, as well. For example, they discard milk that tests positive for *S. aureus*. When *S. aureus* dies, it is capable of producing *enterotoxins* that remain unaffected by heat treatment. An enterotoxin is a harmful substance that can cause food poisoning-like symptoms such as diarrhea and nausea (USFDA 2005). Enterotoxins in milk may pose risks to medically fragile babies.

Researchers continue to investigate the best method of milk storage. Length of storage time and storage temperature affect milk integrity (Ogundele 2002, Hanna 2004). Changes in milk antioxidant activity occur from chilling and freezing. This may be important in populations of preterm infants, who are at increased risk of tissue damage from oxygen free radicals. Anti-oxidant activity of human milk may be one of the mechanisms that protect preterm infants from NEC, chronic lung disease, and

intraventricular hemorrhage (Shoji 2004). Freezing somewhat diminishes the antioxidant activity of human milk. The optimal methods for human milk storage constitute an important area for future research.

Cytomegalovirus

Newborn exposure to cytomegalovirus (CMV) may occur during delivery or afterward through virus shed in breast milk (Meier 2005). Very low birth weight infants may be more susceptible to the virus, because they are born before the transfer of protective immunoglobulins, and they have extremely immature immune systems.

While freezing milk can diminish the viral load, it does not kill CMV in human milk. Hamprecht (2004) reported that viral infectivity of CMV was preserved in frozen milk. Maschmann (2006) reported a case of a preterm infant who developed symptomatic postnatal CMV while receiving milk from his CMV positive mother that had been frozen for 2 months at -20 C. Heat treatment with pasteurization kills CMV; therefore, mothers donating milk that will be pasteurized are not specifically tested for the virus.

Peer-to-peer milk sharers should be informed that women with reactivated CMV infection and even some women with primary cases may be asymptomatic or only mildly ill. Because CMV is often mistaken for a common cold, a peer-to-peer donor may not think to withhold her milk from donation during such a mild illness. However, virus is being shed into the milk (Vochem 1998). Unpasteurized milk may thus exposes a recipient infant to acute CMV infection (Meier 2005). CMV is sometimes fatal in extremely low birth weight preterm infants.

In Norway, researchers have demonstrated the benefits of providing immediately frozen, unpasteurized, donor milk to hospitalized infants whose own mothers are temporarily unable to produce sufficient milk. However, the donors are carefully screened for CMV status before donating milk and are rescreened every 3 months (Lindemann 2004). When close screening is impossible, pasteurization is vital.

Nutritional Labeling

In donor milk banks, raw milk is thawed for processing on regularly scheduled pasteurization days. In some milk banks, milk from several mothers is randomly pooled in hopes of assuring homogeneous fat content and a wide variety of immune factors. However, because of pronounced variation in milk fat content between mothers, random pooling may result in low calorie milk that is not adequate for the infant's nutritional needs.

It is important to note that individual variations in the caloric value of a mother's own milk are insignificant for the normal breastfeeding baby. Breastfeeding babies are able to regulate their milk intake to accommodate variations in milk fat content that arises owing to time of day, relative breast fullness, or any other factor (Daly 1993, Kent 2006). Consequently issues related to the calorie value of pumped milk are only relevant for the non-breastfeeding infant, who cannot self-regulate intake.

In Texas, the Mothers' Milk Bank at Austin (MMBA) sought more specific control of the milk pooling process in order to produce batches of milk with adequate caloric values to protect the growth needs of low birthweight preterm infants. This goal led to the purchase of a Foss MilkoScan™ (**Fig. 339**), a machine used in the dairy industry to conduct a full spectrum infrared nutritional analysis. MMBA neonatologists re-calibrated the instrument to analyze human milk.

Use of the MilkoScan™ permits targeted pooling of donor milk. In other words, the milk in each pool is specifically selected for optimal nutritional values. Each bottle of pooled milk is then labeled with the total caloric and protein content. This method also identifies milk that cannot meet optimal nutritional levels, and therefore is not adequate for use in populations of hospitalized infants with high growth requirements.

Nutritional labeling permits the dispensing of milk to special care nurseries with labeled caloric values of 20, 22, and 24 calories per ounce. Labeling assists in the feeding of hospitalized infants with differing nutritional requirements. Outpatients are generally able to receive milk that is 17 calories per ounce or higher. Controlling for variations in calorie and protein may prevent reported growth problems sometimes seen in infants receiving human donor milk (Slusher 2003).

Short Term Use of Donor Milk in Other Special Situations

While most banked human milk in the US is targeted for preterm infants, if supplies could be increased, short-term use of donor milk could be employed to feed a baby for a day or so until a woman's own milk came in. It would be wonderful to have enough available human donor milk to be able to provide temporary feeds for all breastfeeding infants who need to be supplemented. Certainly, access to small volumes of donor milk would prevent exposing vulnerable populations of infants to formula. For example, infants born small for gestational age (SGA) experience increased risk of developing metabolic syndrome if exposed to formula (Nobilli 2008). Additionally, formula

exposure is associated with neurodevelopmental deficits in female infants born SGA (Morley 2004). SGA infants have immediate needs for calories to prevent postnatal growth faltering, hypoglycemia, and lethargic feeding (Lawrence 2011). Having the option to stabilize them with physiologic volumes of human donor milk extends meaningful protection to these infants. The amount of milk needed for each infant is small and temporary.

In **Fig. 340** pasteurization workers at the MMBA have performed targeted pooling of the milk of 3 mothers. The milk of these 3 donors was selected for pooled processing because the caloric and protein content of their milk will complement each other to satisfy minimum requirements.

The workers shown in **Fig. 340** pour pooled milk from large, sterilized, glass beakers into sterilized bottles. Then capped bottles are placed into pasteurizers (**Fig. 341**) for Holder pasteurization. In the Holder process, the milk will be held in a shaking water bath at a carefully monitored temperature of 62.5°C for 30 minutes (**Fig. 342**). Following heat treatment, the bottles are plunged into an ice slurry to cool quickly.

Prior to refreezing the milk, the worker shown in **Fig. 343** withdraws small samples of milk for post-pasteurization bacteriological testing. Bottles are labeled with the date of pasteurization, a coded number identifying the donors in the pool, and information about caloric and protein values. The processed bottles are frozen to await the results of bacterial testing (**Fig. 344**). Records are carefully maintained. The milk is not available to be dispensed until bacteriological results are reviewed, and the milk is verified to be sterile.

After bacteriological results are received, each bottle is labeled with an expiration date one year from the earliest pumping date of the milk in that batch. Freezers are equipped with sensors that signal on and off-site during power outages (**Fig. 345**). Emergency generators protect the integrity of the frozen milk.

Fig. 346 shows a bottle of high calorie donor human milk from the Mothers' Milk Bank at Fort Worth labeled with specific nutritional information.

Processed milk is transported by car to hospitals within the city or region. Other batches are packed to prevent thawing and tampering and are shipped by air for 24-hour delivery. Computerized batch-tracking records are carefully maintained, providing a record of the chain of control of the milk from donor drop off to the time the hospital or recipient family receives the shipment.

Cost Issues

Developing a donor human milk bank is a rewarding undertaking with wide-reaching benefits to the community. While cost is often cited as a reason not to provide human donor milk, a single case of NEC increases the length of a preterm baby's hospital stay and adds cost to the care provided to that infant. Using human donor milk as a strategy to prevent NEC is cost-effective (Ganapathy 2011, Vaidyanathan 2012, Carroll 2013).

Disclaimer: Barbara Wilson-Clay is a founding board member and served as the Vice President of the board of directors of the Mother's Milk Bank of Austin. She received no financial compensation and has no conflicts of interest to declare with regard to the information presented here.

American Academy of Pediatrics, Section on Breastfeeding. Breastfeeding and the use of human milk. *Pediatrics* 2012; 129(3):e827-e841.

Andersson Y, Savman K, Blackberg L, et al. Pasteurization of mother's own milk reduces fat absorption and growth in preterm infants. *Acta Paediatrica* 2007; 96(10):1445-1449.

Arnold LD. Global health policies that support the use of banked donor human milk: a human rights issue. *International Breastfeeding Journal* 2006; 1:26.

Azema E, Callahan S. Breast milk donors in France: a portrait of the typical donor and the utility of milk banking in the French breastfeeding context. *Journal of Human Lactation* 2003; 19(2):199-202.

Baumgartel KL, Conley YP. The utility of breastmilk for genetic or genomic studies: a systematic review. *Breastfeeding Medicine* 2013; 8(3):249-256.

Bertino E, Coppa GV, Guiliani F, et al. Effects of Holder pasteurization on human milk oligosaccharides. *International Journal of Immunopathological Pharmacology* 2008; 21(2):381-385.

Bielicki J, Huch R, von Mandach U. Time-course of leptin levels in term and preterm human milk. *European Journal of Endocrinology* 2004; 151(2):271-276.

Butte N, Garza C, Johnson C, et al. Longitudinal changes in milk composition of mothers delivering preterm and term infants. *Early Human Development* 1984; 9(2):153-162.

Carroll K, Hermann K. The cost of using donor human milk in the NICU to achieve exclusively human milk feeding through 32 weeks postmenstrual age. *Breastfeeding Medicine* 2013; 8(3):286-290.

Chuang C, Lin S, Lee H, et al. Free amino acids in full-term and pre-term human milk and infant formula. *Journal of Pediatric Gastroenterology and Nutrition* 2005; 40(4):496-500.

Cohen RS, Xiong SC, Sakamoto P. Retrospective review of serological testing of potential human milk donors. *Archives of Diseases in Childhood Fetal Neonatal Edition* 2010; 95(2):F118-F120.

Czank C, Simmer K, Hartmann P. Design and characterization of a human milk product for the preterm infant. *Breastfeeding Medicine* 2010; 5(2):59-66.

Daly SE, Owens RA, Hartmann PE. The short-term synthesis and infant-regulated removal of milk in lactating women. *Experimental Physiology* 1993; 78(2):209-220.

Diehl-Jones W, Askin D. Nutritional modulation of neonatal outcomes. *AACN Clinical Issues* 2004; 15(1):83-96.

Dvorak B, Fituch C, Williams C, et al. Increased epidermal growth factor levels in human milk of mothers with extremely premature infants. *Pediatric Research* 2003; 54(1):15-19.

Fattal-Valevski A, Kesler A, Sela B, et al. Outbreak of life-threatening thiamine deficiency in infants in Israel caused by defective soy-based formula. *Pediatrics* 2005; 115(2):e233-238.

Fildes V. *Breasts, Bottles and Babies: A History of Infant Feeding.* Edinburgh, Scotland: Edinburgh University Press, 1986.

Fildes V. The culture and biology of breastfeeding: an historical review of Western Europe, in P Stuart-Macadam, K Dettwyler (ed), *Breastfeeding: Biocultural Perspectives.* New York, NY: Aldine de Gruyter, 1995; pp. 101-126.

Ganapathy V, Hay JW, Kim JH. Costs of necrotizing enterocolitis and cost-effectiveness of exclusively human milk-based products in feeding extremely premature infants. *Breastfeeding Medicine* 2011; 7(1):29-37.

Geraghty S, Davidson B, Warner B, et al. The development of a research human milk bank. *Journal of Human Lactation* 2005; 21(1):59-66.

Goedhais D, Rossouw I, Hallbauer U, et al. The tainted milk of human kindness. *Lancet* 2012; 380(9842):702.

Hale T. Medications in breastfeeding mothers of preterm infants. *Pediatric Annals* 2003; 32(5):337-347.

Hanson LA. *Immunobiology of human milk: how breastfeeding protects babies.* Amarillo, TX: Pharmasoft Publishing; 2004.

Hamprecht K, Maschmann J, Muller D, et al. Cytomegalovirus (CMV) inactivation in breast milk: reassessment of pasteurization and freeze-thawing. *Pediatric Research* 2004; 56(4):529-535.

Hanna N, Ahmed K, Anwar M, et al. Effect of storage on breast milk antioxidant activity. *Archives of Disease in Childhood Fetal and Neonatal Edition* 2004; 89(6):F518-520.

Hartmann BT, Pang WW, Kell AD, et al. Best practice guidelines for the operation of a donor human milk bank in an Australian NICU. *Early Human Development* 2007; 83(10):667-673.

Irmak MK, Oztas Y, Oztas E. Integration of maternal genome into the neonate genome through breast milk mRNA transcripts and reverse transcriptase. *Theoretical Biology & Medical Modeling* 2012; 9(1):20

Iversen C, Lane M, Forsythe SJ. The growth profile, thermotolerance and biofilm formation of *Enterobacter sakazakii* grown in infant formula milk. *Letters in Applied Microbiology* 2004; 38(5):378-382.

Jones F. History of North American donor milk banking: one hundred years of progress. *Journal of Human Lactation* 2003; 19(3):313-318.

Kent JC, Mitoulas LR, Cregan MD, et al. Volume and frequency of breastfeedings and fat content of breast milk throughout the day. *Pediatrics* 2006; 117(3):e387-395.

Landers S, Hartmann BT. Donor human milk banking and the emergence of milk sharing. *Pediatric Clinics of North America* 2013; 60(1):248-260.

Lawrence RA, Lawrence RM. *Breastfeeding: a guide for the medical profession* (7th ed). Maryland Heights, MO: Elsevier Mosby, 2011. pp. 542-543.

Lemons J, Moye L, Hall D, et al. Differences in the composition of preterm and term human milk during early lactation. *Pediatric Research* 1982; 16(2):113-117.

Lindemann P, Foshaugen I, Lindemann R. Characteristics of breast milk and serology of women donating breast milk to a milk bank. *Archives of Disease in Childhood Fetal and Neonatal Edition* 2004; 89(5):F440-441.

Lording RJ. A review of human milk banking and public health policy in Australia. *Breastfeeding Reveiw* 2006; 14(3):21-30.

Lucas A, Cole TJ. Breast milk and neonatal necrotising enterocolitis. *Lancet* 1990; 336(8730):1519-1523.

Luig M, Lui K, NSW & ACT NICUS Group. Epidemiology of necrotizing enterocolitis - Part I: changing regional trends in extremely preterm infants over 14 years. *Journal of Paediatric Child Health* 2005; 41(4):169-173.

Maschmann J, Hamprecht K, Weissbrich B, et al. Freeze-thawing of breast milk does not prevent cytomegalovirus transmission to a preterm infant. *Archives of Disease in Childhood Fetal Neonatal Edition* 2006; 91(4):F288-F290.

McGuire W, Anthony M. Donor human milk versus formula for preventing necrotizing enterocolitis in preterm infants: systematic review. *Archives of Disease in Childhood Fetal and Neonatal Edition* 2003; 88(1):F11-F14.

Meier J, Lienicke U, Tschirach E, et al. Human cytomegalovirus reactivation during lactation and mother-to-child transmission in preterm infants. *Journal of Clinical Microbiology* 2005; 43(3):1318-1324.

Morley R, Fewtrell MS, Abbott RA, et al. Neurodevelopment in children born small for gestational age: a randomized trial of nutrient-enriched versus standard formula and comparison with a reference breastfed group. *Pediatrics* 2004; 113(3 Part I):515-521.

Navarro-Blasco I, Alvarez-Galindo J. Aluminium content of Spanish infant formula. *Food Additives and Contaminants* 2003; 20(5):470-481.

Ng D, Lee S, Leung L, et al. Bacteriological screening of expressed breast milk revealed a high rate of contamination in Chinese women. *Journal of Hospital Infection* 2004; 58(2):146-150.

Nobilli V, Alisi A, Panera N, et al. Low birthweight and catch-up growth associated with metabolic syndrome: a ten-year systematic review. *Pediatric Endocrinology Review* 2008; 6(2):241-247.

Obed JY, Agida ET, Mairiga AG. Survival of infants and children born to women who died from pregnancy and labour related complications. *Nigerian Journal of Clinical Practice* 2007; 10(1):35-40.

Oddy W, Sherriff J, de Klerk N, et al. The relation of breastfeeding and body mass index to asthma and atopy in children: a prospective cohort study to age 6 years. *American Journal of Public Health* 2004; 94(9):1531-1537.

Ogundele MO. Effects of storage on the physicochemical and antibacterial properties of human milk. *British Journal of Biomedical Science* 2002; 59(4):205-211.

Osbaldiston R, Mingle L. Characteristics of human milk donors. *Journal of Human Lactation* 2007; 23(4):350-357.

Ozkan H, Tuzun F, Kumral A, et al. Milk kinship hypothesis in light of epigenetic knowledge. *Clinical Epigenetics* 2012; 4(1):14-16.

Pimenteira Thomaz AC, Maia Loureiro LV, da Silva Oliveira T, et al. The human milk donation experience: motives, influencing factors, and regular donation. *Journal of Human Lactation* 2008; 24(1):69-76.

Quigley MA, Henderson G, Anthony MY, et al. Formula milk versus donor breast milk for feeding preterm or low birth weight infants. *Cochrane Database System Review* 2007; 17(4):CD002971.

Ronnestad A, Abrahamsen T, Medbo S, et al. Late-onset septicemia in a Norwegian national cohort of extremely premature infants receiving very early full human milk feeding. *Pediatrics* 2005; 115(3):e269-276.

Ronayne de Ferrer P, Baroni A, Sambucetti M, et al. Lactoferrin levels in term and preterm milk. *Journal of the Americal College of Nutrition* 2000; 19(3):370-373.

Shoji H, Shimizu T, Shinohara K, et al. Suppressive effects of breast milk on oxidative DNA damage in very low birthweight infants. *Archives of Disease in Childhood Fetal and Neonatal Edition* 2004; 89(2):F136-F138.

Slusher T, Hampton R, Bode-Thomas F, et al. Promoting the exclusive feeding of own mother's milk through the use of hindmilk and increased maternal milk volume for hospitalized, low birth weight infants (<1800 grams) in Nigeria: a feasibility study. *Journal of Human Lactation* 2003; 19(2):191-198.

Stout G, Lambert DK, Baer VL, et al. Necrotizing enterocolitis during the first week of life: a multicentered case-control and cohort comparison study. *Journal of Perinatology* 2008; 28(8):556-560.

Terpstra FG, Rechtman DJ, Lee ML, et al. Antimicrobial and antiviral effect of high-temperature short-time (HTST) pasteurization applied to human milk. *Breastfeeding Medicine* 2007; 2(1):27-33.

Tully MR. Donating human milk as part of the grieving process. *Journal of Human Lactation* 1999; 15(2):149-150.

Underwood MA. Human milk for the premature infant. in Morrow AL, Chantry CJ. Breastfeeding updates for the pediatrician. *Pediatric Clinics of North America* 2013; 60(1):189-207.

Updegrove K. Necrotizing enterocolitis: the evidence for the use of human milk in prevention and treatment. *Journal of Human Lactation* 2004; 20(3):335-339.

US Food & Drug Administration (USFDA/), Center for Food Safety & Applied Nutrition. *Foodborne Pathogenic Microorganisms and Natural Toxins Handbook (The Bad Bug Book)*, 2005. www.cfsan.fda.gov/~mow/chap3.html. Accessed on July 31, 2008.

US Food & Drug Administration (US FDA). Use of donor human milk. Nov. 30, 2010. www.fda.gov. Accessed June 2013.

Vaidyanathan G, Hay JW, Kim JH. Costs of necrotizing enterocolitis and cost effectiveness of exclusively human milk-based products in feeding extremely premature infants. *Breastfeeding Medicine* 2012; 7(1):29-37.

Vochem M, Hamprecht K, Jahn G, et al. Transmission of cytomegalovirus to preterm infants through breast milk. *Pediatric Infectious Disease Journal* 1998; 17(1):53-58.

World Health Organization (WHO). Melamine-contaminated powdered infant formula in China-Update. Sept. 22, 2008. www.who.int/csr/don/2008_0922/en/ Accessed June, 2013.

Wilson-Clay B. Roundtable and response on peer-to-peer milk sharing: rebuttal response to "Biomedical ethics and peer-to-peer milk sharing," by Karleen D. Gribble, PhD, BRurSC. *Journal of Clinical Lactation* 2013; 4(1):28-35.

Breastfeeding in Special Circumstances

Human milk provides superior nutrition while reducing infant energy expenditure (Lubetzky 2003), making it especially important for the compromised infant. The entire health care team must possess sufficient assessment skills to identify infants who need special breastfeeding assistance (Hall 2002, Hill 2007, Mannel 2011). When direct breastfeeding is delayed, health care providers should work together to ensure human milk feeds for the infant (AAP 2012).

Far too many mothers receive suboptimal lactation care, and suffer the loss of lactation through no fault of their own. This can be especially devastating when the mother knows how important her milk is for her compromised infant. While it is commonly recognized that women grieve over infertility or the loss of a pregnancy, grief over the loss of the breastfeeding experience is seldom acknowledged in cultures where bottle-feeding is prevalent. This striking observation was first made by Karen Pryor (1973), but lack of acknowledgment of this form of grief continues, and may contribute to postpartum depression.

Whether it is the infant, the mother, or both who require assistance, research demonstrates that excellent breastfeeding support results in increased maternal self-esteem and strengthens the bond between mother and baby (Ekstrom 2006). It also appears to confer resilience against psychosocial stress and postpartum depression (Montgomery 2006, Dennis 2009).

Breastfeeding provides unique physical benefits for the mother as well. For example, short- and long-term decreases in maternal blood pressure have been observed during lactation (Jonas 2008). Lactation appears to be a modifiable behavior that improves maternal metabolic profile in ways that may positively affect women's future risk of cardiovascular and metabolic diseases (Gunderson 2007). Thus, effective breastfeeding support protects women both physically and emotionally. These are important goals when mothers are already stressed or physically challenged following the birth of a child with special needs.

Continuity of care is particularly essential for the at-risk dyad. Referrals to community-based lactation care and to mother support groups should be routinely provided at the time of hospital discharge in compliance with Step 10 of the Baby Friendly Hospital Initiative. An overview of conditions that require extra assistance to protect and preserve successful breastfeeding follows.

Down Syndrome

Down Syndrome (Trisomy 21) is a chromosomal abnormality that occurs approximately once in every 1000 births. Growth and development are affected to varying degrees. Most affected individuals develop as do other children, though on a delayed timetable. Down Syndrome (DS) is marked by certain distinctive physical traits, low muscle tone, and mental retardation that ranges from mild to severe. It is common for infants with DS to have cardiac defects, and to be more susceptible to respiratory infections and otitis media (Davenport 1990). For information and resources available for families in the US, contact the National Down Syndrome Society: www.ndss.org.

Breastfeeding positively affects neurological development, attainment of gross motor skills, and enhances facial and dental formation (Romero 2011). This information should be shared with parents so that they can make an informed choice about how to feed their child with DS. In a research study that matched 560 children with Down Syndrome with 2 groups of healthy control infants, Pisacane (2003) reported that infants with DS were significantly less likely to be breastfed. The main reasons their mothers reported for chosing to bottle feed were: infant illness, maternal frustration and depression, perceived milk insufficiency, and infant sucking problems. Families may be more motivated to persevere if they receive specific information about how breastfeeding maximizes health and neurological outcomes and improves physical appearance.

A group of Dutch infants was studied to examine the effect of breastfeeding on neurological development (Lanting 1994). Newborn neurological examinations classified the infants at birth as normal, slightly abnormal, or frankly abnormal. At 9 years of age, the children were reexamined, and their mothers described their infant feeding practices. Researchers identified a small but significant beneficial effect of breastfeeding on neurological status, even after the data were adjusted for confounding issues. Kramer (2008) reported the results of the largest randomized trial ever conducted in the area of human lactation and provided evidence that prolonged and exclusive breastfeeding significantly improves the cognitive development of children.

Gross motor skill attainment was improved in infants who breastfed or who received human milk feeds (Sacker 2006). Sacker suggests that the protective effect is "attributable to some component(s) of breast milk or feature of breastfeeding and is not simply a product of [the mother's] advantaged social position, education or of parenting style..."

Some infants with Down Syndrome breastfeed well from the start. Others may be slow, inefficient feeders who need extra time at the breast and careful postural support. Ultrasonographic images reveal that sucking deficiencies in infants with DS result from hypotonicity of the perioral muscles, lips, and masticatory muscles, and from deficiencies in the smooth tongue movement (Mizuno 2001). These sucking problems appear to be related to developmental lag, and improve over time.

Hopman (1998) noted that infants with DS experienced a delay in the age at which solid food was introduced. It may be helpful to initiate pre-speech therapy for babies who appear to be experiencing oral motor deficits that interfere with acceptance of solids.

Severely affected infants with Down Syndrome, especially those with cardiac problems, require a comprehensive program of feeding interventions to protect normal growth and development.

These interventions include:

- Careful evaluation of the infant's feeding capabilities
- Decisions about how to supplement, if needed
- Protection of the milk supply with pumping
- Growth monitoring with growth charts specifically designed for the baby with DS (Cronk 1988)
- Periodic reassessment to normalize feeding as the baby matures

The infant in **Fig. 347** demonstrates some of the facial characteristics common in children with Down Syndrome. Note the flat face, the low, flat nasal bridge, and low-set ears positioned below the lateral canthal eyeline. The eyes have an almond shape with an epicanthal fold and slant upward. The tongue appears to protrude and may be flat and unable to adequately cup the breast. The baby has a "pear-shaped" trunk (**Fig. 348**). Other characteristics include: small nose, short neck, small oral cavity, and high palate. Due to muscular hypotonia, the face may appear expressionless.

Breastfeeding encourages appropriate use of the infant's facial muscles (Labbok 1987) and assists in improving facial tone and development. Because facial development affects social acceptance, parents should be informed about the positive impact of breastfeeding on facial appearance and dental health. A Brazilian study looked at feeding, non-nutritive (NNS) sucking habits,

and dental development in children with DS. The prevalence of open bite and crossbite was associated with use of bottle feeding, pacifier sucking for more than 24 months, and breastfeeding for less than 6 months (Oliveira 2010). Even weakly feeding infants should be put to the breast and allowed to enjoy comfort sucking. Improved orofacial development impacts speech and may assist in minimizing the tongue protrusion seen in some children with DS. Normalizing physical appearance may improve social interactions, and thus is an important issue for families of children with this condition.

Fig. 349 shows a palmar crease. A single crease on the palm is another characteristic trait of Trisomy 21. A single plantar crease is sometimes seen on the soles of the feet as well. Some individuals who do not have DS may also have single creases on the hands and feet.

Both male babies in **Fig. 350** are 4 months old. The hypotonic infant with Down Syndrome pictured on the right cannot stabilize his head, while the neurologically healthy infant on the left can maintain head control when pulled to a sitting position. Hypotonia in the body extends to the muscles of the face, mouth, and throat, and may result in a weak suck. The baby's lips may lack the strength and tone to form a proper seal. The tongue may be unable to sustain the muscular effort needed to create suction. If the baby tires, discontinuing the feed too soon, intake will suffer. The mother can compensate for this by providing careful postural support, including supporting the breast in the baby's mouth using the Dancer hand position (Danner 1990) seen in **Figs. 351** and **352**.

Gentle counter pressure applied to the cheeks is an element of the Dancer hand position (**Fig. 352**). Counter pressure on the cheeks decreases the intraoral space. Reducing the size of the oral cavity means the baby does not have to suck as hard to create a vacuum. Mothers can also use breast compression during breastfeeding (**Fig. 353**) to increase both the volume and caloric value of the feed (Stutte 1988).

Short, frequent feeds are easier for a weak baby to manage. The baby may feed well at some feedings and poorly at others, depending upon fatigue level or behavioral state (see Ch. 3). Mothers should be instructed to express milk accordingly since effective milk removal is an essential factor in protecting full milk production.

Low Tone and Feeding Problems

Feeding involves the coordination of sucking, swallowing, and breathing. Weakness and lack of coordination of these activities in low-tone babies increase the risk of aspiration. Low tone may prevent the epiglottis from sealing tightly, increasing the risk of milk spilling into the lungs (McBride 1987). The soft palate is a muscle. If the muscle tone of the soft palate is too poor to support tight closure at the base of the nasopharynx, nasal regurgitation may occur during feeding. Milk that enters the naso-pharynx creates nasal congestion and impairs breathing. Aspiration into the nasopharynx or the lungs increases the risk of respiratory illness, including, in severe cases, aspiration pneumonia. The LC should always listen to an infant's breathing. If an infant is congested or appears to have blocked nasal passages, this may indicate increased risk of a swallowing problem.

To facilitate safe swallowing and protect respiration in low-tone infants, use external pacing techniques when supplementing (see Ch. 14). Avoid hyperflexing or hyperextending the baby's neck during bottle feeding. Maintenance of a *patent* (open) throat protects swallowing and breathing. Allow the baby to come off the breast for a few moments during the let-down if the milk ejection is forceful or appears to overwhelm the baby. Breastfeeding positions that permit extension of the head help stabilize low tone babies.

Reflux

Spitting up milk is common in infants. It is typically not considered to be a medical problem unless infant growth is affected or the infant frequently appears to be in pain. Low muscle tone can affect the lower esophageal sphinc-ter and contribute to gastric reflux. To reduce spitting up, avoid bending the baby forward in a "V" position during burping (winding) as shown in **Fig. 354**. Bending the baby in this manner compresses the abdomen and increas-es intra-abdominal pressure causing reflux, especially if the baby's stomach is full.

Infants suffering from gastroesophageal reflux disease (GERD) grow poorly. They often cough between feeds and may fuss when placed in car seats or in positions that cause the baby to slump (Wolf and Glass 1992). Whenever a tight waistband pushes on the abdomen below the lower esophageal sphincter, compression can push the stomach contents into the esophagus.

Babies with GERD are assisted when placed in open, elongated body positions or in baby seats that allow them to lean back. Some affected infants (Fig. **355**) may benefit from being diapered while lying on their sides. Diapering on the side avoids abdominal com-pression that may occur when the baby's legs are lifted and pressed back toward the belly.

Sudden Loss of Muscle Tone as a Marker for Infant Illness

Sometimes a baby who has previously breastfed well develops hypotonia and feeding-related prob-lems. This is a marker for illness. Infants with Rett Syndrome, for example, may breastfeed normally for several months before progressive encephalopathy and loss of purposeful motor activity begin to interfere with feeding (Percy 2005).

The mother of the 9 month-old baby in **Fig. 356** became concerned about her baby, who previously breastfed well. His worsening body tone and weak suck prompted the mother to seek medical evaluation. Her baby was subsequently diagnosed and treated for a brain tumor.

Hydrocephalus

The 4 month-old baby in **Fig. 357** has hydrocephalus, a condition that results when an obstruction prevents the normal circulation and drainage of cerebrospinal fluid. Hydrocephalus is one of the most common birth defects, with an average occurrence similar to that of Down Syndrome (1 in 1000 births). The condition can be congenital (present at birth) or acquired as the result of head trauma, brain tumor, or infection. Hydrocephalus may occur as an aspect of a syndrome. Some individuals with the condition live normal lives, and function with normal intelligence. Others experience motor and learn-ing disabilities, memory deficits, and sensitivity to sound, pressure, and bright lights. The condition cannot be cured, but it can be treated. A nonprofit organization called the Hydrocephalus Foundation, Inc. maintains a website that provides families with information, support, and resources: www.hydrocephalus.org.

Treatment of hydrocephalus involves draining excess cerebrospinal fluid from the brain through an artificial shunt to another part of the body, usually the abdominal cavity or the atrium of the heart, where it can then be eliminated. This prevents build-up of fluid, enlargement of the ventricles of the brain, and dangerously increased pressure inside the skull (Eastwood 1986).

The baby pictured in **Fig. 357** was referred because at 3 months of age he suddenly refused to breastfeed from his mother's left breast. The LC concluded that pres-sure from the mother's forearm on the shunt caused the baby discomfort. Because the baby previously had been willing to breastfeed on both sides, the mother had not considered that pressure on the shunt was the problem. The LC explained that around the age of 3 months, many babies begin to develop opinions about things. This baby had decided that feeding from the left breast was uncomfortable. The LC demonstrated upright feeding positions that avoided putting pressure on this area of the baby's head. The baby then resumed feeding from both breasts.

Abnormal Posturing

Abnormal posturing of the limbs or body can reveal a temporary or enduring problem. Drug exposure, birth trauma, or neurological dysfunction can affect how a baby moves his body. Inability to move freely in utero (as in breech presentations) may result in atrophied muscles and torticollis (see Ch. 3 and **Figs. 53** and **54**). Similarly, restricted movement in utero may cause the newborn baby to move a limb abnormally.

Odd posturing is sometimes the result of injury caused by child abuse. Child abuse must be reported to the appropriate authorities; however, the LC first carefully assesses the situation and rules out other causes. The LC then should discuss concerns about abuse with the family's health care providers.

Excessive Tone and Feeding Problems

Hypertonicity (high muscle tone) caused the 6 week-old infant in **Fig. 358** to assume hyperextended body postures. His arching behavior made him difficult to position for feeding, and prompted his mother to seek help from an LC for painfully damaged nipples. The LC explained that arching contributes to jaw clenching. Hip flexion helps reduce arching and generally improves jaw stability. In the case of the infant pictured in **Fig. 358**, hip flexion also helped the mother bring the baby in closer to the breast, preventing jaw closure on the nipple shaft.

In the event of abnormal infant posturing, the LC should be aware of other conditions such as as *laryngomalacia* and *tracheomalacia*. Both conditions relate to collapse of the airway owing to structural malformation or muscular weakness. Infants with narrow or obstructed airways may assume a hyperextended neck position in order to hold the airway open (Genna 2013). Affected infants may have *stridor* (a high-pitched wheezing sound made during breathing). Unusual or noisy breathing should be reported to the infant's doctor.

Sensory Integration Issues

Some babies have difficulty integrating sensory stimulation. Light touch, sudden sounds, bright lights, and motion appear to startle and overwhelm them. The arching baby in **Fig. 358** exhibited sensory defensiveness in addition

to excessive muscle tone. Too much stimulation while feeding caused his arching to become more severe and worsened his tendency to clamp down on his mother's nipples (see Ch. 2).

The LC advised the mother to rest her nipples for a few days so they could heal. During this time, a hospital grade electric pump maintained her milk supply. The mother's doctor prescribed a topical antibiotic ointment to treat a superficial skin infection on one of her nipples. As her nipples began to heal, the mother alternated breastfeeding with pumping. Eventually, she was able to discontinue pumping. Although breastfeeding became tolerable, it was never completely comfortable. The mother noticed that her baby breastfed better in a quiet environment and when she paid careful attention to his postural stability.

Bonding Issues

During the months that they worked together, the mother of the arching baby in **Fig. 358** confided to the LC that she felt as if her baby did not love her because he was so difficult to cuddle. His stiff, rejecting body language jeopardized their bonding. It helped the mother to deal with her own feelings of rejection when the LC explained that hypertonicity was the underlying issue. Over time, the mother became more sensitive about how best to assist her son. Cobathing in a warm tub and increased skin-to-skin contact helped to relax the baby.

A different baby is pictured in **Fig. 359** being carried in the so-called "colic hold." Being held in a flexed position seems to soothe some tense infants. Carrying babies in slings can also promote physiological flexion.

At age 4, about 6 months after weaning, the child pictured in **Fig. 358** experienced a seizure that temporarily weakened his left arm. The mother speculated to the LC that perhaps his abnormal posturing in infancy was an early indication of an underlying neurological problem.

Failure to Thrive

Lawrence (2011) describes failure to thrive (FTT) in the exclusively breastfeeding baby under 6 months of age. The baby "continues to lose weight after 10 days of life, does not regain birth weight by 3 weeks of age, or gains at a rate below the 10th percentile for weight gain beyond one month of age." A weight gain of 20 g per day assigns an infant to the fifth percentile if observed between 2 and 6 weeks of age. Infants gain approximately 20 to 35 g a day (Hill 2007), with the fastest rate of growth occurring in the first 2 months, and a decrease after 3 months (Dewey 1996).

FTT presents complex issues that may be related to milk production problems, to illness or disorder in the mother or child, or to management and psychosocial problems. Typically, a combination of factors interact to cause FTT. Identifying them is vital in developing a plan to assist the infant who experiences growth faltering.

The infant with FTT differs from the slow gaining baby, who will appear thin, but alert and healthy, and whose growth is slow but consistent. An infant who is FTT may be apathetic, with a weak cry, poor muscle tone, or poor skin turgor. Such infants produce few diapers, and their urine may be dark in color and have a strong smell. They stool infrequently and fail to produce adequate numbers of yellow milk stools by the end of the first week (see Ch. 4).

Because poor growth results in poor energy, the infant with FTT may have difficulty breastfeeding owing to lack of stamina. They may conserve energy by sleeping too much. Weak feeding behavior generally persists until catch-up growth is achieved. Many infants who appear at first to have serious sucking problems feed normally once they recover lost weight and energy. Feeding the baby generously becomes the top priority; however, simultaneous attention must be directed to improving milk production.

Recovery from malnutrition ideally is achieved with human milk feeds (Graham 1996). Supplementation with donor milk or formula may be temporarily or permanently required if the mother has an insufficient milk supply. An infant with FTT who has never experienced a full feeding may not initially be able to consume all the supplement offered. It may take several days before the baby is able to take in appropriate volumes at each feeding. Small, frequent feedings will improve the baby's physiologic capacity (Powers 2001).

Increase in Breastfeeding Malnutrition and the Risks of Dehydration

Hypernatremic dehydration is a potentially devastating and life-threatening disorder that can damage the central nervous system. Breastfeeding infants who lose excessive weight after delivery are at risk. Lawrence (2011) states that: "A loss of 7 percent is average for breastfed infants... when this occurs in the first 72 hours of life, a clinician should be alert to breastfeeding problems and should review the process. A loss of 10 percent is the maximum for breastfed baby." Unal (2008) retrospectively identified a 4.1 percent incidence of hypernatremic dehydration secondary to inadequate breastfeeding in a group of 169 hospitalized term infants.

Dehydration poses serious risks to the neonate including brain shrinkage, venous thrombosis, and subdural capillary hemorrhage. Unsupervised rehydration of the severely dehydrated infant without balancing electrolytes may cause cerebral edema, subsequent seizures, and death (Rand 2001). The US National Library of Medicine - National Institutes of Health (NIH) website describes signs and symptoms of dehydration in infants (www.nlm.nih.gov 2013):

- Sunken eyes
- Sunken fontanelles (the soft spot on the head)
- Poor skin turgor (the skin lacks elasticity and when pinched does not spring back into place)
- Dry mouth; absence of tears
- Dark colored urine
- Lack of wet diapers over many hours
- Lethargic appearance, low blood pressure
- Cold limbs
- Rapid heart rate

Mothers are sometimes unable to recognize acute conditions such as dehydration, or chronic issues such as FTT. They may think that they have a very "good" baby, when, in fact, the baby is lethargic (Neifert 1996). Some parents mistake poor stooling for constipation and hunger cries for colic.

Risk Factors for Failure to Thrive

- Prematurity/SGA
- Multiple births
- Physical anomalies of mother or baby
- Maternal or infant illness
- Breast surgery
- Retained placental fragment
- Transient or enduring infant neurological issues
- Difficulty latching and painful feedings
- Psychosocial or psychophysiologic issues
- Long labor
- History of sexual abuse
- Lack of social support
- Poor lactation management
- Scheduling and/or time-limited feedings

A careful history of both the mother and the baby must be taken to rule out organic reasons for poor growth. Failure to thrive beyond 1 month of age is associated with organic illness of the mother or the baby (Lukefahr 1990).

Telephone counselors must be alert to questions that may indicate that a baby is feeding poorly. Mothers who complain of sore nipples or severe engorgement may have infants who are not breastfeeding well. Some mothers express concerns that their diet does not agree with the baby, causing fussiness that they blame on "gas" or reflux rather than hunger. Other mothers call to ask how to help the baby sleep more or sleep less. Parents who request help to deal with excessive crying should be encouraged to seek a weight check, especially if inquiries about the infant's voiding and stooling pattern reveal low output (Neifert 1996). Test weights provide accurate milk intake information (Hill 2007).

The use of galactagogues such as domperidone (where available) or metoclopramide may be considered to assist the woman's milk supply (da Silva 2001). However, blood tests may be prudent to first document low prolactin levels. If prolactin is not deficient, a prolactin enhancing drug is unlikely to enhance milk production.

Because many breastfeeding mothers are released from the hospital on Day 2, before their milk supply has been established, it is important for all babies to receive appropriately timed post-discharge follow-up. Hospitals should provide clear instructions for parents describing the warning signs of poor intake (scant stooling, excessive crying, lethargy). At-risk dyads should be promptly referred for breastfeeding support from their pediatricians (AAP 2012). Pediatricians must document the recovery of infants who lose excessive weight, utilizing weighing and referral to lactation support (Iyer 2008).

A reporting tool was designed to facilitate early follow-up of at-risk, breastfeeding dyads (Wilson-Clay 2002). The one-page checklist may be faxed at the time of hospital discharge to alert the pediatrician. The *High Risk Report Form* is obtainable from www.BreastfeedingMaterials. com at no cost, and may be reproduced.

Ethical Issues Related to FTT

The LC who encounters an infant with apparent growth failure has an ethical obligation to refer the baby for medical evaluation. The LC assists by sharing information about the infant's feeding behavior and the mother's health history, which may be relevant and often is unknown to the baby's doctor. The LC shares information about the impact of difficult delivery on infant breastfeeding behavior (Chen 1998), and on conditions that affect milk production such as: maternal anemia (Henly 1995), postpartum hemorrhage (Willis 1995), previous breast surgery (Neifert 1990, Hughes 1993, West 2001), breast and nipple anatomy (Neifert 1985), maternal illness (Neifert 1990), medications, and acute or chronic conditions (Neubauer 1993, Betzold 2004).

Consequences of FTT

A group of British researchers compared a group of 6 year olds who had failed to thrive in infancy. These children were below the third percentile for at least 3 months. At age 6, the children who had FTT were "considerably smaller than matched comparisons, in terms of body mass index, and height and weight." (Boddy 2000). Results correspond to past research indicating that non-organic failure to thrive is associated with persistent limitations in physical stature. Consequently, supplementation may be critical. Williams (2002) suggests that LCs should praise the mother's efforts while validating her grief over not being able to exclusively breastfeed. The LC should help the mother find additional methods of nurturing. For example, to promote intimacy, the mother may use a feeding tube worn at the breast, co-bathe, and wear the baby in a cloth carrier.

Management Strategies for the Infant with FTT

The infant in **Fig. 360** is 35 days old. He was examined by his pediatrician on the day the photo was taken. The baby had gained only 5 oz (142 g) above his birth weight of 8 lb (3629 g). The LC was called to assist with supplementation at the breast and to help the mother increase her milk supply. The LC showed the mother how to improve positioning and taught her how to use a feeding tube device. Her weak baby needed constant stimulation to continue sucking, but in this case, the feeding tube device improved his intake. After brief practice, the baby took 2.5 ounces (71 ml) of formula at the breast from the device. This supplementation plan was followed until the baby regained sufficient strength to breastfeed without the feeding tube. Pumping and more effective breastfeeding resulted in improved milk production.

A similar situation occurred with an 18 day-old baby seen by KH, who weighed 1 pound (454 g) below his birth weight of 6 lb 11 oz (3033 g). Someone advised his mother to offer the baby a little water each day. She began feeding him 6 ounces of water daily. The LC speculated that excessive water intake decreased his appetite for milk. The mother was advised to discontinue water supplementation. She briefly used formula supplements to help stabilize the baby's growth. The LC helped the mother improve her breastfeeding technique and milk supply. Her baby then gained weight.

BWC worked with another infant with FTT who was 18 days old. Born at 38 weeks, his birth weight was 7 lb 3 oz

(3260 g). He weighed 6 lb 12 oz (3058 g) at a pediatric check-up on Day 10. When the LC weighed him on Day 19, he had lost another 3 oz (85 g). The baby was visibly jaundiced on his face, trunk, and extremities. The LC observed white lesions in the baby's mouth characteristic of infant thrush. The mother (who had an obsessive-compulsive disorder and who showered 4 to 5 times each day) did not develop sore nipples.

The baby in **Fig. 361** is 75 days old, and 2 oz (60 g) below birth weight. The mother had a history of insufficient milk with her first baby. This baby rarely cried, and when she did, the cry sounded weak. Notice the skin folds on the baby's arm and her worried look which is characteristic of infants who are failing to thrive. The mother had just begun using a feeding tube device, and had called the LC to ask for other suggestions to improve her situation. The LC called the doctor to discuss the the baby's condition, and the mother became upset and discontinued the relationship with LC. The LC was advised by a colleague to carefully document her role in the case, but never had any additional contact with either the mother or the baby's physician.

The baby in **Fig. 362** also is FTT. Observe the worried-alert expression, This first-time mother adhered to a rigid feeding schedule. She limited the baby to 10 minute feeds on each breast. The mother reported that her baby cried a lot with "colic" during his first week. Since then, he had appeared lethargic and was difficult to rouse for feedings. The picture shows marked lip retraction, a sign of poor lip tone. (See also **Fig. 29**). The baby typically closed his eyes early in the breastfeeding session, often a sign of weak or stressed feeding or lack of milk transfer. The infant's jaw excursions were short, choppy, and irregular. He was unable to sustain 10 to 30 sucks before pausing, and he paused more than he sucked. These are markers both of weakness and of an immature, disorganized suck (Bu'Lock 1990, Palmer 1993).

A test weight revealed that the baby ingested less than 1 ounce (24 ml) of milk in a 15-minute feeding before becoming exhausted and falling asleep. The LC calculated that the baby needed a minimum of 19 oz (537 ml) of milk per 24 hours to regain his birth weight. If fed 8 times per 24 hours, milk intake volumes would average 2.3 ounces (66 ml) at each feeding. If a baby is below birth weight, the LC should calculate the volume of milk needed using the baby's birth weight, not the baby's present weight. This allows for catch-up growth. Powers (2010) provides guidelines for determining appropriate volumes of supplementation for the infant with low intake and poor growth. To determine the total

volume of milk (or formula) required from 1 week to 3 month, take the baby's weight in pounds and multiply by 2.5. This gives the number of ounces of milk the baby needs during each 24 hours. Using grams, calculate 150-200 ml per kilogram (kg) per 24 hours.

The LC devised an intervention designed to simultaneously increase the infant's daily caloric intake and to improve maternal milk production. The mother of this FTT infant was a heavy smoker. The LC suggested she cut back to 10 daily cigarettes, and to smoke immediately after breastfeeding. Such timing allows nicotine metabolites to decrease in breast milk prior to the next breastfeeding, theoretically reducing the exposure to the infant (Labrecque 1989).

In order to stimulate milk production, the mother was instructed to double pump with a hospital grade electric pump for 15 minutes after at least 6 daily breastfeeding sessions. She was told to feed 2 oz of pumped milk or formula by bottle at each feed in an effort to achieve catch-up growth. The baby had previously averaged 7 breastfeeds per 24 hours. The LC recommended increasing the frequency to 10 breastfeeds per 24 hours. Half of the supplement was offered at the beginning of each feed to give the baby energy to effectively breastfeed. The second ounce (28 g) was offered when the baby appeared to tire at the breast, or if he acted unsatisfied after breastfeeding. The mother was taught to use deep breast compression whenever the the baby paused longer than 10 seconds while breastfeeding (see **Fig. 353**).

A follow-up appointment was scheduled to take place in 36 hours to weigh the infant. The infant gained 6 ounces (170 g) by the next visit and was more alert. His color, tone, and skin turgor had improved, and he breastfed with greater stamina and better coordination. Test weights performed during the visit verified improved intake. The mother reported that post-feed pumping had resulted in her breasts feeling fuller. She had reduced her cigarette consumption, although not to the desired level, and was pleased at the improvements in her situation.

Follow-up and Outcome Monitoring

The LC maintained telephone contact with this mother for several weeks in order to monitor the effectiveness of the interventions. The baby's bilirubin level dropped quickly as his milk intake increased and stooling became more frequent. The mother was soon able to discontinue formula, but continued using pumped milk to supplement the baby until he regained and surpassed his birth weight. At this point, the baby was fully breastfed and gaining weight normally.

Follow-up is critical when an infant presents with FTT. Close monitoring and communication with the pediatrician permits the LC to revise interventions as needed. If the infant does not begin to gain weight with improved breastfeeding management and increased milk intake, further diagnostic evaluation is required to rule out illness.

Case Management of an Infant with Turner Syndrome

The baby whose unusually-shaped foot is pictured in **Fig. 363** has Turner Syndrome (TS), a chromosomal disorder of females. Girls with TS typically experience growth stunting and most do not achieve normal stature without growth hormones. Ovarian failure is a notable characteristic of TS. Most affected girls are infertile and require estrogen supplementation to stimulate puberty (Hagman 2010). Other problems may be associated with TS, such as cardiac and renal disorders, hearing loss, and hypothyroidism. Physical malformations associated with TS include neck webbing, puffy feet and toes without toenails, unusually shaped palates, and micrognathia. Weak muscle tone is common in infancy. Infants with TS typically experience feeding problems (Skuse 1994a), generally thought to result from palate abnormalities and low tone.

Fig. 364 shows a grooved (channel) palate. While some grooved palates are the result of erosion from intubation (see **Fig. 408**), many syndromes, such as TS, affect palatal formation. Abnormally formed hard palates may create feeding problems similar to those associated with cleft palate (see Ch. 18). Once babies become old enough for solids, parents should check the palatal grove to remove accumulated food. BWC worked with a baby with TS who had just learned to crawl. The baby's mother phoned to report a nursing strike. BWC advised the mother to check the palatal groove. A wad of soggy paper was wedged in the groove. Once it was removed, the baby breastfed normally.

The infant whose foot is pictured in **Fig. 363** is also pictured in **Fig. 21**. Note the tape covering her ear. Another characteristic of TS is rotated ears that fold over on themselves. The baby's pediatrician recalled hearing a lecture on the subject of *auricular* (ear) malformation. He contacted a plastic surgeon who splinted the baby's ears with a soft material (dental compound) held in place by tape. Because ear cartiledge is very malleable in the neonatal period, auricular splinting for several weeks produces excellent cosmetic results in correcting malformed

ears (Brown 1986). The parents of this infant wanted to normalize her appearance in every possible way, because girls with TS often suffer from low self-esteem owing to their short statures (Skuse 1994b, Nabhan 2011).

The infant with TS pictured in **Figs. 21** and **363** was the second child of a mother who had successfully breastfed her first baby. After a difficult birth, the baby was delivered vaginally at 38 weeks, weighing 5 lb 14 oz (2665 g). Preterm and late preterm births occur more often in TS pregnancies, and these babies are typically smaller for gestation age than controls (Hagman 2010). These little girls are going to be small in stature, so it makes sense that they would be smaller at birth; however, girls with TS share many of the characteristics and risk factors of SGA.

Infants who are SGA have special nutritional and energy requirements. At 9 months, girls who were SGA (but not boys) fed enriched formula had a significant developmental disadvantage compared to a breastfed comparison group (Morley 2004). Breastfed infants of both sexes had scored significantly higher on mental and psychomotor assessment compared to formula fed infants at both 9 and 18 months of age, and at school age (Slykerman 2005). Breastfeeding is especially beneficial for cognitive development of children who are born SGA. Children born SGA are at risk for development of the metabolic syndrome, and girls with TS are also at increased risk for abnormal lipid profiles and obesity (Nabhan 2011).

The baby in **Fig. 363** had additional challenges. Her head was engaged in the mother's pelvis for some weeks prior to birth, creating some cranial misshaping. The difficult delivery contributed to the formation of large, bilateral cephalohematomas (seen in **Fig. 21**). Because of cranial bruising, the baby had elevated bilirubin levels and jaundice-related lethargy. She required aggressive suctioning at delivery owing to meconium aspiration. Her vocal chords were temporarily injured, resulting in hoarse vocalizations that persisted for several months. In adults, such injury typically causes a sore throat that may interfere with swallowing.

The day before the LC visit, the baby was fitted for a hip harness to correct hip dysplasia, which the pediatrician attributed to low muscle tone caused by TS. The hip harness further complicated breastfeeding. It was difficult for the mother to find a comfortable feeding position that allowed her to draw the baby close. The baby is seen in **Fig. 365** breastfeeding in the cross-cradle position. This feeding position and a firm nursing pillow helped the mother hold the baby more comfortably.

Like many babies with TS, this baby had a heart defect; a *coarctation* (narrowing) of the aorta and a malformation of the aortal valve. The heart defect required surgery to correct. The doctor informed the parents that excellent early growth was necessary to stabilize the baby prior to surgery. Unfortunately, owing to the many risk factors in her case, the baby breastfed poorly. She fell asleep at breast after a few minutes, and her intake was low.

Luckily, this mother was extremely motivated to breastfeed. She was willing to follow the multi-faceted intervention plan to preserve exclusive human milk feeding until unassisted breastfeeding could be achieved. The mother had a history of milk oversupply. While this had been a problem for her first child, robust milk production and a strong milk ejection reflex compensated for the new baby's weak suck. A nipple shield was occasionally used to block the forceful milk spray, especially during the time when the baby's hoarse crying suggested a sore throat. The nipple shield increased the baby's oral responsiveness, and seemed to stimulate her to suck longer.

Careful attention to positioning and good postural support compensated for this baby's weak muscle tone and the interference caused by the hip harness. The mother used deep breast compression while she breastfed to help improve milk transfer. She pumped after some of the feedings to protect her milk supply. Hindmilk was used to supplement breastfeeding. A rental scale allowed the parents to carefully track the baby's growth, and helped them know how much supplemental milk to provide. The infant was diagnosed with reflux, not unusual in low tone babies. Frequent, small feeds appeared to be more comfortable for her than large, widely-spaced feeds.

At the 2 month pediatric check-up the baby had grown at the rate of one ounce (28.35 g) per day on exclusive human milk feeds. This achievement surprised both the pediatrician and the endocrinologist who was working with the family. The baby nearly doubled her birth weight by 4 months. At 5 months the baby had surgery to repair the aortic arch. The baby weighed 13 lb 7 oz (6095 g) at 6 months, and was 26 inches long. After the surgery, her energy improved significantly and she was able to breastfeed with no further need for supplementation with pumped milk. Girls with TS demonstrate differences in mandibular growth (Simmons 1999). Because the activity of breastfeeding positively benefits orofacial development, extended breastfeeding may benefit the child with TS.

Finally, because growth normally slows in the breastfed baby between 5 and 6 months, it is important for infants

with conditions that impact physical stature to achieve excellent early growth. This may help such children realize their maximum growth potential.

BWC has maintained contact with the mother of another girl with TS for many years. This child, while challenging to feed in infancy, achieved excellent early growth with exclusive human milk feeds. She was breastfed for 5 years. When the girl was 8 years old, her mother wrote: "Our daughter continues to surprise her endocrinologist by growing. She is in the 50th percentile. So far there is still no talk of growth hormones." The mother wrote again 6 years later when her daughter started high school to say: "...she has never been the shortest in her class. She is very healthy in general, doing very well in all her classes, and is maturing in her body, but has not begun having periods yet."

While TS is rare, the LC will encounter other types of complicated cases. Such cases remind the LC that lactation assessment must be thorough. All relevant issues must be identified, reported to the entire health care team, and managed in an integrated way to achieve optimal outcomes.

Infant Surgery

Human milk provides optimal nutrition and immune protection for the infant who is ill or who requires surgery in the neonatal period. Anti-inflammatory properties (Diehl-Jones 2004) and epidermal growth factor (Dvorak 2003) accelerate healing. Thus, human milk feeds are important for the 14 day-old infant pictured in **Fig. 366**, who is recovering from heart surgery performed on Day 4. Cardiac problems create risks for poor feeding before and after surgery. Babies with heart defects require careful monitoring to assure adequate intake.

Infant cardiac patients commonly display poor stamina for feeding. It is important to ensure that they are consuming sufficient calories; however, often their fluid intake is medically restricted. Their care requires careful medical supervision. Communication between the doctor and the LC is critical. It is important to protect the milk supply with post-feed pumping until the baby is stronger.

Maternal stress may affect milk production (Chatterton 2000) or impair the milk ejection reflex. Such stress is common whenever an infant is hospitalized. Oxytocin spray or prolactin-stimulating drugs may assist the mother whose milk supply temporarily falters. Social support and relaxation techniques may also help. Temporary use of banked donor milk, if available, is an option until the stituation stabilizes.

Prematurity and Breastfeeding

The US Centers for Disease Control (2013) reports that 1 of every 9 infants in the US is born prior to 37 weeks gestational age. Preterm births cost the health care system $26 billion each year, and accounted for 35 percent of all infant deaths in the US in 2008. Preterm birth has been described as a "social disease," occurring at higher rates when the mother is poor, has a low educational level, is isolated, single, or too young (Snyder 2004). The percentage of incidence of preterm birth is also increasing in affluent women, owing to advanced maternal age at the time of conception and multi-fetal pregnancies conceived with reproductive technology. These highly vulnerable infants and their mothers require specialized interventions to protect breastfeeding.

The benefits of human milk for preterm infants are reviewed in Ch. 15, and have been well-documented. In spite of increased awareness of these benefits, the percentage of preterm infants who are discharged breastfeeding is low. Siddell (2003) noted that 30 to 70 percent of mothers with babies in the NICU discontinue their efforts to breastfeed prior to the infant's hospital discharge. The period of time shortly after hospital discharge is especially difficult for families. Transitioning to full breastfeeding may be complicated, and mothers require specific help to achieve the goal. Women often report a lack of confidence in their own abilities to determine whether the baby is "getting enough."

The preterm infant has likely been separated from his mother and experiences stressful interventions such as intubations, that might result in the development of oral aversion (Abadie 2001). Bonding opportunities are interrupted, creating the potential for attachment disorders. This may explain the higher reported rates of child abuse and abandonment in preterm infants. In one study, 30 mothers who delivered preterm infants all displayed at least one symptom of post-traumatic stress (Holditch-Davis 2003). Breastfeeding is protective against child abandonment (Mata 1988) and appears to lessen the severity of maternal post-traumatic stress disorders and maternal depression (Kendall-Tackett 2013).

Evidence-based models exist that demonstrate how NICU staff may provide optimal breastfeeding support (Meier 2013). Education about the benefits and protective aspects of breastfeeding can change the knowledge and attitudes of NICU nurses (Siddell 2003). However, supporting breastfeeding in the neonatal intensive care setting should not be optional, based on culture, or be solely the responsi-

bility of the lactation consultant. All staff must be trained to deliver consistent information, and be held accountable for executing policies that provide individualized care based on established best practices (Meier 2013).

Storing and Pumping Milk for Preterm Infants

Clear instructions on hygiene are important to prevent infection in the special care nursery environment. Mothers should be instructed to wash their hands and gently scrub under their fingernails prior to pumping. Pump exteriors should be disinfected between users. Sterilizing wipes should be placed on the pump carts, and each mother using the pump should be taught to clean the exterior prior to use. Pump kits should be washed carefully in soap and water after use. Bottles should be turned upside down to dry and covered with a clean towel (D'Amico 2003). Mothers should rinse off their nipples with clear water prior to pumping (Hurst 2004). These practices help prevent the spread of infection and prevent milk contamination.

Pumping to protect the milk supply is the *key intervention* in preserving the option to breastfeed for mothers with preterm infants. Even when preterm infants are given early access to the breast, which should be encouraged, they are seldom capable of initiating and maintaining a full milk supply. Nyqvist (2008) explored the breastfeeding behavior of very preterm infants and documented rooting and short sucking bursts in infants of 29 weeks. Full breastfeeding was attained between 32 and 38 weeks. Time to attainment of full breastfeeding may not occur until 40 weeks for some preterm infants. Palmer (1993) identified transitional sucking patterns in preterm infants that differ from those of term infants. Mothers should be counseled to maintain reasonable expectations of infant feeding behavior until the infant matures. Outcomes obviously depend on many factors. Careful growth monitoring is vital.

Mothers should begin pumping as soon as their own condition permits, ideally within an hour of birth (Meier 2013). Hill (1999) found that expressing milk a minimum of 6 times per day was associated with maintenance of 500 ml/day milk production. This volume is considered to be the minimum level of production to sustain a preterm infant at discharge, but it is unlikely to be adequate as the infant grows. Mothers who pumped at lower frequencies were unlikely to produce adequate milk supplies. Hill observed that the level of milk production reached by week 3 is likely to be maintained in subsequent weeks. It is therefore optimal for pump-dependent women to achieve an early *bountiful* supply, not just the small volumes needed by the preterm infant in the first days.

Mothers should be instructed to pump 8 to 10 times per day so that they are making a normal volume of milk when the infant is discharged.

Staff and parents should be trained to recognize normal and expected milk production volumes and to employ pumping schedules that mimic physiologic norms. Under ideal circumstances, a healthy, term infant removes 6-15 ml of colostrum during the first 24 hours after birth in 10 breastfeedings. By Day 4 to 7, milk volumes increase to 500 to 600 ml/day. This information should be used to create production targets for mothers. Pumping logs help mothers remember when to pump, and provide records of pumped milk volumes and hours spent in skin-to-skin care (Hoover 2010). Deviations from expected volumes should prompt immediate investigation and intervention.

Jones (2001) identified a significant increase in milk production with double pumping. Breast massage and hand expression combined with pumping increases milk volumes (Morton 2009). Hill (2001) reported that average pumping time per session was less significant in influencing milk production than was frequency of pumping.

The preterm infant seen in **Fig. 367** is being held skin-to-skin, also called "kangaroo care." Hill (1999) identified time spent in kangaroo care and frequency of pumping as being significantly related to improved milk production.

Evidence-based Interventions to Support Mothers of Preterm Infants

Programs such as the Rush Mothers' Milk Club (Rush-Presbyterian St. Luke's Medical Center, Chicago, Ilinois) have devised effective, evidence-based interventions to help mothers of preterm infants establish full milk supplies (Meier 2003, 2013). Although the low income, predominantly African American mothers in this urban hospital have significant risk factors for weaning, they achieve the most positive breastfeeding outcomes for preterm infants reported in the literature. Lactation initation rates in this program are 98 percent, with an average daily dose of human milk that exceeds 60 ml/k/day. The postnatal timing of high doses of human milk is important because of the need to promote optimal gut colonization and to protect the preterm infant from exposure to bovine products associated with higher morbidity and mortality.

The Rush interventions (Meier 2013) include:

- Consistent, standardized information from all staff that includes the message: "Your milk is a medicine that helps protect your baby from health problems and complications during and after the NICU hospitalization."
- Weekly educational luncheons for mothers that include scientific explanations about how human milk protects the baby, and a forum for families to share concerns.
- Free transportation so that mothers may attend the weekly meetings.
- Specially trained peer counselors available 7 days a week who interact with and teach the mothers in the NICU, by phone, and during home visits after discharge.
- Early initiation of breast stimulation with hospital grade pumps to establish a milk supply of approximately 1000 ml/day.
- Instruction of mothers in methods of safely pumping, handling, warming and feeding their milk, and techniques on how to separate foremilk from hindmilk, perform creamatocrits, and perform test weights to determine infant intake during breastfeedings.
- Skin-to-skin holding as the standard of care.
- Providing 0.2 ml of freshly expressed colostrum to the infant in the NICU (preferably fed by the father) as soon as feasible.
- Providing initial enteral feedings by gavage (intermittent bolus feedings rather than continuous to minimize bacterial growth and optimize delivery of nutrients.)
- Providing extubated infants opportunities to taste milk from the breast and to suck on an emptied breast while held skin-to-skin.
- Adjusting the size of pump flanges as needed
- Using nipple shields to assist with latch and to increase milk intake during breastfeeding sessions.
- Verbal and printed instruction on how to transition to cue-based feeding, with continued test weights on home-rental scales to permit careful monitoring of growth until the infant reaches term.
- Discharge instructions about pumping to protect the milk supply until the infant is competent to maintain production.
- Individual supervision until all interventions can be discontinued on a time table that is based on the individual infant's progress.

Because of infants' physiological immaturity and owing to maternal concerns about milk adequacy, the transition from special care nursery to the home can be stressful for the breastfeeding mother. Special support is required to overcome challenges and mothers may be motivated by information about specific benefits of at-breast feedings for these babies (Buckley 2006). If this support is deficient, the demands of pumping and supplementing often result in the abandonment of lactation.

Test Weighing

Because preterm infants lack predictable feeding behaviors and manifest indistinct behavioral cues, they require vigilance regarding their growth. Concern about adequacy of feeding is a source of anxiety for their mothers. Families worry about milk intake during the vulnerable period of transition from hospital to home (Kavanaugh 1995). Clinical observation of breastfeeding (audible swallowing, changes in breast fullness, etc.) does not provide accurate or reliable information on the milk intake of preterm infants (Meier 1996). Weighing on sensitive, reliable scales permits appropriate calculation of supplementation, and assists in the management of the preterm infant, especially after hospital discharge.

Test weighing does not undermine maternal confidence (Hill 2007). Hurst (2004) examined maternal reactions and breastfeeding outcomes in a group of mothers performing in-home test weights compared to a matched group who did not use test weights in the 4 weeks following discharge. All of the women in the test weight group reported that in-home measurement of milk intake had been "very" or "extremely" helpful to them. Approximately 35 percent stated that the use of the scale made them "somewhat" nervous; however, they reported that weighing helped them transition to cue-based breastfeeding. In the group of mothers who did not weigh, 75 percent indicated that in-home measurement of milk intake would have been "somewhat" to "extremely" helpful to them. These women felt that weighing would have relieved the stress of trying to decide how much extra milk to provide.

Kavenaugh (1995) reported that in the absence of real information about intake, mothers gave extra bottles "just to be sure." The lack of evidence documenting increased maternal stress or anxiety as the result of test weighing indicates that the prejudice against it should be reexamined. Test weights are a crucial tool for practitioners and parents. They can be used to evaluate intake when infants are immature, ill, or when they exhibit ambiguous feeding cues.

Abadie V, Andre A, Zaouche A, et al. Early feeding resistance: a possible consequence of neonatal oro-oesophageal dyskinesia. *Acta Paediatrica* 2001; 90(7):738-745.

American Academy of Pediatrics Section on Breastfeeding (AAP). Breastfeeding and the use of human milk. *Pediatrics* 2012; 129(2):e827-841.

Betzold C, Hoover K, Snyder C. Delayed lactogenesis II: a comparison of four cases. *Journal of Midwifery and Women's Health* 2004; 49(3):132-137.

Boddy J, Skuse D, Andrews B. The developmental sequelae of nonorganic failure to thrive. *Journal of Child Psychology and Psychiatry* 2000; 41(8):1003-1004.

Brown F, Colen L, Addante R, et al. Correction of congenital auricular deformities by splinting in the neonatal period. *Pediatrics* 1986; 78(3):406-411.

Bu'Lock F, Woolridge MW, Baum JD. Development of co-ordination of sucking, swallowing and breathing: ultrasound study of term and preterm infants. *Developmental Medicine and Child Neurology* 1990; 32(8):669-678.

Buckley KM, Charles GE. Benefits and challenges of transitioning preterm infants to at-breast feedings. *International Breastfeeding Journal* 2006; 1:13.

Chatterton R, Hill P, Aldag J, et al. Relation of plasma oxytocin and prolactin concentrations to milk production in mothers of preterm infants: influence of stress. *Journal of Clinical Endocrinology & Metabolism* 2000; 85(10):3661-3668.

Chen D, Nommsen-Rivers L, Dewey K, et al. Stress during labor and delivery and early lactation performance. *American Journal of Clinical Nutrition* 1998; 68(2):335-345.

Cronk C, Crocker AC, Pueschel SM, et al. Growth charts for children with Down Syndrome: 1 month to 18 years of age. *Pediatrics* 1988; 81(1):102-110.

Danner S, Cerutti E. *Nursing Your Neurologically Impaired Baby* (2nd edition) Waco, TX : Childbirth Graphics, 1990.

da Silva O, Knoppert D, Angelini M, et al. Effect of domperidone on milk production in mothers of premature newborns: a randomized, double-blind, placebo-controlled trial. *Canadian Medical Association Journal* 2001; 164(1):17-21.

D'Amico C, DiNardo C, Krystofiak S. Preventing contamination of breast pump kit attachments in the NICU. *Journal of Perinatal and Neonatal Nursing* 2003; 17(2):150-157.

Davenport S. The child with multiple congenital anomalies. *Pediatric Annals* 1990; 19(1):23-33.

Dennis CL, McQueen K. The relationship between infant-feeding outcomes and postpartum depression: a qualitative systematic review. *Pediatrics* 2009; 123(4): e736-751.

Dewey KG, Cohen RJ, Rivera LL, et al. Do exclusively breastfed infants require extra protein? *Pediatric Research* 1996; 39(2):303-307.

Diehl-Jones W, Askin D. Nutritional modulation of neonatal outcomes. *AACN Clinical Issues* 2004; 15(1):83-96.

Dvorak B, Fituch CC, Williams CS, et al. Increased epidermal growth factor levels in human milk of mothers with extremely premature infants. *Pediatric Research* 2003; 54(1):15-19.

Eastwood S (editor). *About Hydrocephalus: A Book for Parents*. San Francisco: University of California Press, 1986.

Ekstrom A, Nissen E. A mother's feelings for her infant are strengthened by excellent breastfeeding counseling and continuity of care. *Pediatrics* 2006; 118(2):e309-314.

Genna CW. The influence of anatomic and structural issues on sucking skills. In *Supporting Sucking Skills in Breastfeeding Infants*, ed. CW Genna. Burlington, MA: Jones and Bartlett Learning, 2013; p, 232-234.

Graham G, MacLean W, Brown K, et al. Protein requirements of infants and children: growth during recovery from malnutrition. *Pediatrics* 1996; 97(4):499-505.

Gunderson EP, Lewis CE, Wei GS. Lactation and changes in maternal metabolic risk factors. *Obstetrics and Gynecology* 2007; 109(3):729-738.

Hagman A, Wennerholm UB. Kallen K, et al. Women who give birth to girls with Turner syndrome: maternal and neonatal characteristics. *Human Reproduction* 2010; 25(6):1553-1560.

Hall R, Mercer A, Teasley S, et al. A breast-feeding assessment score to evaluate the risk for cessation of breast-feeding by 7 to 10 days of age. *Journal of Pediatrics* 2002; 141(5):659-64.

Henly S, Anderson C, Avery M, et al. Anemia and insufficient milk in first-time mothers. *Birth* 1995; 22(2):87-92.

Hill P, Aldag J, Chatterton R. Effects of pumping style on milk production in mothers of non-nursing preterm infants. *Journal of Human Lactation* 1999; 15(3):209-216.

Hill P, Aldag J, Chatterton R. Initiation and frequency of pumping and milk production in mothers of non-nursing preterm infants. *Journal of Human Lactation* 2001; 17(1):9-13.

Hill PD, Johnson TS. Assessment of breastfeeding and infant growth. *Journal of Midwifery and Womens Health* 2007; 52(6):571-578.

Holditch-Davis D, Bartlett T, Blickman A, et al. Posttraumatic stress symptoms in mothers of premature infants. *Journal of Obstetric, Gynecologic, and Neonatal Nursing* 2003; 32(2):161-171.

Hoover K, Wilson-Clay B. *Pumping Milk for Your Preterm Baby*, Manchaca, TX :BreastfeedingMaterials.com, 2010.

Hopman E, Csizmadia C, Bastiani W, et al. Eating habits of young children with Down Syndrome in The Netherlands: adequate nutrient intakes but delayed introduction of solid food. *Journal of the American Dietetic Association* 1998; 98(7):790-794.

Hughes V, Owen J. Is breast-feeding possible after breast surgery? *Maternal Child Nursing* 1993; 18(4):213-217.

Hurst N, Meier P, Engstrom J, et al. Mothers performing in-home measurement of milk intake during breastfeeding of their preterm infants: maternal reactions and feeding outcomes. *Journal of Human Lactation* 2004; 20(2):178-187.

Iyer NP, Srinivasan R, Evans K. Impact of an early weighing policy on neonatal hypernatraemic dehydration and breastfeeding. *Archives of Disease in Childhood* 2008; 93(4):297-299.

Jones E, Dimmock P, Spencer S. A randomized controlled trial to compare methods of milk expression after preterm delivery. *Archives of Diseases in Children* 2001; 85(2):F91-F95.

Jonas W, Nissen E, Ransjo-Arvidson AB. Short- and long-term decrease of blood pressure in women during breastfeeding. *Breastfeeding Medicine* 2008; 3(2):103-109.

Kavanaugh K, Mead L, Meier P, et al. Getting enough: mothers' concerns about breastfeeding a preterm infant after discharge. *Journal of Obstetric, Gynecologic, and Neonatal Nursing* 1995; 24(1):23-32.

Kendall-Tackett K, Cong Z, Hale TW. Depression, sleep quality, and maternal well-being in postpartum women with a history of sexual assault: a comparison of breastfeeding, mixed-feeding, and formula-feeding mothers. *Breastfeeding Medicine* 2013; 8(1):16-22.

Kramer M, Aboud F, Mironova E, et al. Breastfeeding and child cognitive development. *Archives of General Psychiatry* 2008; 65(5):578-584.

Labbok M, Hendershot G. Does breastfeeding protect against malocclusion? An analysis of the 1981 child health supplement to the national health interview survey. *American Journal of Preventative Medicine* 1987; 3(4):227-232.

Labrecque M, Marcoux S, Weber J, et al. Feeding and urine cotinine values in babies whose mothers smoke. *Pediatrics* 1989; 83(1):93-97.

Lanting C, Fidler V, Huisman M, et al. Neurological differences between 9-year-old children fed breast-milk or formula-milk as babies. *Lancet* 1994; 344(8933):1319-22.

Lawrence RA, Lawrence RM. *Breastfeeding: A Guide for the Medical Profession* (7th edition), Maryland Heights, MO: Elsevier Mosby, 2011; pp. 338; 343-349.

Lubetzky R, Vaisman N, Mimouni F, et al. Energy expenditure in human milk -versus formul-fed preterm infants. *Journal of Pediatrics* 2003; 143(6):750-753.

Lukefahr J. Underlying illness associated with failure to thrive in breast-fed infants. *Clinical Pediatrics* 1990; 29(8):468-470.

Mannel R. Defining lactation acuity to improve patient safety and outcomes. *Journal of Human Lactation* 2011; 27(2):163-170.

Mata L, Saenz P, Araya JR, et al. Promotion of breastfeeding in Costa Rica: the Puriscal study, in *Programmes to Promote Breastfeeding*, ed. DB Jelliffe, EFP Jelliffe, Oxford, England: Oxford University Press. 1988, pp. 55-69.

McBride M, Danner S. Sucking disorders in neurologically impaired infants: assessment and facilitation of breastfeeding. *Clinics in Perinatology* 1987; 14(1):109-130.

Meier P. Supporting lactation in mothers with very low birth weight infants. *Pediatric Annals* 2003; 32(5):317-325.

Meier P, Engstrom J, Fleming B, et al. Estimating milk intake of hospitalized preterm infants who breastfeed. *Journal of Human Lactation* 1996; 12(1):21-26.

Meier PP, Patel AL, Bigger HR, et al. Supporting breastfeeding in the neonatal intensive care unit: Rush Mother's Milk Club as a case study of evidence-based care. *Pediatric Clinics of North America* 2013; 60(1):209-226.

Mizuno K, Ueda A. Development of sucking behavior in infants with Down's Syndrome. *Acta Paediatrica* 2001; 90(12):1384-1388.

Montgomery S, Ehlin A, Sacker A. Breast feeding and resilience against pyschosocial stress. *Archives of Disease in Childhood* 2006; 91(12):990-994.

Morley R, Fewtrell M, Abbott R, et al. Neurodevelopment in children born small for gestational age: a randomized trial of nutrient-enriched standard formula and comparison with a reference breast-fed group. *Pediatrics* 2004; 113(3):515-521.

Morton J, Hall JY, Wong RJ, et al. Combining hand techniques with electric pumping increases milk production in mothers of preterm infants. *Journal of Perinatology* 2009; 87(11):757-764.

Nabhan ZM, Eugster EA. Medical care of girls with Turner syndrome. *Endocrine Practice* 2011; 17(5):747-752.

National Down Syndrome Society. www.ndss.org. Accessed June 2013.

Neifert M. Early assessment of the breastfeeding infant. *Contemporary Pediatrics* 1996; 13(10):142-166.

Neifert M, DeMarzo S, Seacat J. The influence of breast surgery, breast appearance, and pregnancy-induced breast changes on lactation sufficiency as measured by infant weight gain. *Birth* 1990; 17(1):31-38.

Neifert M, Seacat J, Jobe W. Lactation failure due to insufficient glandular development of the breast. *Pediatrics* 1985; 76(5):823-828.

Neubauer S, Ferris S, Chase C, et al. Delayed lactogenesis in women with insulin-dependent diabetes mellitus. *American Journal of Clinical Nutrition* 1993; 58(1):54-60.

Nyqvist KH. Early attainment of breastfeeding in very preterm infants. *Acta Paediatrica* 2008; 97(6):776-781.

Oliveira AC, Pordeus IA, Torres CS, et al. Feeding and nonnutritive sucking habits and prevalence of open bite and crossbite in children/adolescents with Down syndrome. *The Angle Orthodontist* 2010; 80(4): 748-753.

Palmer M. Identification and management of the transitional suck pattern in premature infants. *Journal of Perinatal and Neonatal Nursing* 1993; 7(1):66-75.

Percy AK, Lane JB. Rett Syndrome: model of neurodevelopmental disorder. *Journal of Child Neurology* 2005; 20(9):718-721.

Pisacane A, Toscano E, Pirri I, et al. Down Syndrome and breastfeeding. *Acta Paediatrica* 2003; 92(12):1479-1481.

Powers N. How to assess slow growth in the breastfed infant, in RJ Schanler (ed.). *The Pediatric Clinics of North America Breastfeeding* 2001. Part II The Management of Breastfeeding 2001; 48(2):345-363.

Powers N. Low intake in the breastfed infant: maternal and infant considerations, in J Riordan, K Wambach ed. *Breastfeeding and Human Lactation* (4th edition), Sudbury, MA: Jones and Bartlett, 2010, pp. 325-363.

Pryor K. *Nursing Your Baby*. New York: Simon and Schuster, 1973; p. 7.

Rand S, Kolberg A. Neonatal hypernatremic dehydration secondary to lactation failure. *Journal of the American Board of Family Practice* 2001; 14(2):155-158.

Romero CC, Scavone-Junior H, Garib DG, et al. Breastfeeding and non-nutritive sucking patterns related to the prevalence of anterior open bite in primary dentition. *Journal of Applied Oral Science* 2011; 19(2):161-168.

Sacker A, Quigley MA, Kelly YJ. Breastfeeding and developmental delay: findings from the Millennium Cohort study. *Pediatrics* 2006; 118(3):e682-689.

Siddell E, Marinelli K, Froman R, et al. Evaluation of an educational intervention on breastfeeding for NICU nurses. *Journal of Human Lactation* 2003; 19(3):293-302.

Simmons K. Growth hormone and craniofacial changes: preliminary data from studies in Turner's Syndrome. *Pediatrics* 1999; 104(4):1021-1024.

Skuse D. Feeding difficulties among infants and older children with Turner Syndrome, in J Rovet (ed.) *Turner Syndrome Across the Lifespan: Proceedings from the 3rd International Turner Syndrome Contact Group Meetings*, Toronto, Canada, 1994a; pp. 17-26, 151-164.

Skuse D, Percy E, Stevenson J. Psychosocial functioning in the Turner Syndrome: a national survey, in B Stabler, L Underwood (eds). *Growth, Stature, and Adaptation: Behavioral, Social, and Cognitive Aspects of Growth Delay*. Chapel Hill: University of North Carolina Press, 1994b; pp. 151-164.

Slykerman RF, Thompson AM, Becroft DM. Breastfeeding and intelligence of preschool children. *Acta Paediatrica* 2005; 94(7):832-837.

Snyder U. Preterm birth as a social disease. *Medscape Ob/Gyn & Women's Health* 2004; 9(2):1-6.

Stutte P, Bowles B, Morman G. The effects of breast massage on volume and fat content of human milk. *Genesis* 1988; 10(2):22-25.

Unal S, Arhan E, Kara N. Breast-feeding-associated hypernatremia: retrospective analysis of 169 term infants. *Pediatrics International* 2008; 50(1):29-34.

US Centers for Disease Control (CDC): www.cdc.gov/reproductive-health/MaternalInfantHealth/PretermBirth.htm. Accessed June 2013.

Willis C, Livingstone V. Infant insufficient milk syndrome associated with maternal postpartum hemorrhage. *Journal of Human Lactation* 1995; 11(2):123-126.

Williams N. Supporting the mother coming to terms with persistent insufficient milk supply: the role of the lactation consultant. *Journal of Human Lactation* 2002; 18(3):262-263.

Wilson-Clay B, Maloney B. A reporting tool to facilitate community-based follow-up for at-risk breastfeeding dyads at hospital discharge, in K Auerbach ed. *Current Issues in Clinical Lactation* 2002; pp. 59-67.

Wolf L, Glass R. *Feeding and Swallowing Disorders in Infancy*. Tucson, AZ: Therapy Skill Builders, 1992; pp. 340-343.

Ankyloglossia

The tongue plays an important role in breastfeeding, speech, and dental health. Anatomical variations that affect how the tongue moves may interfere with successful breastfeeding (Ramsay 2004a, Geddes 2008a, Hazelbaker 2010).

Ankyloglossia is a congenital abnormality of the tongue, commonly called *tongue-tie*. The *lingual frenulum* is a mucous membrane connecting the tongue with the floor of the mouth. When the lingual frenulum is short, tight, or positioned too far forward, it limits the normal range of motion of the tongue. Tongue-tie may occur in isolation, or may be associated with a range of malformation syndromes (Gorski 1994, Coryllos 2004, Lalakea 2003, Olivi 2012). Ankyloglossia often runs in families.

Ankyloglossia occurs in approximately 2 to 5 percent of newborns, affecting males more commonly than females by a 3:1 ratio (Ballard 2002, Lalakea 2003, Ricke 2005, Wallace 2006, Olivi 2012). Tongue-ties may be characterized as *anterior* or *posterior*. Anterior ankyloglossia is defined as a tongue-tie with a visable lingual frenulum. The tongue tip is tethered and appears distorted when protruded or lifted. Posterior tongue-tie, felt to be less common, may be less well recognized. It is not so apparent when visualized, but manual palpation reveals a short, thick, or fibrous cord of tissue at the base of the tongue that limits the ability of the tongue to lift (Hong 2010). Hong also reported a female predominance in posterior tongue-tie.

The lingual frenulum may be short, but not always tight or fibrotic. This means that some tongue-tied infants are able to breastfeed without difficulty. However, it is clear that other tongue-tied infants experience significant breastfeeding difficulties (Ballard 2002). Messner (2000) observed breastfeeding difficulties in 25 percent of the mothers of tongue-tied babies as compared with only 3 percent of the mothers whose infants were not tongue-tied. Tongue-tie affects individuals to varying degrees (Amir 2005), and the problems it causes are often underestimated (Wright 1995). A restricted tongue may contribute to poor latch, reduced milk transfer, prolonged feedings, poor infant weight gain, and maternal nipple pain (Hogan 2005, Wallace 2006, Geddes 2008b).

Some tongue-tied infants slide off the breast frequently. Mothers may report a sensation like a "snap-back" of the tongue as the baby releases the breast (Hazelbaker 1993). These abrupt releases may be painful to the mother and can be observed when the baby breastfeeds. Instead of wide, regular jaw excursions, the chin seems to jerk. Flicking of the tongue as it snaps back can be abrasive to the underside of the nipple shaft. When the baby loses suction, clicking sounds may be heard.

Ultrasound permits visualization of the tongue while infants are breastfeeding. Infants with tongue-tie suck differently when compared with infants who have unrestricted tongue mobility (Geddes 2008b).

Assessment

Classification protocols to describe the presence and degree of ankyloglossia are not yet consistent, but provide helpful ways of thinking about the degree of impairment caused by a tongue-tie.

Lalakea (2003) described a method of determining tongue mobility in children who were old enough to cooperate with assessment. Measurements of tongue protrusion were calculated in millimeters of tongue-tip extension past the lower teeth. Tongue elevation was measured by recording the distance between the incisors with the tongue tip lifted as high as the child could manage, ideally touching the upper teeth. The researchers used a series of such measurements to help define degrees of tongue restriction. They found that protrusion and elevation values are typically in the range of 15 mm or less in children with ankyloglossia, and 20 to 25 mm or greater in normal children.

The Hazelbaker Assessment Tool for Lingual Frenulum Function (HATLFF) was developed to screen the total population of infants, and to make the distinction between affected and non-affected infants (2009).

Kotlow (1999) assessed tongue-tie based on the distance from the tip of the tongue to the place where the frenulum attaches. A distance of greater than 16 mm was defined as normal. Attachment at lesser distances determined the degree of ankyloglossia.

- Class I: Mild ankyloglossia (12-16 mm)
- Class II: Moderate (8-11 mm)
- Class III: Severe (3 to 7 mm)
- Class IV: Complete (less than 3 mm)

Because few lactation consultants have access to ultrasound or even to tools that would allow them to measure the distance between the tongue tip and the frenulum attachment site, a functional assessment is also important in terms of identifying tongue-tie. Olivi (2012) proposed criteria for recommending surgical release of the tongue:

- Breastfeeding difficulty
- Speech impediment
- Atypical swallowing
- Difficulty licking upper and/or lower lip
- Difficulty lifting tongue to upper gum ridge while mouth is open wide
- Distorted tongue shape/notched tongue tip

The Mechanics of Breastfeeding Affected by Tongue-tie

Milk can be removed from the breast using positive pressure alone (hand expression). Milk can also be removed from the breast using negative pressure alone (breast pumping). During breastfeeding, the baby uses a combination of positive and negative pressure. Full range of motion of the tongue permits effective milk removal.

During breastfeeding, the baby's lips and cupped tongue seal the oral cavity. Once it is tightly sealed, suction draws the breast tissue into an elongated teat that extends nearly to the junction of the hard and soft palates. The edges of the tongue curl around the breast, forming a channel that controls the direction of the milk flow.

During milk ejection, the downward movement of the baby's posterior tongue and lower jaw creates negative pressure that facilitates milk flow from the breast. When the tongue rises, it compresses the teat between the tongue and hard palate. When the teat is maximally compressed, milk flow slows or is interrupted (Ramsay 2004b). It is during this phase of the cycle that the infant pauses to take a breath (Meier 2003). When the tongue drops again like a piston, the level of negative pressure increases and the mouth refills with milk. 3D ultrasound studies have observed a peristaltic wave of the tongue that assists in moving milk to the back of the mouth for swallowing (Burton 2013).

Given the complexity of these oral maneuvers, it is clear that if the tongue cannot move freely, breastfeeding may become difficult and exhausting for the infant.

During routine exams of infants, the LC should observe the lift of the tongue while the infant's mouth is wide open. If the tongue cannot lift past the mid-line plane of the mouth and the tip notches or distorts, impairment of mobility is present.

Because the forward position of the tongue pads the breast, protecting it from the full force of lower jaw compression, the degree of tongue extension impacts sore nipples. A

light tap to the tongue tip elicits tongue extension. The tongue normally extends beyond the infant's lower gum ridge, and ideally extends beyond the lower lip line. The infant should be able to maintain tongue extension without effort and without frequent release that produces a snap-back sensation.

Inability to form a central groove with the tongue suggests that the tongue cannot lateralize or cup normally. Lack of mobility in this dimension impairs the infant's capacity to organize fluids for safe swallowing. Milk may spill over the edges of the tongue, pooling in the vestibule of the mouth, creating an aspiration risk. Breastfeeding and, if applicable, bottle-feeding should be directly observed for milk spilling, swallowing difficulty, and noisy or wet breathing. Wet breathing may be an indication of aspiration (Meier 2003). External pacing techniques may be used to make feeding safer during alternative feeding. The mother should allow the breastfeeding infant to pull off the breast to reorganize breathing if necessary.

Nipple Distortion and Variant Sucking Patterns Associated with Tongue-tie

Using ultrasound, Geddes (2008a) demonstrated that minimal distortion of the nipple occurs during successful, established breastfeeding. Infants with ankyloglossia display visable differences in sucking (Ramsay 2004a). Two "distinct patterns of sucking" were observed in tongue-tied infants prior to frenotomy (Geddes 2008b). One group of tongue-tied infants positioned the tip of the nipple farther from the hard and soft palate junction (HSPJ). They humped the posterior tongue, pinching the nipple to a point. This group appeared to have difficulty sustaining enough suction to form an adequate seal.

A second group of infants in Geddes's ultrasound studies appeared to hold the nipple tip closer to the HSPJ, but compressed or bit the base of the nipple. Both patterns of sucking appear to be compensations employed by infants who were unable to latch normally or perform normal sucking mechanics. Both variant sucking patterns were associated with higher maternal pain scores and ineffective infant milk transfer.

After frenotomy, ultrasound revealed that the variant sucking patterns resolved or lessened. The infants in the study displayed significantly increased rates of milk transfer in shorter feeds and their mothers reported improved comfort during breastfeeding (Geddes 2008b). While only ultrasound permits direct visualization of variant suck patterns, published case series have also reported improved maternal comfort and improved infant feeding following frenotomy (Srinivasan 2006, Wallace 2006). Four randomized controlled trials (using sham proceduces in the control groups) have been published showing improvements in breastfeeding following frenotomy (Berry 2012, Buryk 2011, Dollber 2006, Hogan 2005).

Images of the Tongue

Fig. 368 shows normal range of motion of the tongue. Note how this adolescent girl can lift her tongue tip to touch her upper teeth with her mouth open wide. Tongue lift is assessed with the mouth open because the baby has to open wide to latch to the breast. Compare the appearance of a normal tongue to that of the woman in **Fig. 369** whose frenulum attaches near the tip of her tongue. Because her tongue tip is tethered to the floor of the mouth, the woman cannot lift her tongue to touch her upper teeth. Note that the tongue tip assumes a distorted, heart-shape as she tries to elevate it.

The man in **Fig. 370** is the father of a tongue-tied infant who was being assessed by an LC. Note how his tongue tip curls under as he attempts to lift it. Distortions of the tongue that create an unusual appearance may result in social problems such as bullying and teasing, especially during adolescence. This man is unable to touch the tip of his tongue to his upper teeth. Inability to move the tongue and place it behind the upper teeth inhibits, in some individuals, the formation of certain sounds, and is implicated in speech disorders, including lisp (Marchesan 2004).

Both authors have had numerous conversations with parents of tongue-tied infants who had their own tongues clipped as children to remediate speech or dental problems.

In spite of the fact that studies have identified ankyloglossia in adults (Lalakea 2003, Marchesan 2012), physicians may delay interventions to remediate tongue-tie in infants because they believe that the condition will resolve spontaneously. Parents may be told that a tongue-tie will "disappear."

Ranly (1998) described the rapid forward growth of the mandible during the first 4 months after birth. Changes in the orientation of the lower jaw may indeed explain some cases when breastfeeding a tongue-tied baby becomes less painful over time. The forward jaw growth may stretch the frenulum or pull the tongue slightly forward, assisting the infant's ability to latch.

What more commonly occurs is accidental cutting of the frenulum. Toddlers may tear the frenulum in a fall, often biting through it with their sharp, new teeth, or a

toy. BWC has worked with several families who have described toddlers tearing a frenulum.

Photos of adults with tongue-ties, as pictured in **Figs. 369** and **370**, serve to document that ankyloglossia can persist beyond infancy.

The belief that time or fate will resolve tongue-tie frequently causes delays in correcting ankyloglossia. Concerns about the social implications of speech disorders, dental problems, or facial appearance often result in frenotmy as the individual matures, but impairment of the ability to breastfeed may not receive the same level of attention.

While some infants appear to have sore tongues following the procedure, frenotomy does not cause excessive bleeding (Amir 2005), and is considered to be "simple, safe, and effective" (Hong 2010). During the first 3 months, frenotomy is generally performed as an office procedure. Delaying remediation past early infancy increases health risks owing to the loss of the protection of breastfeeding. Infants older than 3 months, toddlers, and most pre-school age children cannot be depended upon to remain still during frenotomy. Tongue-tie revisions in the older baby or toddler typically require general anesthesia, increasing the risk of the procedure.

Fig. 371 pictures a tongue-tied infant. Note how the baby's tongue tip forms a distorted, notched "V" shape. The heart-shaped tongue tip is characteristic of tongue-tie. Restriction at the tip of the tongue prevents the individual from adequately forming a central groove. Fernando (1998) documents tongue-tied older children with excessive salivation and difficulties managing solids as the result of poor organization of swallowing.

Fig. 372 illustrates the variability of tongue lengths. The photo shows a married couple. The woman (on the left) has normal tongue extension. The man has a short tongue which limits his range of motion. For instance, he could not lick an ice cream cone.

Frenotomy is a relatively common procedure in orthodontia patients, where the influence of the tongue on teeth spacing is widely appreciated (Palmer 1998). Other aspects of dental health may be negatively affected by tongue-tie. When tongue mobility is restricted, the tongue cannot perform normal oral mechanics such as removing food particles from side or back teeth, contributing to development of caries.

The 12 year-old boy in **Fig. 373** is tongue-tied, with a lingual frenulum that attaches just behind his lower gum ridge. The extreme forward placement of the lingual frenulum caused his tongue tip to roll under when he tried to stick it out. In spite of the fact that he cannot extend his tongue, and has an unusual appearance, he breastfed without problems. At age 17, the boy's othodontist performed a frenotomy to preserve the beneficial effect of braces used to correct his malformed teeth and open bite, which the orthodontist attributed to ankyloglossia. While the frenotomy was not painful, the boy complained that his recovery was more uncomfortable than he had been led to expect. For a week after his frenotomy, his tongue hurt at the site of the incision.

The baby in **Fig. 374** has an unusually long tongue. Her siblings nicknamed her "Giraffe Tongue." The length of the baby's tongue may have contributed to her mother's sore nipples, which persisted in spite of interventions to adjust positioning and latch. The mother described breastfeeding this infant as very different from what she had experienced with her other 2 children, suggesting that differences in tongue length may impact breastfeeding comfort.

Note the bunching and distortion as the tongue-tied infant in **Fig. 375** attempts to extend her tongue. The LC should observe and report such distortions.

Fig. 376 illustrates normal tongue lateralization in an adolescent girl. Her younger sister, seen in **Fig. 377**, has a tight lingual frenulum that attaches at the mid-section of the tongue. Note how the tongue-tied girl demonstrates a limited ability to lateralize. Her tongue distorts as she attempts to move it toward her lateral incisors. Such impairment may also restrict the ability to efficiently clear food from the tongue during swallowing. This girl complained that she often had a white, coated tongue and bad breath. She observed that food caught in her tonsils, and wondered if this contributed to her frequent episodes of sore throat.

The infant pictured in **Fig. 378** demonstrates normal tongue mobility. She is able to easily move her tongue from side to side. To assess lateralization, the LC lightly touches the side of the tongue. This should produce a lateral tongue-seeking response.

Fig. 379 shows a baby girl with a tongue-tie. Note the mother's nipple damage. The LC assisted with improving the latch, but the baby was unable to draw in enough breast tissue for her mother to experience pain-free breastfeeding. Once the baby's frenulum was clipped, breastfeeding became comfortable.

Contrast the limited lift of the tongue in the baby shown in

Fig. 379 with that of the baby pictured in **Fig. 380**. Note how this infant can position her tongue tip behind her upper gum ridge.

Positioning Interventions for the Tongue-tied Infant

Breastfeeding positions that pull the chin very close to the breast shorten the distance the tongue must reach to draw in, cup, and hold the breast. An extended head position that brings the chin close helps the tongue-tied infant breastfeed. Prone positions that help drop the tongue forward may also be useful.

Mothers may find it helpful to support the breast with their hand to help the baby stabilize and hold onto the breast. Breast support may be especially useful for infants who bite the base of the nipple (Geddes 2008b). When the baby's nose is tipped away from the breast (as in **Fig. 116**), it indicates that the chin is sufficiently close.

Fig. 381 shows a normal infant breastfeeding. The mother pulls back on the breast to reveal the wide gape of a well-latched infant. The tongue is seen cupping the underside of the breast. Note how the curled lateral edges of the tongue assist the lips in forming a seal around the breast. The sides of the tongue fill the gaps at the corners of the mouth when it is wide open. When the tongue cannot seal the gap at the corners of the mouth, suction is impaired. Any impairment in the infant's ability to create negative pressure makes breastfeeding more effortful.

Frenotomy and Frenuloplasty

Numerous breastfeeding experts recommend evaluation and correction of tongue-tie if breastfeeding is painful or infant growth is affected (Neifert 2001, Powers 2001, Wight 2001, Lawrence 2011).

Frenotomy and frenuloplasty are terms that describe procedures to free the tongue from the restriction of ankyloglossia, permitting it to move normally. Jain (2013) produced a video to instruct pediatricians in the procedure of frenotomy.

Lalakea (2003) describes frenotomy as a simple release of the tongue, generally performed in newborn infants and older individuals without anesthesia or topical analgesia. The procedure is performed by pediatricians, ear, nose and throat specialists (ENTs), dentists, oral surgeons, and other physicians. Two gloved fingers or a tool called a grooved director are placed below the tongue to lift the tongue and expose the frenulum. Small, sterile scissors make a cut directly adjacent to the tongue to avoid injuring the submandibular ducts in the floor of the mouth. Occasionally, more than one cut is needed to fully release the tongue. Bleeding is slight, although because blood mixes with saliva, it may sometimes seem as if there is more bleeding than really occurs. Slight pressure for a minute or so generally causes bleeding to subside.

Sometimes the genioglossus muscle requires resectioning to obtain an adequate release of the tongue. Frenuloplasty is performed in these cases. It is a more invasive procedure involving more of the underside of the tongue, and requires general anesthesia. The wound is closed with sutures. Following the surgery, older patients are asked to perform tongue exercises to strengthen the tongue. The activity of breastfeeding, itself, provides physical therapy for the tongue, and infants and older babies should be encouraged to breastfeed immediately after the procedure, or as soon as they can tolerate sucking.

The Genetics of Ankyloglossia

Research into the nature of orofacial abnormalities has uncovered an association between the location of the gene for ankyloglossia, cleft palate, and other mid-line defects seen as part of a cluster of symptoms in syndromic conditions (Forbes 1996). Japanese researchers (Mukai 1991) have noted an association of tongue-tie with abnormalities of the epiglottis and larynx. Infants whose mid-line defects extend to the throat may experience breathing problems (apnea) as well as feeding difficulties.

Because of the role that the tongue plays in shaping the palate during the prenatal period, there is speculation that disorders of the tongue may contribute to unusually shaped palates. Certainly it is often the case that infants with severely restricted tongues present with high, narrow, or arched palates.

BWC consulted with the family of a 2 month-old infant who was experiencing breastfeeding problems. A digital assessment identified a high, bubble-shaped palate, causing BWC to comment that she seldom felt such a palate unless the baby was tongue-tied. When the infant subsequently began to cry, a tongue-tie was observed.

Because mid-line defects may be linked with other genetic syndromes that have the potential to affect an infant's general health, it is crucial to look at the whole baby, not just the tongue-tie. Sucking impairment often has more than one cause, and some tongue-tied babies continue to have feeding problems even after the tongue is released.

Hypospadias is another mid-line defect that sometimes appears in families with a history of tongue-tie or as part of a cluster of defects in an individual. Hypospadias refers to an atypical location of the urethral opening on the shaft or base of the penis, scrotum, or perineum (Stokowski 2004). Hypospadias is a common developmental disorder of the urogenital tract occurring in approximately 1 in 125 male births.

The boy in **Fig. 382** breastfed well after the LC corrected positioning and latch problems. His case was interesting because he had a midline defect involving his urethral opening. It was located at the base of the penis. While the infant was not tongue-tied, his father and a male cousin were, suggesting a family history of such defects. The child underwent successful surgical repair of the urethra at one year of age. Because the infant faced surgery and there were general concerns about his urogenital health, the low renal solute load of breast milk was considered to be beneficial for him.

Case Study of a Tongue-Tied Infant With FTT

Failure to thrive in exclusively breastfed tongue-tied infants has previously been reported (Forlenza 2010). **Fig. 383** shows a 10 day-old infant one pound (452 g) below birth weight as she attempts to latch onto her mother's breast. Note her expression of distress. Her lips are retracted. Even though her chin is placed close to the breast, she seems unable to draw in enough breast tissue to latch on. Her mother told the LC that each breastfeeding session was marked by frustration. If the baby managed to latch, the mother heard a few minutes of noisy sucking during milk ejection. As soon as the milk ejection subsided, the baby's eyes closed, and she fell asleep. When the mother tried to lay her down, the baby would awaken, cry frantically, and the cycle would begin again. Because she was born weighing slightly over 10 pounds (4535 g), her family did not appreciate the impact that her excessive early weight loss had on her energy and ability to feed.

Fig. 384 reveals a tight, fleshy lingual frenulum attached to the infant's tongue tip. Such a thick membrane is unlikely to stretch. Note how flat the tongue appears. During the initial evaluation, the LC observed that the baby had difficulty forming a central groove with her tongue. This affected her ability to feed from a cup and bottle, as well as to breastfeed. When offered a bottle, the baby struggled, spilling milk. She appeared to have difficulty swallowing and occasionally coughed while feeding. The baby became very agitated when cup fed, spilling more milk than she swallowed.

The LC recommended that the mother ask the baby's pediatrician about a referral to a pediatric ENT. Three days later, after continuous struggle to supplement her, the baby had gained only 2 ounces (57 g). The pediatrician referred the infant for evaluation by a pediatric ENT.

Fig. 385 shows the pediatric ENT manipulating the baby's tongue. He agreed that the frenulum was unlikely to stretch on its own, and observed that the baby had poor ability to lift, cup, or extend her tongue. The baby was now 18 days old, still feeding poorly, and was still significantly below her birth weight. The ENT recommended frenotomy to release the tongue. The infant was seated on her mother's lap, and her head was held still by the mother and a nurse. The doctor, wearing a visor with a spotlight carefully visualized the frenulum to locate any blood vessels. He lifted the tongue with his fingers and snipped the frenulum twice (**Fig. 386**).

In **Fig. 387** the doctor applies pressure on the underside of the tongue with a gauz ' pad. Within a few minutes of the procedure, the infant began rooting for the breast. Within 10 minutes she latched onto the breast more deeply than ever before (**Fig. 388**), and breastfed until she fell asleep.

Fig. 389 shows the underside of the tongue almost a week after the frenotomy. Note the small white lesion, which has not yet fully healed. Unlike many babies who have their tongue-ties clipped and immediately feed well, this baby continued to have problems gaining weight. It is apparent in the photo that the tongue still does not lift past the midline plane of the tongue. The release of the tongue may not have been fully achieved.

Within 2 weeks of the frenotomy (**Fig. 390**) the tongue completely healed. The tongue, which had previously been unable to cup, is now able to assume a more cupped shape. **Fig. 391** shows the baby breastfeeding 3 weeks after the procedure. She was better able to coordinate swallowing fluids from both breast and bottle. Her stamina improved, allowing her to sustain longer, more effective feedings. Her growth rate improved, although she continued to gain more slowly than expected unless her mother provided pumped hind milk supplementation. This provided additional evidence suggesting either that the tongue had not been fully released, or that the baby had additional, as yet undiagnosed, feeding problems.

More Case Studies: Tongue-tied Babies with Very Different Breastfeeding Experiences

Fig. 392 shows a tight frenulum that distorts a baby's tongue into the characteristic heart shape so often seen in tongue-tied individuals. However, this baby was able to breastfeed without causing his mother discomfort. His weight gain was appropriate. This case emphasizes

how difficult it is to predict the breastfeeding ability of a tongue-tied infant.

The 9 day-old baby in **Fig. 393,** is also tongue-tied. Her 33 year-old, first-time mother, phoned her obstetrician's office, complaining of sore nipples. The mother reported severe deep breast pain, a burning sensation, and white material on the surface of her nipples. Without being examined, she was advised by the nurse to phone BWC to discuss remedies for a yeast infection.

BWC insisted on seeing the mother and the infant in person. She immediately observed that the infant was tongue-tied and could not lift her tongue past the mid-line plane of the mouth. When the baby tried to lift her tongue, her thick lingual frenulum pulled against it, notching the tongue tip (**Fig. 393**). The infant had regained birth weight by Day 9 when first evaluated by the LC, but the mother was supplementing with formula by bottle, owing to reduced milk supply and painful breastfeeding.

Both nipples were badly abraded; the left nipple (**Fig. 394**) more severely affected than the right. The left nipple was inflamed and red. The red area spread past the areolar margin, onto the breast itself. The Montgomery glands around the left areola were swollen, with white heads. Lesions on both nipples were crusted over with yellow, crystallized material. Blood and pus oozed from open lesions on the left nipple.

BWC and the mother agreed that it would be too painful to practice latching. The mother was willing to express her milk with a hospital grade electric pump for several days to protect her milk supply while allowing the nipples to heal. Milk volumes were low at the first pumping; the mother pumped a total of only 15 ml during a double pumping session lasting approximately 12 minutes. The pumped milk was stained with blood and contained clumps of pus. The appearance of the milk so upset the mother that she refused to feed it to the baby.

BWC phoned the mother's OB to report these symptoms. Even though the mother was afebrile, there were more signs and symptoms of bacterial infection than there were of a fungal infection. Interestingly, this mother stated that she almost never developed an elevated temperature when ill. The OB prescribed an oral and a topical antibiotic. Within several days of beginning antibiotic therapy, the woman's nipples began to heal, and the appearance and volume of her pumped milk returned to normal.

BWC also faxed a written report to the baby's pediatrician, describing the mother's extreme nipple damage. She recommended assessment of the infant by a pediatric

ENT. The ENT evaluated the baby on Day 21 and noted moderate ankyloglossia with poor tongue elevation. In his report to the LC, the ENT stated, "It seemed as if the 2 sides of the tongue were moving in opposition." The ENT performed a frenotomy in his office, and noted immediate improvement in the way the baby moved her tongue.

Fig. 395 shows the baby 15 days after the initial assessment, 2 days after frenotomy. The baby's tongue was able to lift and extend normally.

At this point, the mother had been exclusively pumping for the past 15 days. Her right nipple was healed, and her more damaged left nipple was almost healed (**Fig. 396**). The mother confided during a phone call that she was afraid to latch the baby onto the breast. She requested a follow-up visit from the LC to practice latching. BWC helped the woman find a comfortable position, and the baby self-attached. The relieved mother exclaimed that it was no longer painful to breastfeed. The baby was still breastfeeding at 19 months, when this mother called BWC to refer a cousin whose new baby was also tongue-tied.

Frenotomy at Age Forty

The adult woman whose tongue-tie is seen in **Fig. 369** had considered a frenotomy for some years. She had a slight speech impediment that she disguised well, and she disliked the appearance of her tongue. A speech pathologist gave her a mirror and asked the woman to chew a red pill used by dentists to help patients identify accumulations of dental plaque. The speech pathologist asked the woman to observe how many swallows it took to clear the chewed up red pill from her tongue. In this way, the speech pathologist demonstrated how dysfunctionally the woman's tongue performed routine oral mechanics. After consultation with the speech pathologist, the woman's dentist agreed to perform a frenotomy. Although no topical anesthesia was used, the woman described the procedure as essentially painless. "It felt strange; like dull scissors cutting through wet wool." Because her frenulum was thick and fibrous, it took the dentist 3 snips before the tongue was freed. She felt a slight "burning sensation" on the last clip.

In the weeks following the frenotomy, the woman performed simple exercises suggested by the speech pathologist. She was initially unable to lateralize her tongue. It quivered and became extremely tired when she tried to hold it in an elevated position. One of her exercises involved balancing a small, round plastic ring on the front of her elevated tongue. After several months of exercising, she was able to move her tongue in any direction, and it functioned normally. Her tongue after frenotomy is pictured in **Fig.**

397. Note that while she can now lift it without so much effort, the heart-shaped tongue tip remains.

It may be that some infants experience similar weakness of the tongue muscle following frenotomy as this older woman did. Infants may also require a period of rehabilitation. A parent can imitate some of the simple exercises suggested to the woman in **Fig. 397**.

To trigger lateral tongue movement, place a clean finger at the corners of the lips. Switch back and forth to encourage the baby to move the tongue from side to side. Sucking on a finger or on a soft air- or gel-filled pacifier encourages the infant to do "push-ups" with the tongue. (A hollow, collapsible pacifier is not as useful as it offers too little resistance.) Tap lightly on the tongue tip to elicit tongue protrusion, encouraging the baby to extend the tongue. The activity of breastfeeding, will itself, help strengthen the tongue.

Parents should be reminded that while some babies will breastfeed better immediately following frenotomy, others need time to heal and strengthen, especially if their growth has been compromised and they are weak. It may take a while for some babies to re-pattern the tongue. In general, it appears that the longer the baby waits to have the frenotomy, the longer the period of rehabilitation. Based on maternal observations in regards to feeding difficulties, Steehler (2012) concluded that there is more benefit when frenotomy is performed before, rather than after, the baby is a week old.

Amir LH, James JP, Beatty J. Review of tongue-tie release at a tertiary maternity hospital. *Journal of Paediatric and Child Health* 2005; 41(5-6):243-245.

Ballard J, Auer C, Khoury J, et al. Ankyloglossia: assessment, incidence and effect of frenuloplasty on the breastfeeding dyad. *Pediatrics* 2002; 110(5):e63.

Berry J, Griffiths M, Westcott C. A double-blind, randomized controlled trial of tongue-tie division and its immediate effect on breastfeeding. *Breastfeeding Medicine* 2012; 7(3):189-193.

Burton P, Deng J, McDonald D, et al. Real-time 3D ultrasound imaging of infant tongue movements during breastfeeding. *Early Human Development* 2013; May 18. Ahead of print.

Buryk M, Bloom D, Shope T. Efficacy of neonatal release of ankyloglossia: a randomized trial. *Pediatrics* 2011; 128(2):280-288.

Coryllos E, Genna CW, Salloum D. Congenital tongue-tie and its impact on Breastfeeding. American Academy of Pediatrics, Section on Breastfeeding newsletter, *Breastfeeding: Best for Baby and Mother* Summer 2004; 1-7.

Dollber S, Botzer E, Grunis E, et al. Immediate nipple pain relief after frenotomy in breastfed infants with ankyloglossia: a randomized, prospective study. *Journal of Pediatric Surgery* 2006; 41(9):1598-1600.

Fernando C. *Tongue Tie: From Confusion to Clarity*. Sydney, Australia: Tandem Publications, 1998.

Forbes A, Brennan L, Richardson M, et al. Refined mapping and YAC contig construction of the X-linked cleft palate and ankyloglossia locus (CPX) including the proximal X-Y homology breakpoint within Xq21.3. *Genomics* 1996; 31(1):36-43.

Forlenza GP, Black NMP, McNamara EG, et al. Ankyloglossia, exclusive breastfeeding, and failure to thrive. *Pediatrics* 2010; 125(6): e1500-e1504.

Geddes DT, Kent JC, Mitoulas LR, et al. Tongue movement and intra-oral vacuum in breastfeeding infants. *Early Human Development* 2008a; 84(7):471-477.

Geddes DT, Langton DB, Gollow I, et al. Frenotomy for breastfeeding infants with ankyloglossia: effect on milk removal and sucking mechanism as imaged by ultrasound. *Pediatrics* 2008b; 2(1):e188-194.

Gorski S, Adams K, Birch P, et al. Linkage analysis of X-linked cleft palate and ankyloglossia in Manitoba Mennonite and British Columbia native kindreds. *Human Genetics* 1994; 94(2):141-148.

Hazelbaker A. *The Assessment Tool for Lingual Frenulum Function.* Master's Thesis, Pasadena, CA: Pacific Oaks College, 1993.

Hazelbaker A. *Hazelbaker Assessment Tool for Lingual Frenulum Function Chart Note.* 2009.

Hazelbaker AK. *Tongue-tie: morphogenesis, impact, assessment and treatment.* Columbus, OH: Aidan and Eva Press, 2010.

Hogan M, Westcott C, Griffiths M. Randomized, controlled trial of division of tongue-tie in infants with feeding problems. *Journal of Paediatric and Child Health* 2005; 41(5-6):246-250.

Hong P, Lago D, Seargeant J, et al. Defining ankyloglossia: a case series of anterior and posterior tongue ties. *International Journal of Pediatric Otorhinolaryngology* 2010; 74(9):1003-1006.

Jain E. *Posterior and Anterior Tongue-tie* (DVD) www.drjain.com 2013.

Kotlow LA. Ankyloglossia (tongue-tie): a diagnostic and treatment quandary. *Quintessence International* 1999; 30(4):259-262.

Lalakea M, Messner A. Ankyloglossia: does it matter? *Pediatric Clinics of North America* 2003; 50(2):381-387.

Lawrence RA, Lawrence RM. *Breastfeeding: A Guide for the Medical Profession* (7th edition). Maryland Heights MO: Elsevier Mosby 2011; p. 269.

Marchesan IQ. Lingual frenulum: classification and speech interference. *International Journal of Orofacial Myology* 2004; 30:31-38.

Marchesan IQ. Lingual frenulum protocol. *International Journal of Orofacial Myology* 2012; 38:89-103.

Meier P. Supporting lactation in mothers with very low birth weight infants. *Pediatric Annals* 2003; 32(5):317-325.

Messner AH, Lalakea ML, Aby J, et al. Ankyloglossia: incidence and associated feeding difficulties. *Archives of Otolaryngology - Head & Neck Surgery* 2000; 126(1):36-39.

Mukai S, Mukai C, Asaoka K. Ankyloglossia with deviation of the epiglottis and larynx. *Annals of Otology, Rhinology, and Laryngology Suppl.* 1991; 153:3-20.

Neifert M. Prevention of breastfeeding tragedies. in RJ Schanler (ed.) *Pediatric Clinics of North America* 2001; 48(2):273-297.

Olivi G, Signore M, Olivi MDG. Lingual frenectomy: functional evaluation and new therapoeutical approach. *European Journal of Paediatric Dentistry* 2012; 13(2):101-106

Palmer B. The influence of breastfeeding on the development of the oral cavity: a commentary. *Journal of Human Lactation* 1998; 14(2):93-98.

Powers N. How to assess slow growth in the breastfed infant. in R Schanler, (ed). *Pediatric Clinics of North America* 2001; 48(2):345-363.

Ramsay D, Langton D, Gollow I, et al. Ultrasound imaging of the effect of frenulotomy on breastfeeding infants with ankyloglossia, Abstract of the 12th International Conference of the International Society for Research in Human Milk and Lactation, Sept. 10-14, 2004a; Queen's College, Cambridge, UK, 2004a; p. 52.

Ramsay D, Mitoulas L, Kent J, et al. Ultrasound imaging of the sucking mechanics of the breastfeeding infant. Abstract of the 12th International Conference of the International Society for Research in Human Milk and Lactation, Sept. 10-14, 2004, Queen's College, Cambridge, UK, 2004b; p. 53.

Ranly D. Early orofacial development. *Journal of Clinical Pediatric Dentistry* 1998; 22(4):267-275.

Ricke L, Baker N, Madlon-Kay D, et al. Newborn tongue-tie: prevalence and effect on breastfeeding. *Journal of the American Board of Family Practice* 2005; 18(1):1-7.

Srinivasan A, Dobrich C, Mitnick H, et al. Ankyloglossia in breastfeeding infants: the effect of frenotomy on maternal nipple pain and latch. *Breastfeeding Medicine* 2006; 1(4):216-224.

Steehler MW, Steehler MK, Harley EH. A retrospective reiew of frenotomy in neonates and infants with feeding difficulties. *International Journal of Pediatric Otorhinolaryngology* 2012; 76(9):1236-1240.

Stokowski L. Hypospadias in the neonate. *Advances in Neonatal Care* 2004; 4(4):206-215.

Wallace H, Clarke S. Tongue tie division in infants with breast feeding difficulties. *International Journal of Pediatric Otorhinolaryngology* 2006; 70(7):1257-1261.

Wight N. Management of common breastfeeding issues, in RJ Schanler (ed.) *Pediatric Clinics of North America* 2001; 48(2):321-344.

Wright J. Tongue-tie. Journal of Paediatric Child Health 1995; 31(4):276-278.

Cleft Lip and Cleft Palate

Clefts of the lip and palate are among the most common birth defects. In the US, approximately 1 in 600 babies is born with a cleft defect (Cleft Palate Foundation 2008). Cleft lips and palates occur about twice as often in boys, while cleft palate alone is slightly more common in girls. Clefts are more common among Asian and American Indian races, and whites are almost twice as likely to be affected as blacks. Information and resources for parents and professionals are available from the American Cleft Palate-Craniofacial Association (2013). Special feeding bottles can be ordered from their website.

Clefts form early in pregnancy, often before women are aware they are pregnant. Clefts of the lip appear between the 5th and 8th gestational weeks. Clefts of the palate form during the 6th to 12th weeks when the palate fails to fuse.

No single factor has been identified to explain what causes cleft defects; however, both genetics and environmental exposures are believed to be involved. A positive association has been identified between maternal smoking during the first trimester of pregnancy and cleft lip and palate (Little 2004, Bille 2007). Treatment with excessive amounts of Vitamin A during pregnancy induces fetal malformations in mice, most notably, cleft palate (Inomata 2005). Folic acid supplements and a diet high in folate (fruits and vegetables) seem to reduce the risk of isolated cleft lip (Wilcox 2007). Genetic studies have mapped the chromosomal locus for some forms of cleft palate and ankyloglossia, and have identified these two midline defects in certain families as a recurrent genetic trait (Gorski 1994).

There are isolated clefts, and clefts associated with other birth defects, and more than 300 syndromes. Approximately 10 to 15 percent of individuals with cleft lip with or without cleft palate have a related syndrome. About 40 to 50 percent of individuals with cleft palate alone have an associated syndrome. Most of these are apparent at birth (Cleft Palate Foundation 2008). When clefts occur as part of a broader syndrome, other aspects of the specific condition must also be considered in the feeding plan.

For example, certain syndromes may be associated with muscle weakness that may impact infant tone, thus affecting suck. Cardiac abnormalities may affect infant feeding stamina or require restriction of fluid intake. Feeding a child with a combination of medical issues requires careful planning to ensure that adequate nutritional support is provided in a way that addresses all the child's special needs. A team approach ensures that the LC communicates with other experts and tailors her feeding plan appropriately.

Genetic Counseling

When a couple gives birth to a child with a cleft defect, the risk of delivering another child with similar problems is increased 2 to 5 percent. Parents are typically referred for *genetic counseling*. Genetic counseling includes taking a detailed family history, and may involve laboratory examinations of DNA samples (Cleft Palate Foundation 2008). Such counseling helps determine the odds of bearing another child at risk for a cleft defect. It also helps parents identify whether their child has an isolated cleft, or if the cleft defect has occured as part of a syndrome.

Bonding and Cleft Defects

The relationship between appearance and social stereotyping has been established as one of the most consistent research findings in social science. In earlier times, a bodily difference was referred to as a *stigma*. Cleft disorders have been considered in many cultures to be stigmatizing. Even in more sophisticated eras and locales, the appearance of an infant with an orofacial abnormality may initially be shocking. While intellectually aware that the condition is repairable, on an emotional level, a new mother or father may feel distress at the child's appearance. For a time, until the parents adjust, they may painfully experience the impact of this distress again each time a new person sees the baby.

Parents of children with orofacial abnormalities may experience what has been described as "chronic" grief. They worry about many things, including how to provide the baby and themselves with a normal experience. Over time, most families adjust, but often initially require familial and social support. The parents need specific genetic counseling and help learning how to communicate with all the various members of the infant's care team. They will certainly need emotional nurturing. The degree to which the parents, especially the mother, feel well-supported has implications for the bonding and attachment process. The quality of parental responsiveness has important long-term effects on the baby's cognitive and behavioral outcomes (Ainsworth 1982).

Experts in the field of attachment and bonding observe that the mother provides a "mirror" for her baby (Klaus 1996). Her responsiveness to the baby's appearance, her sensitivity and success in handling, holding, feeding, and how much she smiles at her baby, all influence the baby's responses to her. These mutual responses create an ongoing feedback loop. Because feeding involves both nutrition *and* nurture, it is crucial to consider the bonding implications connected with the activity of feeding. Success in feeding often determines how women judge their competency as mothers (Ramsay 1996).

Parents of children with orofacial abnormalities realize that surgery will correct the facial defect. However, parents of infants who are ill or born with a congenital defect process information anxiously and respond to their children differently. For example, parents of infants who are hospitaltized in special care nurseries smile less at their infants. Their infants, in turn, smile less at 3 months (Minde 1982).

Health care providers may view breastfeeding as too stressful for a mother whose child has special needs. However, helping the mother establish lactation can provide a meaningful way to lessen the burden of additional illnesses for such a child. Knowing she can positively affect her child's health may empower her and help stabilize her mood-state (Mawson 2013). Thus, lactation protects maternal as well as infant health (Groer 2004).

Because the breast may obscure the facial defect, breastfeeding gives the mother a chance to look at the baby without the constant visual intrusion of the facial abnormality. Even though breastfeeding attempts may not produce much milk intake, mothers have shared that the only time their infant looked "normal" was when placed at the breast. Because of the beneficial effect on bonding, such experiences should be encouraged. The LC also models acceptance by commenting on other strengths of the baby.

Active listening and validation of feelings help establish trust and rapport between the mother and the LC. The LC avoids adopting a crisis mentality when helping families of infants with birth defects. Just as tension can be "catching," so can calm. Tone of voice is important. The skillful LC deliberately pitches her voice to help soothe anxious parents. Some parents worry that they will not be able to master special feeding instructions or learn to use the equipment involved in caring for the baby. The LC seeks to reduce parental stress by calmly repeating details, provides written instructions, and establishes a plan for follow-up until feeding stabilizes.

Human Milk for Infants with Cleft Defects

Early failure-to-thrive (FTT) is common in infants with cleft defects (Glenny 2004), and it has generally been attributed to feeding difficulties. However, FTT appears to be linked to cleft type and to the presence of other anomalies (Beaumont 2008). Infants with cleft lip had similar birth weights when compared to the general population. Infants with cleft lip and palate, or those with isolated cleft palate were significantly lighter at birth and had significantly more early growth delay. This difference in weight is perhaps explained by the fact that about half of infants with cleft palate have an associated syndrome. Therefore, infants with cleft palate require more specialized feeding support to protect growth. Their growth often influences the timing of surgical repair. Consequently, more systematic support for these infants could improve nutritional intake and move the schedule for surgical repair forward (Amstalden-Mendes 2007).

The infant with cleft palate is at high risk for poor ventilation of the eustachian tube, a contributing factor for development of *otitis media* (middle ear infection). The eustachian tube is opened and closed by muscles that cross the palate. Because the palatal plates have failed to form normally, these muscles are also abnormally formed. The impaired ventilation of the eustachian tube is not fully corrected by either surgery or tubes in the ears (Aniansson 2002). Thus, the infant with a cleft palate is at risk for chronic ear infections.

No difference in hearing sensitivity per se was found in a study that compared children with cleft lip and palate to children in a control group. However, perhaps because of a greater frequency of middle-ear disease, the children with cleft lip and palate had lower language comprehension scores, and lower scores on tests of cognition and expressive language (Jocelyn 1996). Consequently, it is crucial to identify other preventive methods of reducing episodes of ear infections in this population. Paradise (1994) and Aniansson (2002) identified that longer duration of human milk feeding is significantly correlated with a reduction in acute and secretory otitis media in children with cleft palate.

BWC has worked with 2 infants with clefts of the palate who were exclusively fed human milk for 5 and 6 months respectively. As was periodically verified by test weighing, neither infant was capable of obtaining adequate milk intake from direct breastfeeding. Their mothers comforted them at the breast, but these babies were primarily fed pumped breast milk by bottle. Neither baby experienced any ear infections until formula or solid food was introduced into their diets. Ethically, parents should be informed of the risk of formula in the development of otitis media in infants with cleft defects. If a mother's milk supply is not adequate, donor human milk from an accredited human milk bank is an option.

The Cleft Lip/Cleft Palate Team

In order to advocate for the important protections conferred by lactation (for the mother) and human milk (for the infant), cleft palate care teams should be educated in best practices for initiation of lactation, and should have access to an IBCLC. The LC performs individualized breastfeeding assessments, advises about pumping, milk storing, and alternative feeding methods. She assists the mother with different feeding positions, and encourages skin-to-skin holding as a way to assist milk production and enhance bonding.

Infants with cleft palate defects are challenging to feed no matter what feeding method is used. They may choke, experience nasal regurgitation, and spill milk. These challenges may put the infant at risk for reduced positive social contact during feeding (Morris 1977). Whatever initial difficulties occur, parents can be reassured that feeding skills will most likely improve over time.

An isolated cleft of the lip may not significantly affect breastfeeding; however, there are few documented cases of effective breastfeeding of infants with cleft palate. One study of 20 Thai infants found that only 2 infants with cleft palate were exclusively breastfed for 6 months (Pathumwiwatana 2010). Neither mother worked outside the home, they required extensive follow-up support, and both mothers basically hand-expressed milk into their baby's mouth at every feeding.

The baby with a cleft palate typically cannot create enough suction to transfer sufficient amounts of milk to produce normal growth. Supplementation, ideally with own mother's milk, is generally required. It is doubtful that infants with cleft palate have the ability to empty the breast adequately enough to sustain a full milk supply. Therefore, most mothers will need to express milk to maintain a full supply. Some mothers of infants with cleft palate do not receive this information. Their infants may fail to thrive and their milk supplies may be undermined. The Academy of Breastfeeding Medicine (2007) describes a "...lack of evidence on which to base clinical decisions" in this population with regard to specific breastfeeding strategies.

While being realistic about the need for supplementation with pumped milk, the LC should encourage the mother to experiment with various breastfeeding positions. If a palatal cleft is small and located on the hard palate only, a mother with soft, elastic breasts may find that her breast tissue plugs the cleft. If she has an ample milk supply, a responsive milk ejection reflex, and erect nipples, her

infant may be able to breastfeed better than expected. Older infants may become more adept over time, as has been reported in the anthropological literature.

While many claims are made for various feeding devices and methods, a Cochrane Review of research related to feeding infants with cleft defects (Bessell 2011) found no statistical difference between feeding outcomes in infants who were fitted with maxillary plates compared to no plates. Nor did they discover any statistical difference in growth outcomes when comparing the available bottle types used to feed infants with clefts. The Cochrane Review found no evidence to support any type of current maternal advice and/or support for these babies. Since evidence-based protocols do not yet exist to provide specific guidance for feeding children with clefts, common sense approaches aim to maximize growth while reducing the risk of aspiration.

The LC, along with other feeding specialists such as occupational therapists (OTs), assist in teaching mothers alternative feeding methods. Given the lack of evidence to demonstrate the superiority of one method over another, the team must experiment to discover which method of feeding works best for the individual infant. Cups, spoons (Goval 2012), bottles, disposable syringes (Ize-Iyamu 2011) and feeding tubes are all acceptable methods, but it may take experimentation to find the one that is most suitable. Maternal self-esteem is enhanced when the health care team takes into account the mother's perceptions of how her infant reacts to various feeding interventions.

Cleft Lip

The lips stabilize the breast in the mouth, and help the tongue form a seal (see Ch. 3). Maintenance of a tight seal allows the baby to generate suction (Geddes 2008). Since the ability to create effective suction is critical for milk removal, gaps or breaks in the seal are problematic. A small, incomplete cleft of the lip (**Figs. 398 and 399**) generally does not impede breastfeeding if it can be sealed in some manner. Cleft lip is classified as complete if the cleft extends from the lip into the nasal cavity (as in **Fig. 407**). Complete clefts of the lip are more disfiguring and harder to seal.

To plug or seal a cleft lip, the mother holds the infant close to her breast. She draws up breast tissue between 2 fingers (similar to grasping a cup handle) and presses it into the gap in the lip. The so-called "teacup hold" is demonstrated in **Fig. 400**). Or, the mother may place her finger over the cleft to create a seal. Once a seal is achieved, the baby can create suction. If the cleft lip extends into the nasal cavity, it is more difficult for the mother to help the infant achieve a seal. Surgical repair of a cleft lip usually takes place within a few days, weeks, or months of the birth, depending on the preferences of the surgical team and the family, and on the size and health of the baby. There is moderate to strong evidence that infants can breastfeed immediately following cleft lip surgery (Reilly 2007).

Types of Cleft Palates

Clefts of the palate vary greatly. Some involve small, isolated perforations of the hard or soft palate; other cleft formations are more extensive and create severe facial disfigurement. The size and location of the cleft influence feeding in different ways. Clefts of the palate can be bilateral, that is, affecting both sides of the mouth on each side of the midline. Clefts can be unilateral, on one side only. Clefts can be complete, from uvula to nostrils. They can be incomplete, meaning that the cleft does not extend to the gum ridge.

Figs. 401 and **402** show clefts of the soft palate. Note the absence of the uvula. **Fig. 403** shows an adult woman with a *bifid uvula*. The presence of a bifid (cleft) uvula is often a marker for a *submucousal cleft of the palate* ((Rudolph 2003, Oji 2013).

Submucousal clefts are relatively uncommon. Submucousal clefts of the soft palate consist of a deficiency or lack of muscle tissue or incorrect positioning of the muscles. Symptoms include eustachian tube dysfunction, hypernasal speech, speech problems, and bifid uvula. Deficiencies of the muscles of the soft palate create dysfunctional swallowing. Some infants with submucousal clefts of the soft palate present with nasal regurgitation and most have feeding problems of some degree.

A submucousal cleft of the hard palate is a defect in the center of the bony palate. Because skin covers the cleft, they are not easily detected by casual visualization. A submucousal cleft of the hard palate can be detected by feeling for a notch or depression when palpated gently during a digital exam. They can also be detected by shining a light on the palate, or by a light probe placed within the nose. Submucousal clefts can persist undetected into adulthood (Ha 2013).

It is tempting to assume that small clefts will not affect feeding, but even a small cleft of the hard or soft palate poses considerable problems for feeding, especially in early infancy. The 3 week-old girl in **Fig. 404** has a centrally located cleft of the soft palate similar to the one pictured in **Fig. 401**. She could not seal her oral cavity and was unable to create suction. Her breathing sounded wet after feeding, suggesting aspiration.

Weighing 9 lbs (4075 g) at birth, this baby appeared robust; however, she had severe feeding problems. No matter what oral feeding method was tried, the baby demonstrated distress after consuming approximately one ounce (28 g) of milk. In **Fig. 404**, the baby is being fed in a semi-upright position to prevent aspiration, and flexed at the hips to help stabilize her body. The baby is feeding from a Mead Johnson™ cleft palate feeder, a soft bottle that allows the mother to squeeze milk into the baby's mouth. The baby flared her lips often during feeding, allowing milk to spill out. As the mother had reported to the LC, the baby consumed about one ounce of milk and then began to demonstrate aversive behavior. When arching failed to result in her mother removing the bottle, the baby appeared to fall asleep (**Fig. 405**).

At the time the photos in **Figs. 404 - 406** were taken, this infant was 30 days old and not back to her birth weight. The LC had been working with this dyad and reporting to the pediatrician since Day 4. The mother had tried various types of feeding implements, including spoons, cups, the Medela Special Needs Feeder™, and the Pigeon™ feeder. A feeding tube at the breast was also tried. The baby demonstrated the same tendency to limit her milk intake no matter how she was fed. The LC informed the pediatrician that feeding was not successful for the infant. The pediatrician, concerned about the lack of weight gain, ordered a nasogastric tube (NG) to be placed. The infant is shown in **Fig. 406** sucking on a pacifier (to protect oral feeding skills and to calm her) while being fed fortified human milk via the NG tube. NG tube feeding immediately improved her milk intake and she began to gain weight.

Early Surgical Repair of Cleft Lip

Traditional repair of cleft defects are scheduled for the lip at 3 months; soft palate repairs are usually done around 6 to 8 months. Hard palate repairs typically occur between 12-18 months. Some teams surgically repair cleft lip as early as the first month, and palates as early as 3 months.

Early repair of cleft lip is based on the idea that during the first 28 days after birth, neonates retain fetal wound healing capabilities. Rapid healing is desirable in itself, and enhances cosmetic effect, helping to improve appearance. Additionally, younger babies have enhanced immunologic status as the result of breast milk feeds and transplacentally -acquired immune factors, enabling them to better withstand the stress of surgery (Jiri 2012).

Because surgeries such as hernia repair and bowel resectioning of infants with NEC are now widely performed on newborns, anesthesiologists are experienced in providing sedation for neonates. Greater skill in managing neonatal anesthesia is thought to reduce the level of risk of early repair surgery. Some surgical teams have been performing early repair of cleft lips in neonates for close to a decade. Some teams perform the surgery in the immediate neonatal period, within the first 8 days (Jiri 2012). Jiri et al., commented that early repair had a positive psychological impact on the child and its family.

Hentges (2011) investigated cognitive development in infants with cleft lip who had undergone late repair (3 months) versus those who underwent early repair. The late repair group showed significantly poorer cognitive development at 18 months when compared to a control group of unaffected children. The early repair group had significantly better cognitive outcomes than the late repair group. The researchers attributed this to the quality of early mother-infant interactions. They concluded that social interactions in the first few months are especially critical for child cognitive outcomes, and recommended that interventions for infants with cleft lip should focus on fostering the best parental care.

Breastfeeding is sometimes interrupted after lip surgery for fear the sutures will tear, although there is little clinical evidence to support this. Weatherly-White found evidence of better weight gain, shorter hospital stays, fewer complications, and no apparent difference in the operative results when he compared breastfed infants with cup- or syringe-fed term infants following lip repair (Weatherly-White 1987). In a prospective, randomized trial, Darzi (1996) showed that early postoperative breastfeeding after cleft lip repair is safe, results in more weight gain at 6 weeks after surgery, and is less labor intensive than spoon feeding.

Not all babies are willing to breastfeed immediately following surgery. Some parents report that their infants refused to breastfeed for several days, apparently owing to discomfort. Some infants will put their mouths close to the breast but will not suck. Other babies breastfeed immediately.

Repair of a Cleft Lip: One Mother's Experience

The mother of an infant born with a simple cleft of the lip wrote the following letter to BWC some months after the surgical repair was performed. The infant's surgical team was firm in instructing this mother that damage to the sutured lip would occur if she breastfed her son within 2 weeks of his lip repair.

"It's been nearly a year since I first asked you for help in planning the surgery for my son's cleft lip repair. I guess I didn't realize it would take this long for me to talk about these events.

"His surgery was done at 5 months and was very smooth, but certainly emotionally draining. He looked like a little refugee from a war-torn country when he came to, and stayed like that for about 24 hours. He didn't make any indication for the first 3 days of wanting to nurse, although once on each of those days I did nurse him because I couldn't stand it. He refused the syringe feedings with extreme vigor and never did accept them except at night when he was so sleepy he didn't realize it. I'm sure the little nursing I offered him made it harder for him, but I found I couldn't make a stand either way.

"At 36 hours after surgery, he began to grab food off my plate (although he still didn't try to nurse). At 48 hours, I finally began to mix a little pureed sweet potato with lots of breast milk and spoon-fed him. He wouldn't accept a syringe from the nurses either. Dr. -- witnessed one of the feeding attempts at length at about 48 hours after surgery. And then, at last he very quietly said, "You know, I guess I've never seen a breastfed baby." I could tell it had sunk in that there was something very different going on here. After 72 hours I couldn't pump enough to keep up with feeding, so I began to nurse to build up the supply again. The baby nursed well with no physical complications, although I was nervous for a few days. And it was not until the first long nursing at home that he made eye contact with me – the first time since the surgery.

"It was hard because of my emotional quandary over being instructed not to nurse the baby. I still haven't told Dr. – that we nursed so early on. He wanted me to wait 2 weeks, which would have been impossible for both of us."

Repair of Cleft Palate

Repair of the soft palate can occur between 6 to 8 months, with some cleft palate teams performing the surgery as early as 3 months (Denk 2001). Hard palate repair is typically done in a 2-stage process. Compared to a single surgery to correct the palate at age 1 year or less, the 2-stage approach has been demonstrated to reduce detrimental effects of surgery on palate growth and to enable improved early speech development (Gundlach 2013).

Because the infant pictured in **Figs. 404-406** was unable to feed normally and had a history of poor growth, her pediatrician referred her to a surgical team in another city for evaluation for early repair of her soft palate cleft. Surgery was scheduled to occur when she reached 10 lbs, which happened at approximately 3 months of age.

The infant experienced a successful and uneventful surgical repair of her soft palate. However, while she was recovering in the special care nursery, she suffered a complete bowel rotation. The neonatologists caring for her speculated that her early self-limitation of milk intake may have had more to do with the undetected partial bowel rotation than to her cleft defect. The total bowel rotation required emergency surgery. The infant slowly recovered and began feeding at the breast with a feeding tube device by the time she was 4 months old. Her stressed mother had difficulty maintaining a full milk supply, and the baby was fed donor human milk whenever supplementation was necessary.

Clefts of the Hard Palate and Grooved Palates

Fig. 407 shows an infant with a *complete cleft* of the lip and hard palate. Note the involvement of the nose. Complete clefts of the hard palate create problems with dental formation. These infants not only require surgery to repair the cleft, they will also need extensive dental correction with surgery and orthodontia (Redford-Badwal 2003). Most require speech therapy.

Fig. 408 shows the palate of an infant who was intubated for many weeks, causing reshaping of the palate and the formation of a groove or channel. This palatal formation can mimic many of the feeding problems created by a cleft of the hard palate. The infant may have difficulty positioning the nipple against the palate (Snyder 1997). Some instances of unusual palate formation occur as part of syndromic conditions (Rovet 1995). **Fig. 409** shows the abnormally-shaped palate of a 12 year-old with Down Syndrome. This boy was unable to breastfeed exclusively as an infant. (See also **Fig. 364** and the discussion of Turners Syndrome in Ch. 16.)

Case Study of an Infant With a Cleft of the Lip and Palate

The infant in **Figs. 410-414** was referred by the mother's midwife. The infant had a complete (nose to soft palate) unilateral cleft (**Fig. 410**). His mother had previously breastfed another child and had normal, well-everted nipples. Her breasts were firmly engorged at the time of the LC visit. The hospital nurses helped the mother initiate breastfeeding, and the baby received no supplementation during the first 4 days after birth. The baby's birth weight was 7 lb. 6 oz. (3345 g). He had lost approximately 8 percent of his body weight at the time of the lactation consultation on Day 4. He appeared jaundiced and had produced only one small, dark stool in the past 36 hours (**Fig. 411**).

The hospital staff had taught the mother to use upright feeding positions to protect the baby from choking. They correctly encouraged her to carefully support the weight of her breast in her hand, and to use breast compression to help transfer milk to the baby (**Fig. 412**). The hospital LCs assumed that the baby was breastfeeding well because he made many "swallowing sounds." However, this impression was not validated by test weights on an accurate scale, and the baby was discharged without documentation that he was actually transferring milk.

When BWC visited the mother at home, she also shared an initial impression based on feeding observation that the baby was breastfeeding well. The mother demonstrated good positioning and excellent breastfeeding technique. The baby sounded like he was swallowing milk. However, test weights revealed no evidence of intake. The first weight indicated that the baby actually lost 1 g during the feeding. Three subsequent test weights were performed after positioning changes. All the test weights indicated zero intake.

Based on the lack of measurable intake, reduced stooling, dark, scant urine, rising bilirubin levels, and continued weight loss, the LC advised the mother to begin pumping her breasts and to use her milk to supplement the baby. The mother had a small quantity of hand-expressed colostrum in the refrigerator. The colostrum was warmed and offered to the baby by spoon and then by cup. He seemed unable to organize swallowing from these utensils. In **Fig. 413** the baby is shown drinking this colostrum from a Medela Special Needs Feeder™ (formerly called the Haberman Feeder™). The baby's feeding affect was depressed at this feeding, but improved over the next 24 hours. The baby was soon feeding reasonably well from the special bottle.

The LC discussed the options available to the family, including early repair of the lip. The parents visited the website of a plastic surgeon who specializes in early repair. On Day 18, the family traveled out of state for the surgery. The surgery was uneventful, and the baby is pictured in **Fig. 414** several days after the surgery (photo courtesy of K. Bird). The initial surgery closed the lip and partially repaired the palate. Subsequent surgeries would be required to fully close the hard palate.

One of the factors that motivated the parents to seek early repair was their goal of preserving breastfeeding. However, even this highly motivated mother experienced problems maintaining her milk supply. She took domperidone, took herbs, pumped at recommended levels, and used a feeding tube device at the breast. Because of the hard palate cleft, the baby had great difficulty obtaining milk from any method that required creation of suction, and soon refused to breastfeed.

The mother told the LC, "He gets so angry when I try to nurse him, and I feel really sad and rejected." The mother had problems achieving a milk ejection when she pumped. Shortly after returning home from the hospital where the surgery was performed, both the baby and his older sibling developed *respiratory syncytial virus* (RSV). "Between caring for the baby and the 2 year-old, pumping, doing the nebulizer and oxygen treatments, I felt just a little bit insane." The mother decided to wean. She described feelings of depression as she dealt with the loss of the breastfeeding experience.

This case serves to remind HCPs of the enormous stress involved in caring for such infants. Stress may impact the decision to continue to maintain lactation (Lau 2001). In spite of help from an LC, and good social support, breastfeeding was not successful. However, the infant had the benefit of colostrum and of several weeks of exclusive human milk feeds. In such situations, the LC helps the mother process her feelings, praises her for her efforts, and answers questions accurately, including details about relactation or assistance with weaning.

Nasal Regurgitation

Inability to create suction is only one problem caused by cleft defects. The breach of the barrier between the oral and nasal cavities exposes the nasal tissues to contact with food when the infant swallows. An infant with a cleft palate may experience frequent nasal regurgitation, spilling milk out of the nose with each swallow. The experience worries parents and is uncomfortable and unpleasant for the baby. An upright feeding position may help. The LC reassures parents that feeding ability improves with practice. The baby will eventually learn to swallow more effectively. Human milk is a physiological and non-irritating substance. It contains anti-inflammatory agents (Goldman 1986) and will not irritate sensitive nasal tissue as much as formula will. This issue may be especially important during the time the infant is recovering from surgery, when extensive suturing increases inflammation of the tissues.

Palatal Obturators

Babies with cleft palates may try to obtain milk by compressing with their jaws and tongue because they cannot milk the breast in the normal manner (using suction). While the infant may obtain some milk using compression, many devices have been evaluated to see if breastfeeding might be improved. Some cleft palate teams use a soft silicone prosthesis called an obturator to simulate an intact hard palate (Markowitz 1979, Curtin 1990). Some infants appear to be able to breastfeed more effectively

using such devices, although the evidence for this is weak. Obturators are created from a mold taken of the infant's palate, generally by the pedodontist member of a cleft palate team. New obturators are made as the infant grows.

Another device used in the treatment of infants with clefts is a palatal prosthesis created by an orthodontist to align the palatal segments and nasal cartilage to aid surgical correction. These plates are sized and changed weekly. The baby wears the plate all the time until the repair takes place. The mother removes it for daily cleaning. Bessell (2011) found no statistically significant difference in outcomes for infants fitted with a maxillary plate compared to those with no plate.

Special Bottles

The Medela Special Needs Feeder™ is a bottle with a chambered teat that is controlled by compression rather than suction. Thus, it can be manipulated by an infant who cannot successfully create suction. It is designed to have a controllable flow rate. The soft teat chamber can be squeezed to assist the infant. However, some infants find the flow rate too fast, especially if the teat is squeezed too fast. Three marks (lines) of varying length on the teat indicate flow rate. At the start of the feeding, the feeder inserts the teat so that the shortest line is under the baby's nose. The tip of the teat is positioned under the intact part of the palate. The teat can then be rotated to position the middle or the longest line under the baby's nose. If the infant seems overwhelmed by the milk flow rate, the feeder should rotate the teat until the shortest line is under the nose.

The Pigeon Cleft Palate Nurser™ is a specially designed bottle with a chambered teat that controls the milk flow rate. The Pigeon teat has a Y cut in the tip of the nipple, and a V notched at the base of the nipple. The V indicates an air vent, which must be rotated so that it is positioned under the infant's nose in order to work properly. One side of the Pigeon teat is softer than the other. The soft side is placed in contact with the tongue. Simply touching the teat with the tongue initiates milk flow. If the teat frequently collapses, it may help to slightly enlarge the Y cut, or use a vented bottle system. The mother in **Fig. 415** holds her baby close to her naked breast while he drinks from a Pigeon Feeder™.

Feeding Tube Devices

Feeding tube devices may be useful in feeding some infants with cleft palate. However, in order to work, the infant must be able to create some suction. Some infants with cleft defects become easily exhausted during feedings and will be unable to obtain adequate milk volumes using feeding tube devices. Therefore, intake must be carefully monitored. A gravity feed may increase flow rate and help the infant who is unable to create sufficient suction to draw milk into a feeding tube. If using a Supplemental Nursing System™, for example, the bottle can be elevated (strung on a pole lamp or a hook on the wall) to take advantage of a greater gravity drop. The tube is taped as usual to the mother's breast or to a parent's finger. The device comes with 3 sizes of tubing. The mother can select the largest tubing, providing the flow rate is managable for the baby. The mother can put both tubes into the baby's mouth at the same time (**see Fig. 326**). A parent can also squeeze the device to increase the milk flow rate.

Nipple Shields

Soft silicone nipple shields, which enlarge the diameter of the mother's nipple, may in some sense simulate the effect of a palatal obturator. The extra mass of the shield may help plug a small cleft of the hard palate. The infant will probably not be able to breastfeed normally, but this intervention may help the baby stay on the breast longer, thus assisting the process of bonding. Test weights should be performed to help assess the intake volumes, and no assumptions of intake should be made without empirical verification.

Other Orofacial Issues

As normal growth occurs, the infant skull elongates and the somewhat receding chin pulls forward. However, some infants, for various reasons, have abnormally receding chins. **Fig. 416** shows a baby with a normal chin beside an infant with *retrognathia* (abnormal development) of the lower jaw. A familial tendency toward a receding chin can pose significant, often unrecognized, feeding challenges. The mother of such an infant often experiences sore nipples. While it appears as if the baby is well-positioned at breast, the bottom jaw, being recessed, is not close enough to the breast. Jaw closure occurs on the shaft of the nipple and causes pain for the mother. Poorly positioned jaw closure may also obstruct milk flow to the infant, compromising intake. Because breastfeeding protects against malocclusion (Labbok 1987) it should be encouraged especially for babies with receding chin.

Pierre Robin Sequence (Syndrome)

Pierre Robin Sequence (also referred to as Pierre Robin Syndrome) is an autosomal, recessive, genetic condition marked by significant retrognathia (receding chin). In severe cases, the tongue has a tendency to fall back and block the airway. Serious swallowing disorders, respiratory compromise, and poor feeding may result. Pierre Robin Sequence is often associated with cleft defects that may further compromise feeding.

The Labial Frenum

There are several frena in the human mouth: under the tongue (called the lingual frenulum), between the cheeks and gums, and between the lips and gums. If the upper lip frenum is tight, short, and non-elastic (as in **Fig. 28**), the infant may have difficulty flanging the lips. Rolled-in lips may create abrasion of the nipple. The mother generally can correct this by manually flanging the lips once her baby has latched.

(Wiessinger 1995) reported the case of an infant whose tight upper labial frenum impaired breastfeeding until it was released. There are anectdotal reports from mothers describing breastfeeding problems related to tight labial frena that surgical release resolved. Kotlow (2011, 2013) used the term "lip tie" to refer to tight upper labial frena, and described diagnostic tools for dental practitioners. Treatment options involve laser ablation and do not require hospitalization or anesthesia.

Many children with lip-ties experience no breastfeeding difficulties; however, this midline defect may have a significant effect on dental formation. Dentists know that a tight labial frenum creates a gap between the top 2 teeth, requiring orthodontia to close. **Fig. 417** shows an adult with such a gap. This trait may run in families. The man's daughter had a similar gap caused by a tight labial frenum. She cut her lip-tie when she ran into a backyard clothes line at age 12. The gap between her upper teeth closed during the next 6 months, and she did not require previously planned orthodontia. This man's grandson, seen in **Fig. 418,** was born with a tongue-tie and a tight upper labial frenum. When his teeth errupted, there was a similar gap between the upper incisors.

Ainsworth M. Early caregiving and later patterns of attachment, in M Klaus, M Robertson, (eds), *Birth, Interaction and Attachment: Exploring The Foundations for Modern Perinatal Care*, 1982; Johnson & Johnson, Pediatric Round Table:6, pp. 35-43.

American Cleft Palate-Craniofacial Association: www.acpa-cpf.org Accessed July 2013.

Amstalden-Mendes LG, Magna LA, Gil-da-Silva-Lopes VL. Neonatal care of infants with cleft lip and/or palate: feeding orientation and evolustion of weight gain in a nonspecialized Brazilian hospital. *Cleft Palate and Craniofacial Journal* 2007; 44(3):329-334.

Aniansson G, Svensson H, Becher M, et al. Otitis media and feeding with breast milk of children with cleft palate. *Scandinavian Journal of Plastic and Reconstructive Surgery and Hand Surgery* 2002; 36(1):9-15.

Beaumont D. A study into weight gain in infants with cleft lip/palate. *Paediatric Nursing* 2008; 20(6):20-23.

Bessell A, Hooper L, Shaw WC, et al. Feeding interventions for growth and development in infants with cleft lip, cleft palate, or cleft lip and palate. *Cochrane Database System Review* 2011; Feb. 16(2): CD003315.

Bille C, Olsen J, Vach W, et al. Oral clefts and life style factors - a case-cohort study based on prospective Danish data. *European Journal of Epidemiology* 2007; 22(3):173-181.

Cleft Palate Foundation. *Genetics and You* (2nd edition). 2008. www.aacpa-cpf.org.

Curtin G. The infant with cleft lip or palate: more than a surgical problem. J*ournal of Perinatal & Neonatal Nursing* 1990; 3(3):80-89.

Darzi M, Chowdri N, Bhat A. Breastfeeding or spoon feeding after cleft lip repair: a prospective, randomized study. *British Journal of Plastic Surgery* 1996; 49(1):24-26.

Denk M. Bridging the gap: working with a baby with a cleft. Conference Presentation, ILCA Conference, Acapulco, Mexico, July 18, 2001.

Geddes DT, Kent JC, Mitoulas LR, et al. Tongue movement and intra-oral vacuum in breastfeeding infants. *Early Human Development* 2008; 84(7):471-477.

Goldman A, Thorpe L, Goldblum R. Anti-inflammatory properties of human milk. *Acta Paediatrica Scandia* 1986; 75(5):689-695.

Gorski S, Adams K, Birch P, et al. Linkage analysis of X-linked cleft palate and ankyloglossia in Manitoba Mennonite and British Columbia Native Kindreds. *Human Genetics* 1994; 94(2):141-148.

Goval A, Jena AK, Kaur M. Nature of feeding practices among children with cleft lip and palate. *Journal of Indian Society of Pedodontics and Preventive Dentistry* 2012; 30(1):47-50.

Groer M, Davis M. Health, mood, stress, and immune benefits of lactation. Poster, Proceedings of the12th International Conference of the International Society for Research in Human Milk and Lactation. Sept 10-14, 2004; Queen's College, Cambridge, UK, p. 79.

Gundlach KK, Bardach J, Filippow D, et al. Two-stage palatoplasty, is it still a valuable treatment protocol for patients with a cleft of lip, alveolus, and palate? *Journal of Craniomaxillofacial Surgery* 2013; 41(1):62-70.

Ha KM, Cleland H, Greensmith A, et al. Submucous cleft palate: an often-missed diagnosis. *Journal of Craniofacial Surgery* 2013; 24(3):878-885.

Hentges F, Hill J, Bishop DV, et al. The effect of cleft lip on cognitive development in school-aged children: a paradigm for examining sensitive period effects. *Journal of Child Psychology and Psychiatry* 2011; 52(6):704-712.

Inomata T, Kiuchi A, Yoshida T, et al. Hypervitaminosis A resulting in DNA aberration in fetal transgenic mice. *Mutation Research* 2005; 586(1):58-67.

Ize-Iyamu IN, Saheeb BD. Feeding intervention in cleft lip and palate babies: a practical approach to feeding efficiency and weight gain. *International Journal of Oral and Maxillofacial Surgery* 2011; 4(9):916-919.

Jiri B, Jana V, Michal J, et al. Successful early neonatal repair of cleft lip within first 8 days of life. *International Journal of Pediatric Otorhinolaryngology* 2012; 76(11):1616-1626.

Jocelyn L, Penko M, Rode H. Cognition, communication, and hearing in young children with cleft lip and palate and in control children: a longitudinal study. *Pediatrics* 1996; 97(4):529-534.

Klaus M, Kennell J, Klaus P. *Bonding*. Reading, MA: Addison-Wesley Publishing, 1996; pp. 122-127.

Kotlow LA. Diagnosing and understanding the maxillary lip-tie (Superior Labial, the Maxillary Labial Frenum) as it relates to breastfeeding. *Journal of Human Lactation* 2013; Jul 2. Ahead of print.

Kotlow LA. Diagnosis and treatment of ankyloglossia and tied maxillary fraenum in infants using Er:YAG and 1064 diode lasers. *European Archives of Paediatric Dentistry* 2011; 12(2):106-112.

Lau C. Effects of stress on lactation. in R Schanler, (ed). *Pediatric Clinics of North America* 2001; 48(1):221-234.

Labbok M, Hendershot G. Does breast-feeding protect against malocclusion? An analysis of the 1981 child health supplement to the national health interview survey. *American Journal of Preventative Medicine* 1987; 3(4):227-232.

Little J, Cardy A, Arslan M, et al. Smoking and orofacial clefts: a United Kingdom-based case-control study. *The Cleft Palate-Craniofacial Journal* 2004; 41(4):381-386.

Markowitz J, Gerry R, Fleishner R. Immediate obturation of neonatal cleft palates. *The Mount Sinai Journal of Medicine* 1979; 46(2):123-129.

Mawson AR, Xueyuan W. Breastfeeding, retinoids, and postpartum depression: a new theory. *Journal of Affective Disorders* 2013; June 28, doi: 10.1016/j.jad.2013.05.038. Ahead of print.

Minde K. The impact of medical complications on parental behavior in the premature nursery, in M Klaus, M Robertson (eds), Birth, Interaction and Attachment: Exploring The Foundations for Modern Perinatal Care, 1982; Johnson & Johnson, Pediatric Round Table:6; pp. 98-104.

Morris S. Interpersonal Aspects of Feeding Problems, in J Wilson (ed), Oral Motor Function & Dysfunction in Children, University of North Carolina at Chapel Hill, Division of Physical Therapy, Conference proceedings May 25-28, 1977; pp. 106-113.

Oji T, Sakamoto Y, Ogata H, et al. A 25-year review of cases with submucous cleft palate. *International Journal of Pediatric Otorhinolaryngology* 2013; 77(7):1183-1185.

Paradise J, Elster B, Tan L. Evidence in infants with cleft palate that breast milk protects against otitis media. *Pediatrics* 1994; 94(6):853-859.

Pathumwiwatana P, Tongsukho S, Naratiappakorn T, et al. The promotion of exclusive breastfeeding in infants with complete cleft lip and palate during the first 6 months after childbirth at Srinagarind Hospital, Knon Kaen Province, Thailand. *Journal of the Medical Association of Thailand* 2010; Supple 4:S71-77.

Ramsay M, Gisel E. Neonatal sucking and maternal feeding practices. *Developmental Medicine and Child Neurology* 1996; 38(1):34-47.

Redford-Badwal D, Mabry K, Frassinelli J. Impact of cleft lip and/or palate on nutritional health and oral-motor development. *Dental Clinics of North America* 2003; 47(2):305-17.

Reilly S, Reid J, Skeat J, et al. ABM Clinical Protocol #17: Guidelines for breastfeeding infants with cleft lip, cleft palate, or cleft lip and palate. *Breastfeeding Medicine* 2007; 2(4):243-250.

Rovet J (editor). *Turner Syndrome Across the Lifespan*. Markham, Ontario: Kelin Graphics, 1995; p. iv.

Rudolph C, Rudolph A. *Rudolph's Pediatrics* (21st edition). New York: McGraw Hill, 2003; p. 88.

Snyder J. Bubble palate and failure to thrive: a case report. *Journal of Human Lactation* 1997; 13(2):139-143.

Weatherly-White R, Kuehn D, Mirrett P, et al. Early repair and breast-feeding for infants with cleft lip. *Plastic and Reconstructive Surgery* 1987; 79(6):879-885.

Wiessinger D, Miller M. Breastfeeding difficulties as a result of tight lingual and labial frena: a case report. *Journal of Human Lactation* 1995; 11(4):313-316.

Wilcox AJ, Lie RT, Solvoll K, et al. Folic acid supplements and risk of facial clefts: national population based case-control study. *British Medical Journal* 2007; 334(7591):433-434.

NOTES:

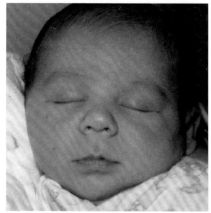

Fig. 1   Deep sleep -- good facial tone

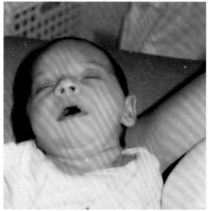

Fig. 2   Deep sleep -- poor facial tone

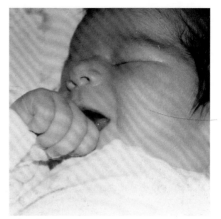

Fig. 3   Light sleep -- early feeding cue

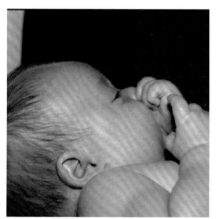

Fig. 4   Pleasurable sucking -- drowsy state

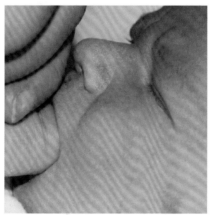

Fig. 5   Facial grimace -- a stress cue

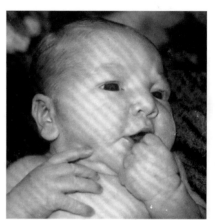

Fig. 6   Quiet alert state

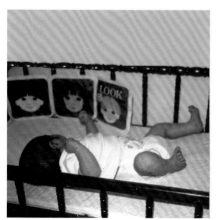

Fig. 7   Active alert state

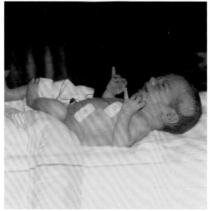

Fig. 8   Motoric stress cues -- finger splaying, stiffening, crying

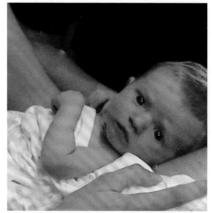

Fig. 9   An infant who is failing to thrive -- worried alert state

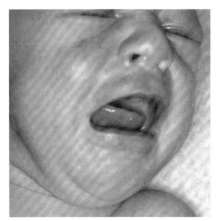

Fig. 10 Crying -- a significant infant stress cue

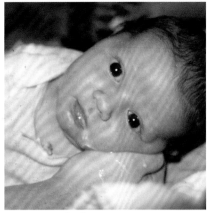

Fig. 11 Satiated appearance (wet burp)

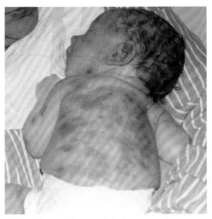

Fig. 12 Normal infant rash

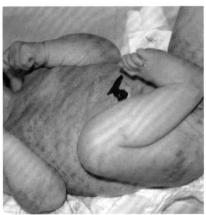

Fig. 13 Infant was ill -- rash may indicate sepsis

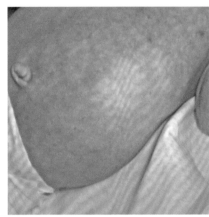

Fig. 14 Mottling on the trunk -- an indication of cold stress

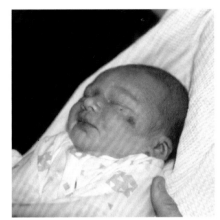

Fig. 15 Forceps bruise

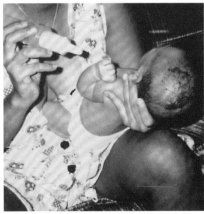

Fig. 16 Vacuum abrasion of the scalp

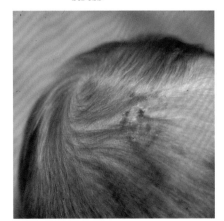

Fig. 17 Fetal monitor scab

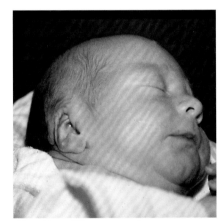

Fig. 18 Flat ear owing to breech position

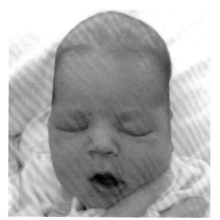

Fig. 19 Cranial molding (narrow head) in a newborn

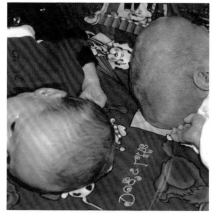

Fig. 20 Cranial asymmetry (premature fusion of cranial sutures)

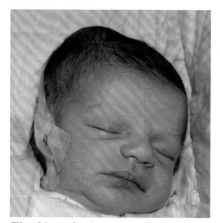

Fig. 21 Cephalohematoma

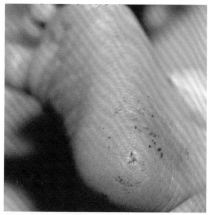

Fig. 22 Heel sticks

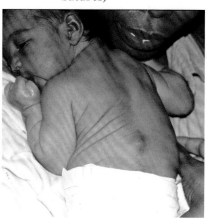

Fig. 23 Spinal tap

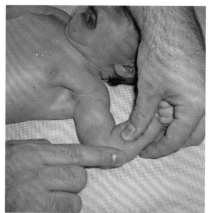

Fig. 24 Identifying jaundice -- press on the skin

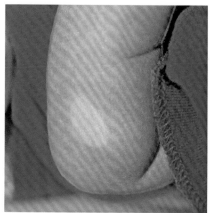

Fig. 25 Identifying jaundice -- observe underlying skin tone

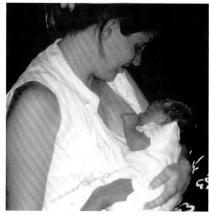

Fig. 26 Fiberoptic bili blanket -- portable phototherapy

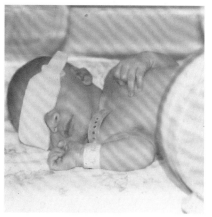

Fig. 27 Traditional phototherapy

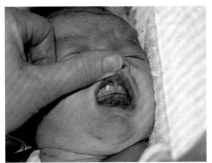

Fig. 28   Tight labial frenum

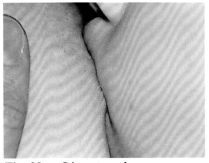

Fig. 29   Lip retraction

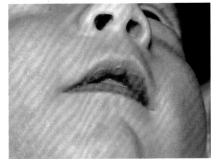

Fig. 30   Sucking blisters on the lip

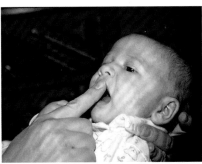

Fig. 31   Facial tone stimulation exercise provided by parent

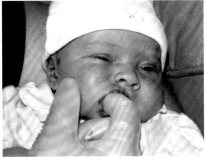

Fig. 32   Assessing thickness of cheek fat pads

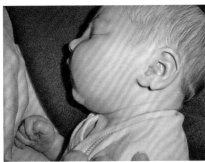

Fig. 33   Receding chin and ear anomaly

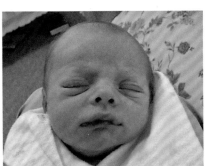

Fig. 34   Jaw asymmetry -- mouth closed

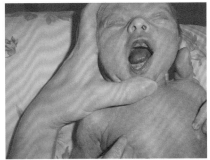

Fig. 35   Jaw asymmetry -- mouth open

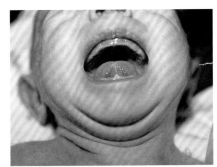

Fig. 36   Bubble palate and Stage 4 tongue-tie

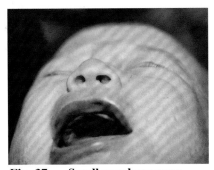

Fig. 37   Small nasal passages

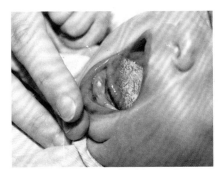

Fig. 38   Newborn with tooth

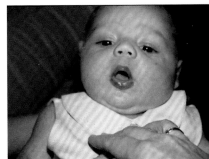

Fig. 39   Lip rounding -- normal lip tone

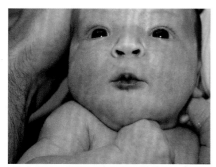

Fig. 40   "Purse string" lips --
           excessive lip tone

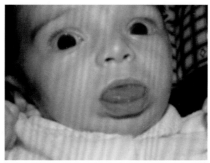

Fig. 41   Low facial tone -- Day 17

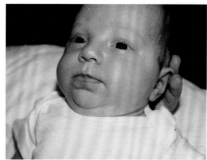

Fig. 42   Lip closure at 5.5 weeks
           after CST

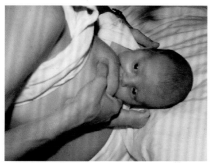

Fig. 43   Breast compression

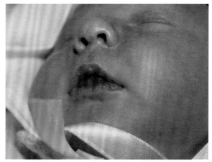

Fig. 44   Low tone -- tongue-tip
           elevation on Day 4

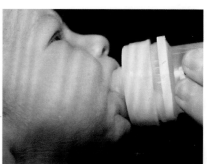

Fig. 45   Lip retraction while
           bottle feeding --
           grimacing

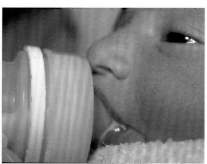

Fig. 46   Poor seal on bottle teat --
           weak lip tone

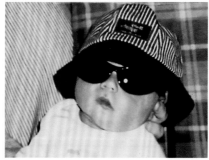

Fig. 47   Jaw asymmetry

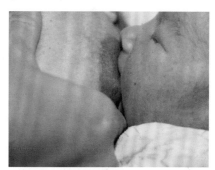

Fig. 48   Jaw support

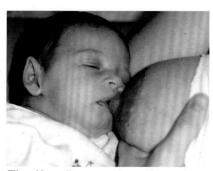

Fig. 49   Depressed rooting reflex

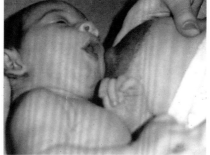

Fig. 50   Remove clothes to rouse

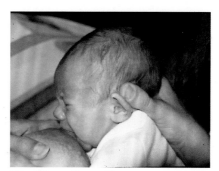

Fig. 51   Gag reflex

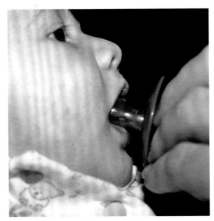

Fig. 52   Therapeutic pacifier use

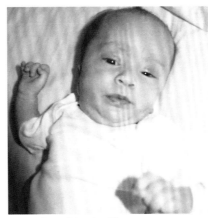

Fig. 53   Torticollis

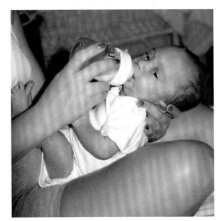

Fig. 54   Hip flexion to assist feeding -- torticollis

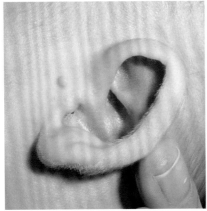

Fig. 55   Ear (auricular) skin tag

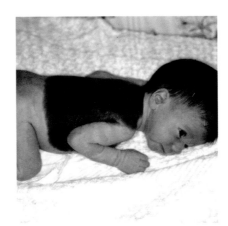

Fig. 56   Nevus

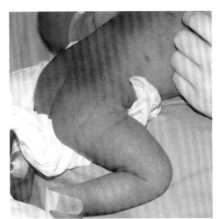

Fig. 57   Congenital dermal melanocytosis

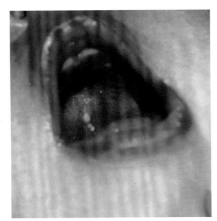

Fig. 58   Epstein's pearls (sometimes mistaken for thrush)

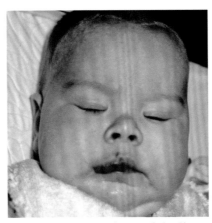

Fig. 59   Hemangioma of the lip

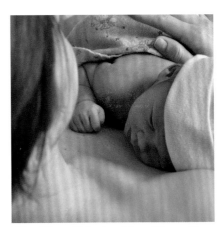

Fig. 60   Skin-to-skin with mother

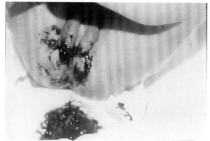

Fig. 61   Meconium stool

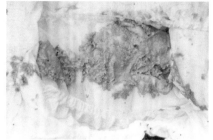

Fig. 62   Transitional stool

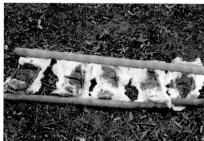

Fig. 63   Bowel output of a 3 day-
                old breastfeeding infant

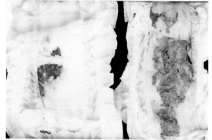

Fig. 64   Size comparison

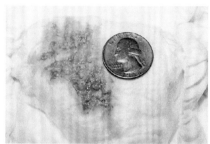

Fig. 65   Coin size comparison --
                A US quarter is 24 mm

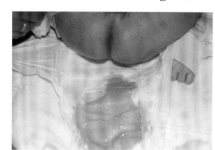

Fig. 66   Watery stool

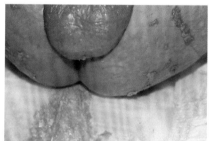

Fig. 67   Seedy stool

Fig. 68   Curd-like stool on Day 6

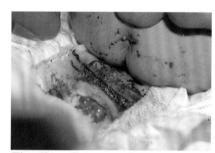

Fig. 69   Green stool

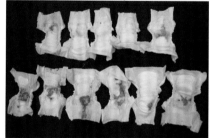

Fig. 70   24-hour output of an
                8 week-old breastfeeding infant

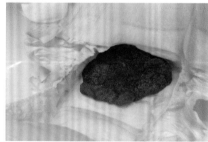

Fig. 71   Stool appearance after
                beginning solid food

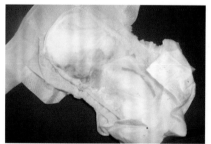

Fig. 72   "Brick dust" urine on
                on Day 2

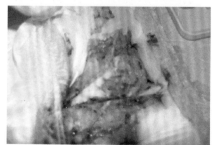

Fig. 73   Blood in stool

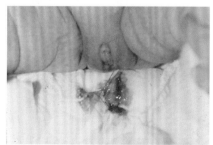

Fig. 74   Bloody vaginal discharge

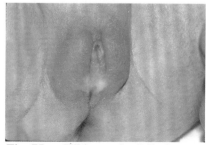

Fig. 75   White vaginal discharge

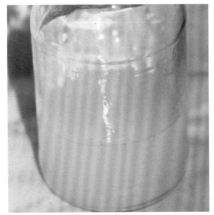

Fig. 76   Clear colostrum

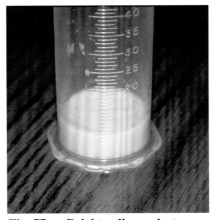

Fig. 77   Bright yellow colostrum

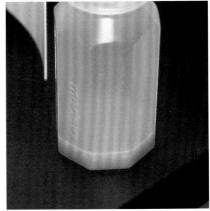

Fig. 78   "Rusty pipe" colostrum

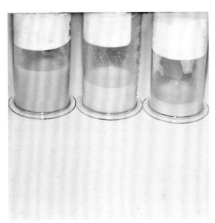

Fig. 79   Light brown colostrum

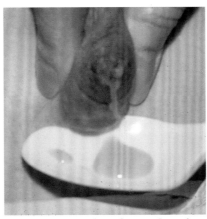

Fig. 80   The size of a newborn's swallow (0.6 ml)

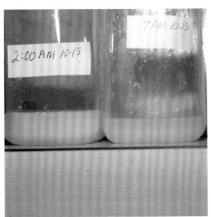

Fig. 81   Milk maturation color changes

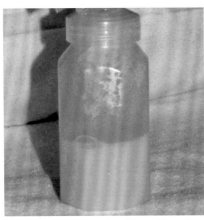

Fig. 82   2.5 oz of milk on Day 3

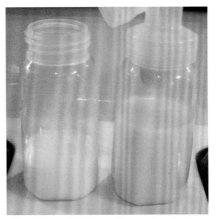

Fig. 83   White milk contrasted with green milk

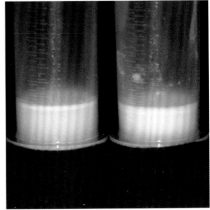

Fig. 84   Foremilk and hindmilk

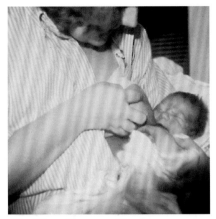

Fig. 85   Poor positioning
frustrates the baby

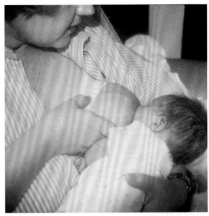

Fig. 86   Improved positioning

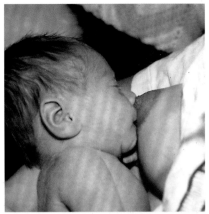

Fig. 87   Line up nose to nipple in
"sniff" position at start
of latch

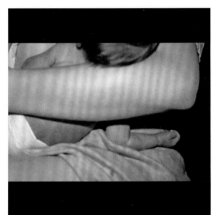

Fig. 88   Poor postural support --
lower arm stress for
baby

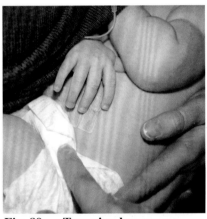

Fig. 89   Trapping lower arm
across the baby's body

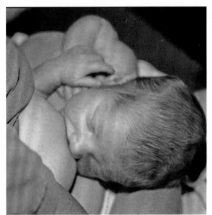

Fig. 90   Both arms are
comfortably positioned
at the midline

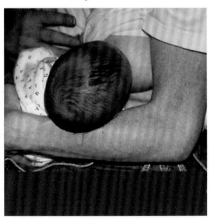

Fig. 91   Baby's head on forearm

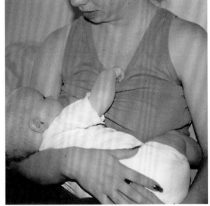

Fig. 92   6 week-old fits in the
crook of the arm

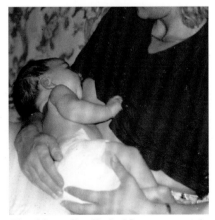

Fig. 93   Cradle hold --
6 week-old

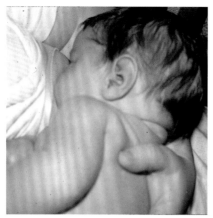

Fig. 94   Over-rotation buries face

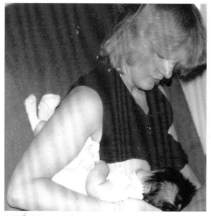

Fig. 95   Football hold

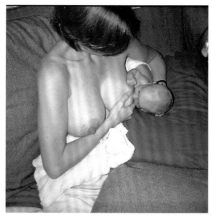

Fig. 96   Variation of football position

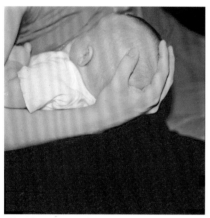

Fig. 97   Avoid hand on head flexing head forward

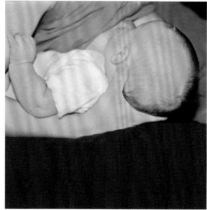

Fig. 98   Improved hand position lessens risk of flexing head

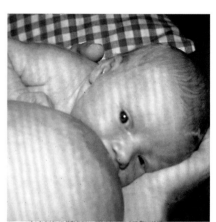

Fig. 99   Cross-cradle position

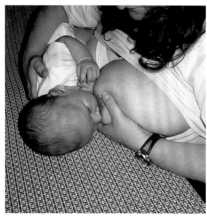

Fig. 100   Cross cradle with table for support

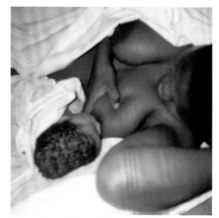

Fig. 101   Side-lying position

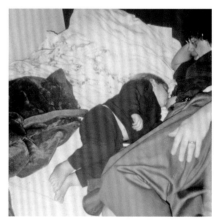

Fig. 102   Side-lying with a 22 month-old

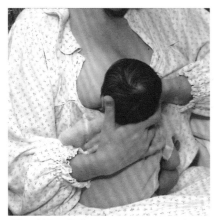

Fig. 103   Seated straddle position

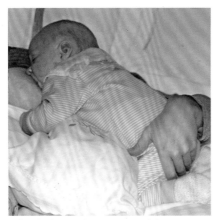

Fig. 104   Laid back position

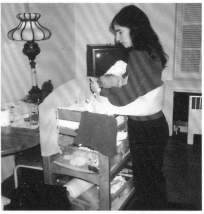

Fig. 105   Breastfeeding while standing

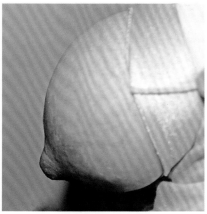

Fig. 106   Nipple located on down-hill slope

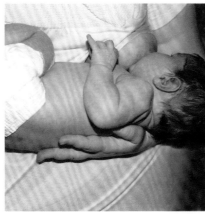

Fig. 107   Supine position to latch

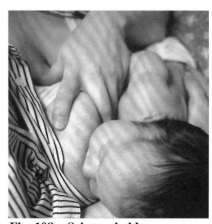

Fig. 108   Scissors hold

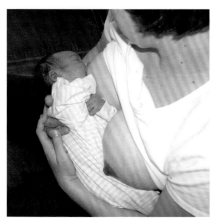

Fig. 109   Alternate cradle postion with a small baby

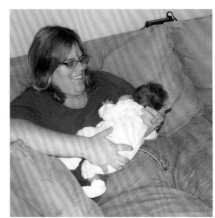

Fig. 110   Alternate cradle position with a larger baby

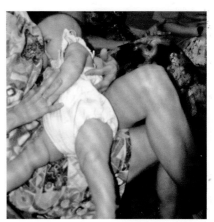

Fig. 111   5 month-old positioning herself

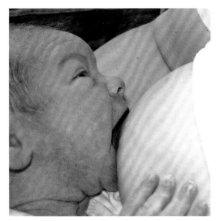

Fig. 112   Chin touches the breast

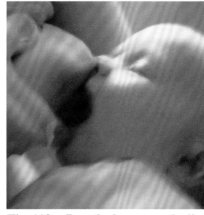

Fig. 113   Rest the breast on the lips and line up nipple to nose

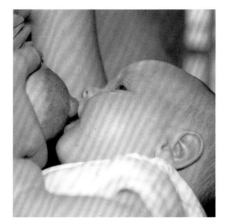

Fig. 114   Tilt the nipple to the palate

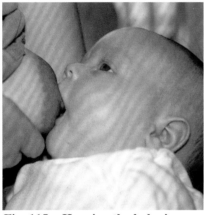

Fig. 115   Hugging the baby in close at the shoulders

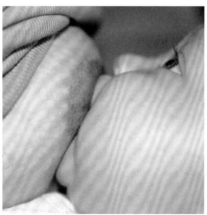

Fig. 116   Asymmetric latch

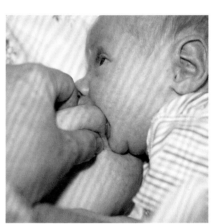

Fig. 117   "Breast sandwich" helps baby latch

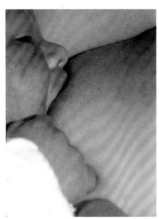

Fig. 118   Start of feed, tight fist

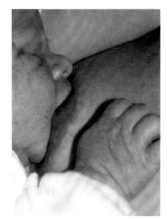

Fig. 119   Gradual relaxation

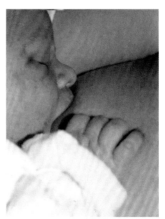

Fig. 120   Hand relaxing

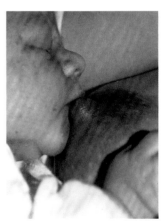

Fig. 121   Baby releases the breast

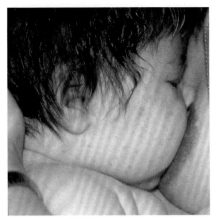

Fig. 122   Chin too close to chest -- face buried

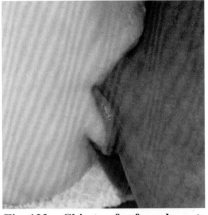

Fig. 123   Chin too far from breast -- jaw will close on nipple shaft

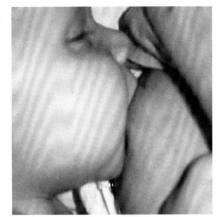

Fig. 124   Shallow latch -- depressed feeding affect

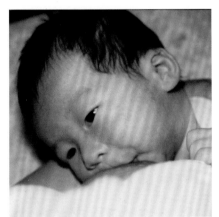

Fig. 125   Lip retraction -- narrow gape

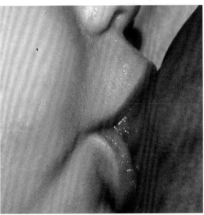

Fig. 126   Narrow gape -- note angle at the corner of the mouth

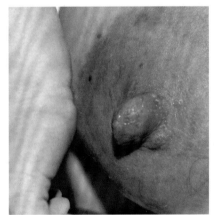

Fig. 127   Pinched nipple -- note angle of the shadow

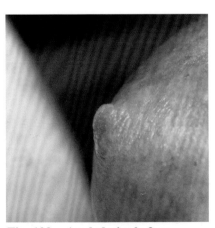

Fig. 128   Angled nipple face

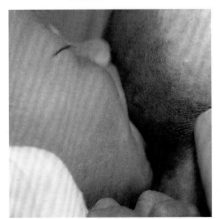

Fig. 129   Well latched newborn -- note wide angle of gape

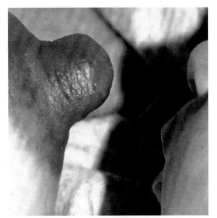

Fig. 130   Nipple undistorted after breastfeeding

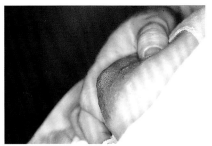

Fig. 131   Flat nipple

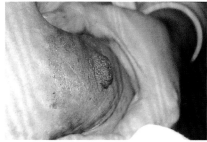

Fig. 132   Sandwich technique

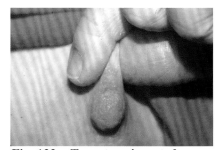

Fig. 133   Teacup or inverted
            nipple hold

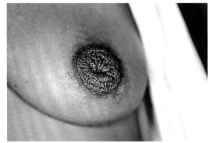

Fig. 134   Inverted nipple at rest

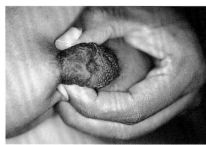

Fig. 135   Inverted nipple when
            compressed

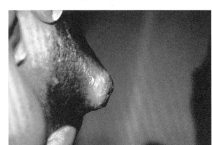

Fig. 136   Inverted nipple after
            mom pulls back on
            areolar tissue

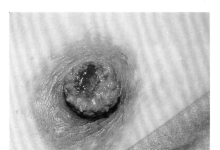

Fig. 137   Dimpled nipple immedi-
            ately after pumping

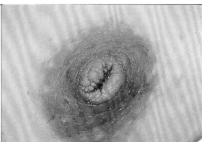

Fig. 138   Dimpled nipple retracted
            2 minutes after pumping

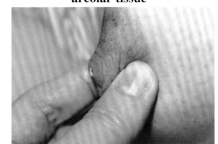

Fig. 139   Lack of breast elasticity
            and a flat nipple

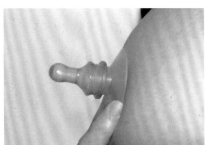

Fig. 140   Antique design of nipple
            shield still being sold

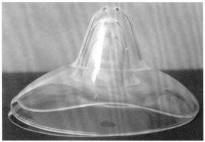

Fig. 141   Size comparison of 3
            nipple shields

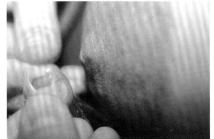

Fig. 142   Applying a nipple shield
            -- turning rim inside out

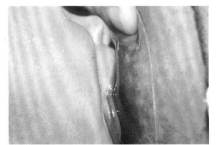

Fig. 143   Well latched on a
            nipple shield

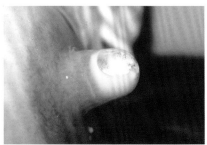

Fig. 144   Nipple drawn into shield
            -- note reservoir of milk

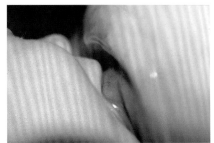

Fig. 145   Poorly latched onto
            a nipple shield

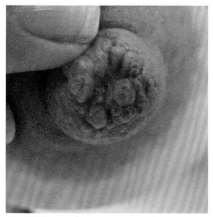

Fig. 146   Raspberry nipple - note individual "drupelets"

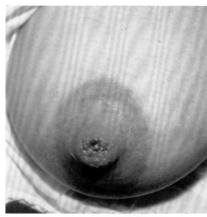

Fig. 147   Inflamed on nipple face - Stage 1 damage

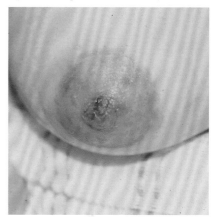

Fig. 148   Suction lesions on flat nipple -- Stage II damage

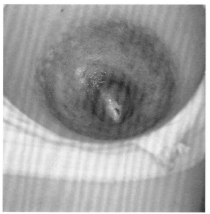

Fig. 149   Pinched nipple -- Stage II damage

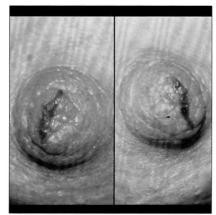

Fig. 150   Scabs from positional stripes -- Stage II damage

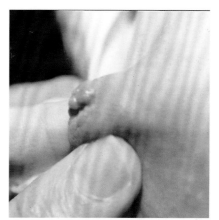

Fig. 151   Fissure 4 weeks postpartum -- Stage III damage

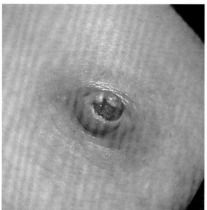

Fig. 152   Partial thickness wound -- Stage III damage

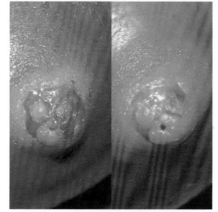

Fig. 153   Eroded and partially healed nipple -- Stage III damage

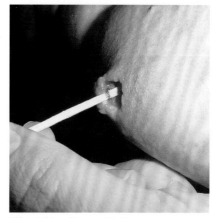

Fig. 154   Stage IV damage

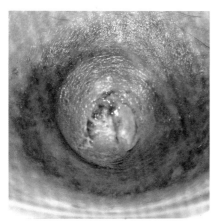

Fig. 155   Infected nipple

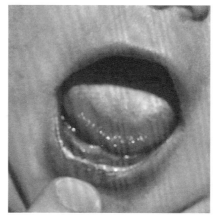

Fig. 156   White tongue

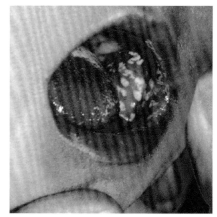

Fig. 157   Thrush on inside
of cheeks

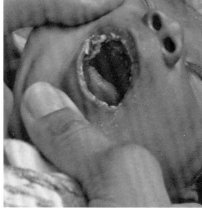

Fig. 158   Oral thrush

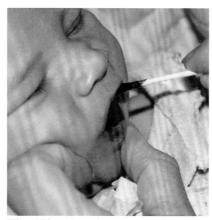

Fig. 159   Treating thrush with
gentian violet

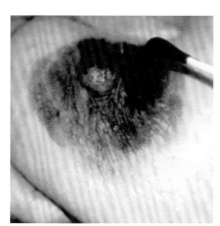

Fig. 160   Gentian violet to treat
nipple yeast

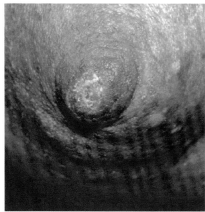

Fig. 161   Nipple yeast -- note
white material on nipple

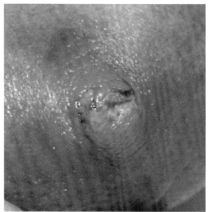

Fig. 162   Bacterial and fungal
infection

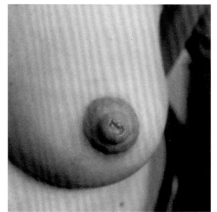

Fig. 163   Tissue breakdown from
untreated infection

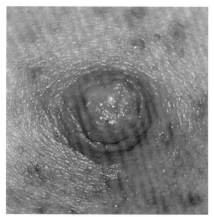

Fig. 164   Allergic reaction to nipple cream

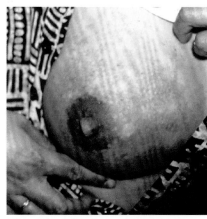

Fig. 165   Hives -- allergic reaction to topical nystatin

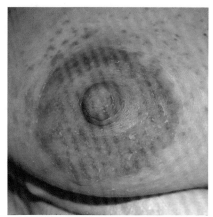

Fig. 166   Eczema

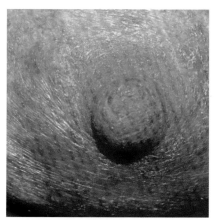

Fig. 167   Psoriasis

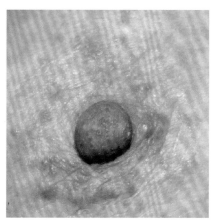

Fig. 168   Poison ivy

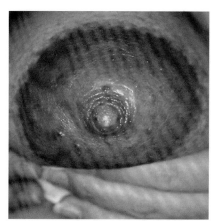

Fig. 169   White spot on nipple - painful blocked nipple pores

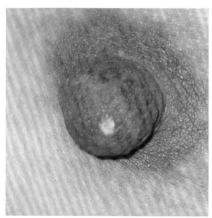

Fig. 170   White spot on nipple - not painful

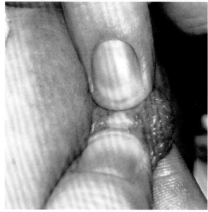

Fig. 171   Sebaceous cyst on shaft of nipple

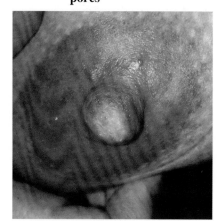

Fig. 172   Vasospasm

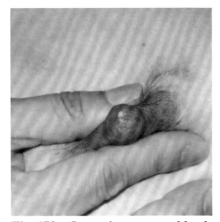

Fig. 173   Squeezing restores blood
            flow and reduces vaso-
            spasm pain

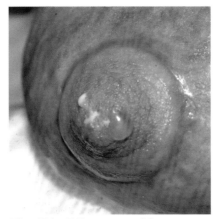

Fig. 174   Blister caused by
            pumping

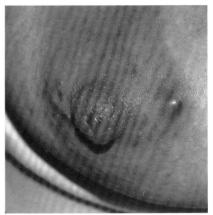

Fig. 175   Infected Montgomery
            gland

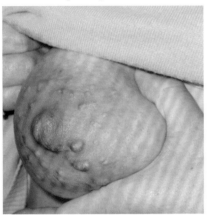

Fig. 176   Swollen areolar tissue
            durring pregnancy

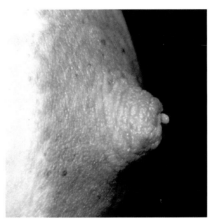

Fig. 177   Skin tag on nipple

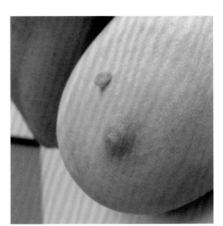

Fig. 178   Skin tag on breast

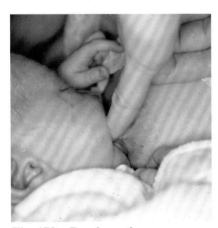

Fig. 179   Break suction
            between gums

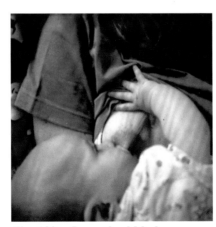

Fig. 180   5 month-old baby

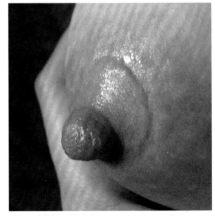

Fig. 181   Babies sometimes leave
            teeth marks on the
            breast

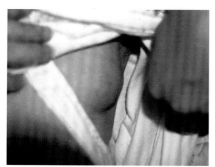

Fig. 182   Engorgement of the
            tail of Spence

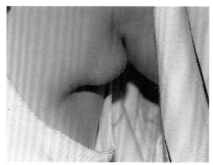

Fig. 183   Accessory breast tissue
            in the axilla 1 month
            postpartum

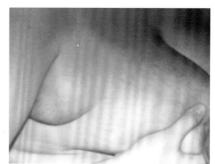

Fig. 184   Accessory breast tissue
            4 days postpartum

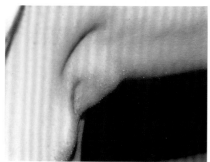

Fig. 185   Engorgement of acces-
            sory breast tissue

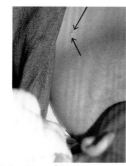

Fig. 186   Ectopic duct

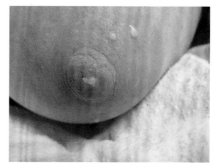

Fig. 187   Milk oozing from
            Montgomery Glands

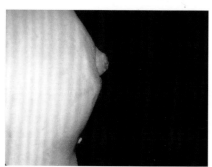

Fig. 188   Accessory (supernumer-
            ary) nipple in profile

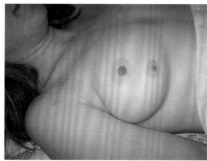

Fig. 189   Bilateral accessory nip-
            ples (Photo S. Gehrman)

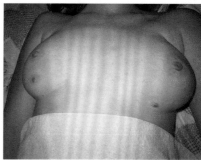

Fig. 190   Bilateral accessory nip-
            ples (Photo S. Gehrman)

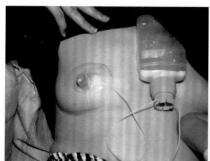

Fig. 191   Underdeveloped breast
            tissue

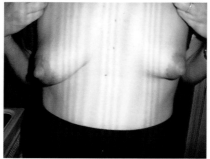

Fig. 192   Underdeveloped breast
            tissue (hypoplasia)

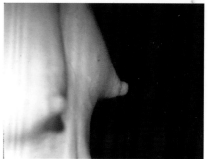

Fig. 193   Underdeveloped breast
            tissue (hypoplasia)

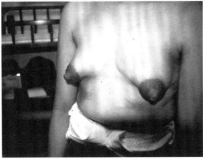

Fig. 194   Tubular breasts --
           impaired milk supply

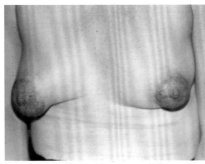

Fig. 195   Unsually shaped breasts
           -- normal milk supply

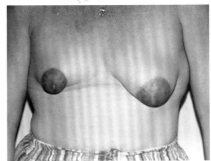

Fig. 196   Breast asymmetry --
           impaired milk supply

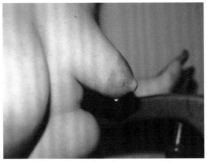

Fig. 197   Tubular breast with
           forward cone areolar
           placement

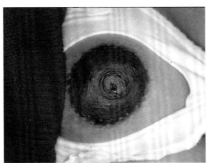

Fig. 198   Periareolar incision --
           impaired lactation

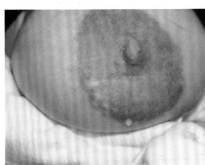

Fig. 199   Periareolar incision --
           evidence of normal MER

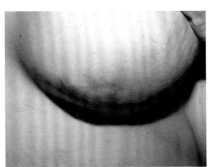

Fig. 200   Abscess at implant site

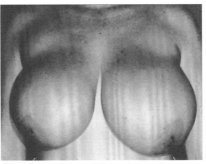

Fig. 201   Large breasts

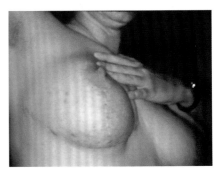

Fig. 202   After reduction
           mammoplasty

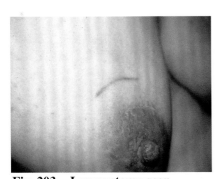

Fig. 203   Lumpectomy scar

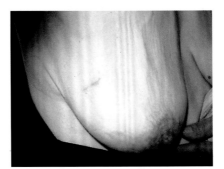

Fig. 204   Weaning breast --
           biopsy scar

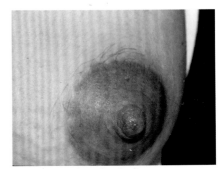

Fig. 205   Areolar hair

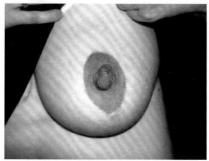

Fig. 206   Unusual nipple shape

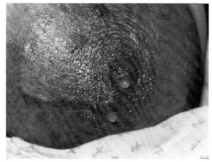

Fig. 207   Double nipple -- oozing milk from both sites

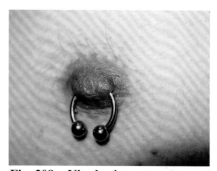

Fig. 208   Nipple ring

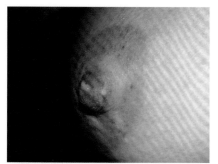

Fig. 209   Oozing milk from nipple ring holes 9 months pp

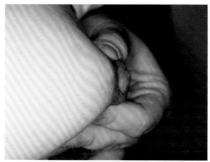

Fig. 210   Nipple at rest

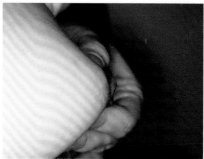

Fig. 211   Nipple inversion revealed when compressed

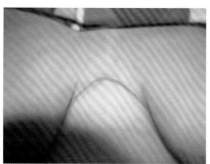

Fig. 212   Open heart surgery scar between her breasts

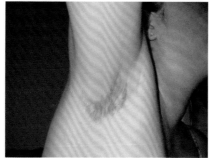

Fig. 213   Axillary scar

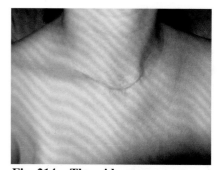

Fig. 214   Thyroid surgery scar

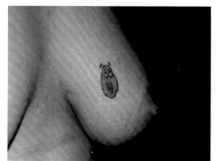

Fig. 215   Tattoo

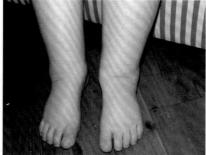

Fig. 216   Swollen ankles during the first week postpartum

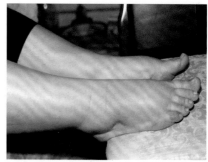

Fig. 217   Swollen feet

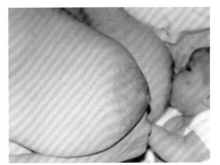

Fig. 218   Large breasts

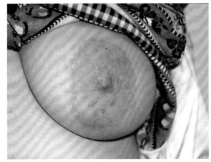

Fig. 219   Large areola

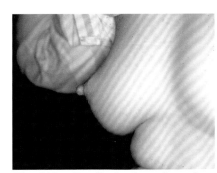

Fig. 220   Small nipple and areola

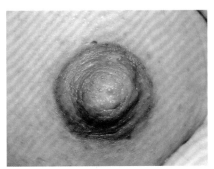

Fig. 221   Small areola

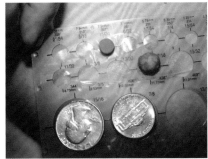

Fig. 222   Engineer's circle template a tool for size comparisons

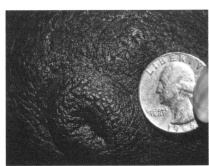

Fig. 223   Quarter-sized nipple

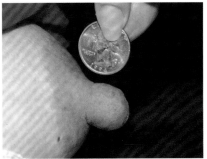

Fig. 224   Coin size comparison - 17 mm long nipple

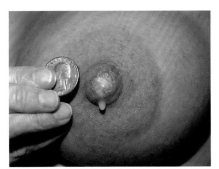

Fig. 225   Large nipple - evidence of infection on Day 6

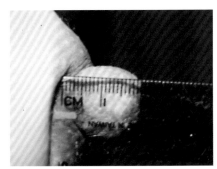

Fig. 226   Nipple length at rest is 2 cm (20 mm)

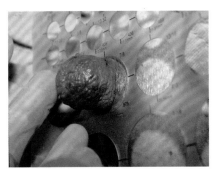

Fig. 227   Large, long nipple (2 cm long)

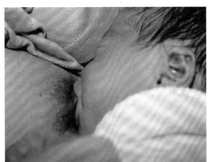

Fig. 228   36-week twin cannot latch onto her large, long nipple

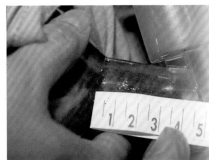

Fig. 229   Nipple 4 cm at full extension

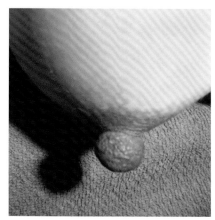

Fig. 230   "Door knob" shaped
            nipple -- note shadow

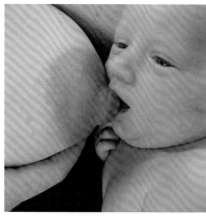

Fig. 231   Nipple size comparison
            with newborn's mouth

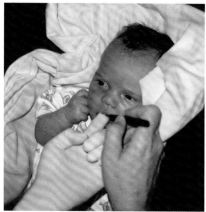

Fig. 232   Measuring oral reach --
            palate length of 7-wk-old

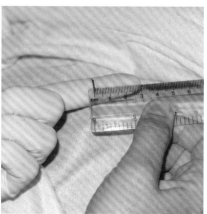

Fig. 233   Palate length of 3 cm

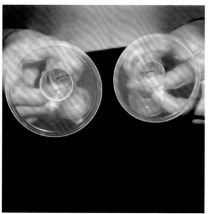

Fig. 234   Medela flange sizes
            30 mm   24 mm

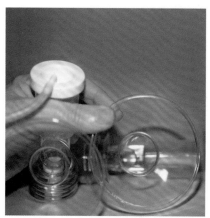

Fig. 235   Ameda (Hollister) flanges
            25 mm   30.5 mm

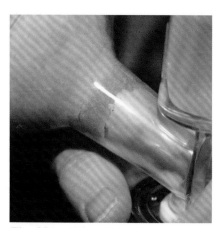

Fig. 236   Tight fit in 25 mm flange

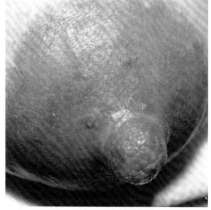

Fig. 237   Tight fit caused cracks
            at base of nipple

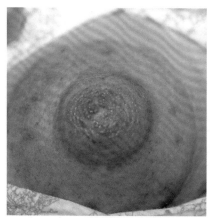

Fig. 238   Tight flange causes
            cracking and abrasion

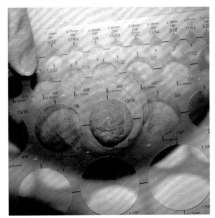

Fig. 239   Pre-pumping nipple
            size 20.64 mm

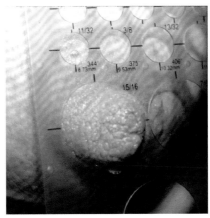

Fig. 240   Post-pumping size swells
            to 23.81 mm

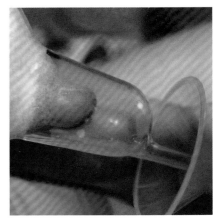

Fig. 241   Glass flange --
            40 mm diameter

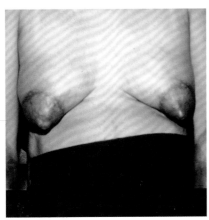

Fig. 242   Woman with PCOS

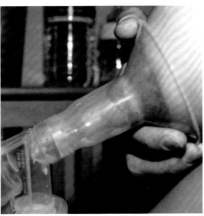

Fig. 243   Woman with PCOS
            pumping with large
            flange

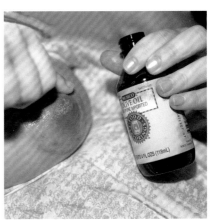

Fig. 244   Lubricating breast with
            olive oil

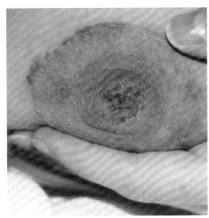

Fig. 245   Abrasions on nipple tip --
            29 mm nipple using
            24 mm flange

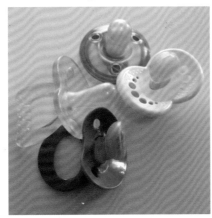

Fig. 246   Various sizes of pacifiers

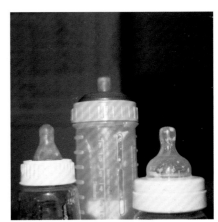

Fig. 247   Bottle teat shapes/sizes
            have clinical implica-
            tions

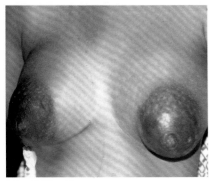

Fig. 248   Breast engorgement
            Day 3

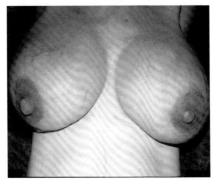

Fig. 249   Breast engorgement
            Day 8

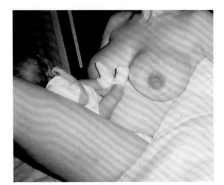

Fig. 250   Breast engorgement
            Day 6

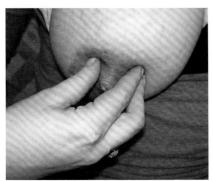

Fig. 251   Reverse pressure
            softening technique

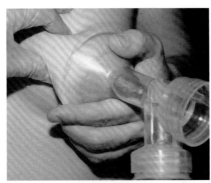

Fig. 252   Flaccid breast Day 12 --
            down regulation of
            supply

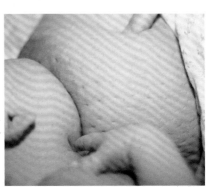

Fig. 253   Peau d'orange

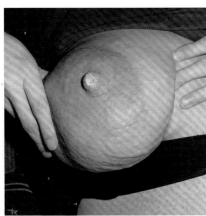

Fig. 254   Infected nipple, mastitis,
            peau d'orange

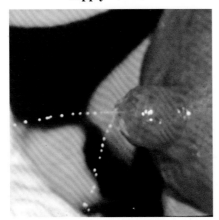

Fig. 255   Milk spray during
            let down

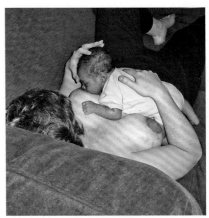

Fig. 256   Prone position
            for managing milk
            oversupply

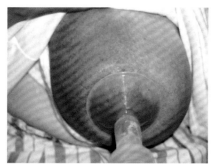

Fig. 257   Breast inflammation
            on Day 4

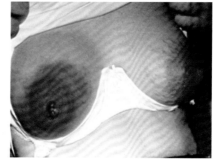

Fig. 258   Bilateral mastitis

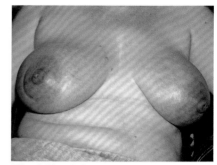

Fig. 259   Bilateral mastitis on
            Day 11

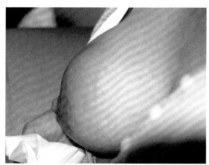

Fig. 260   Ripening abscess with
            induration of the nipple

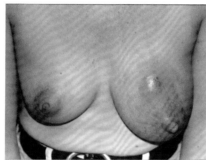

Fig. 261   Ripening abscess

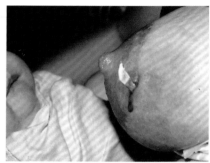

Fig. 262   Subareolar abscess with
            wick

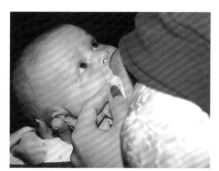

Fig. 263   Holding pad over
            draining abscess wound

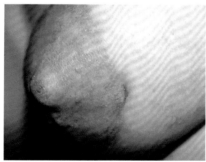

Fig. 264   Healed subareolar
            abscess

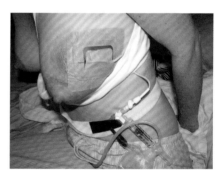

Fig. 265   Percutaneous drain for
            MRSA-related abscess

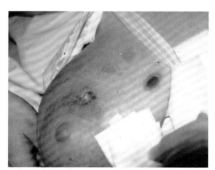

Fig. 266   Multilocular abscesses

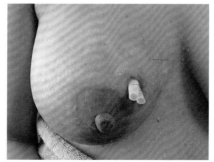

Fig. 267   Abscess drainage tubes

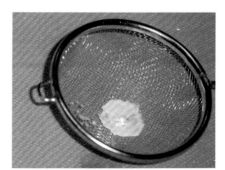

Fig. 268   Clumped milk
            during mastitis

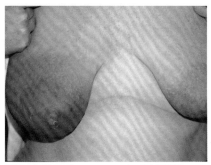

Fig. 269   Case report of MRSA breast infection

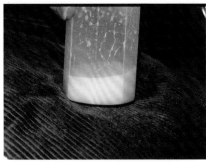

Fig. 270   Yellow milk pumped during MRSA infection

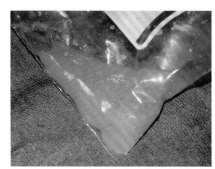

Fig. 271   Orange milk pumped during MRSA infection

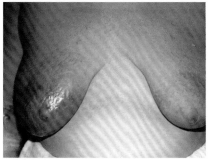

Fig. 272   MRSA infection damages connective tissue and skin

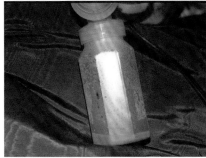

Fig. 273   Red milk pumped during MRSA infection

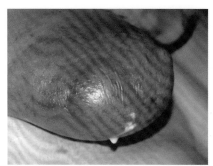

Fig. 274   Milk leaking through broken skin

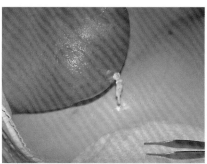

Fig. 275   Congealed milk pulled from original aspiration site

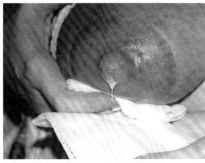

Fig. 276   Congealed milk observed

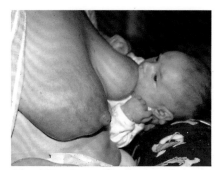

Fig. 277   Breastfeeding on unaffected breast

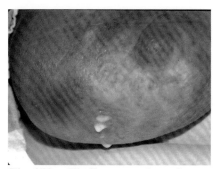

Fig. 278   Healing wound continues to leak milk

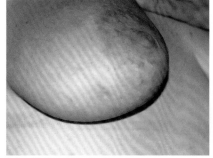

Fig. 279   Healed breast one year later

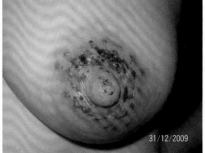

Fig. 280   Herpes infection (Courtesy Sue Cox, IBCLC)

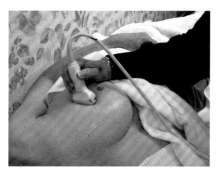

Fig. 281   Ultrasound scan of the breast

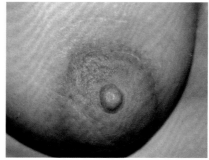

Fig. 282   Incision scars from biopsy and lumpectomy

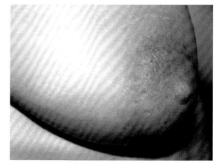

Fig. 283   Bronzed breast during radiation treatment

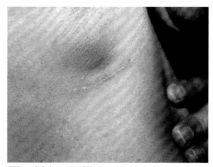

Fig. 284   Axillary node biopsy scar

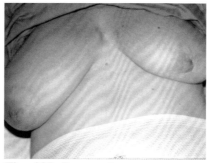

Fig. 285   Lumpectomy

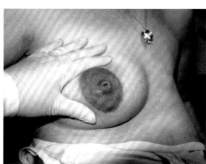

Fig. 286   Sore nipple on remaining breast after mastectomy

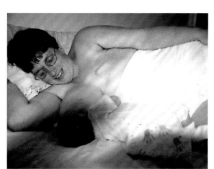

Fig. 287   Breastfeeding after mastectomy

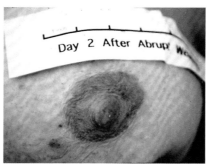

Fig. 288   Needle aspiration bruise on left breast at tumor site

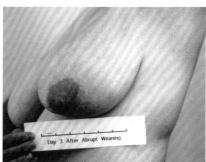

Fig. 289   Induration of the breast above the tumor site

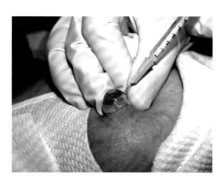

Fig. 290   Lidocaine injection prior to nipple biopsy

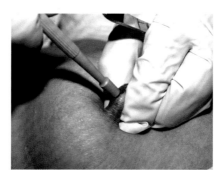

Fig. 291   Punch biopsy tool

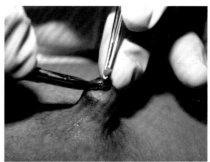

Fig. 292   Core biopsy to rule out Paget's disease of the nipple

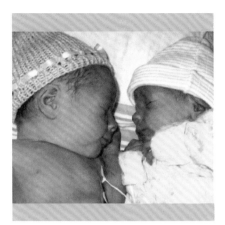

Fig. 293   Discordant Twins (twins of different sizes)

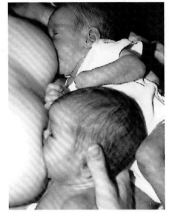

Fig. 294   Poorly positioned twins

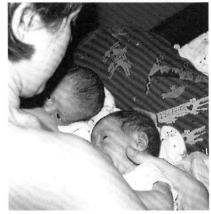

Fig. 295   Improved positioning

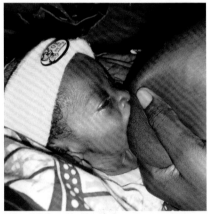

Fig. 296   Guinean mother and preterm twin (1250 g)

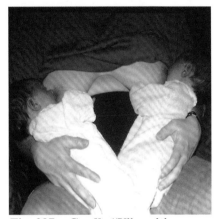

Fig. 297   Cradle "V" position

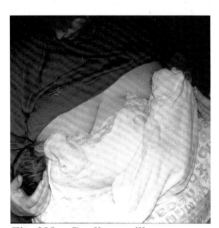

Fig. 298   Cradle on pillow

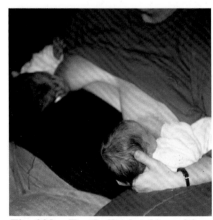

Fig. 299   Football (clutch) position

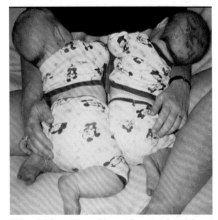

Fig. 300   Kneeling (5 month-old twins with chicken pox)

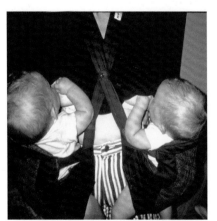

Fig. 301   Twin carrier, 8 months old

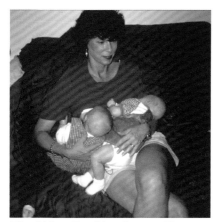

Fig. 302   Combination cradle and football holds, 3 months

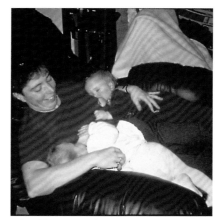

Fig. 303   Reclining along the side, 13 months

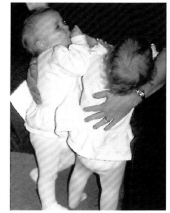

Fig. 304   Twins standing, 13 months old

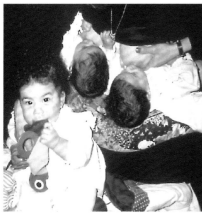

Fig. 305   Triplets, 8 months old

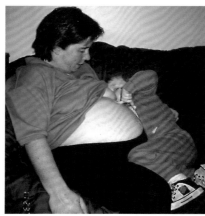

Fig. 306   Breastfeeding during pregnancy

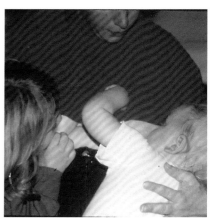

Fig. 307   Tandem breastfeeding 4 year-old and 16 month-old

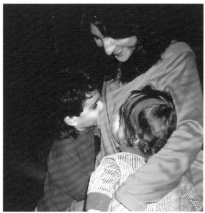

Fig. 308   Tandem feeding 4 year-old and 19 month-old

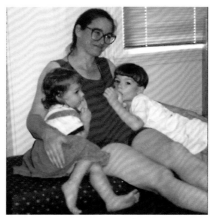

Fig. 309   Tandem feeding 4 year-old and 2 year-old

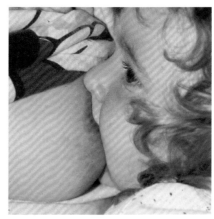

Fig. 310   Breastfeeding 3 year-old

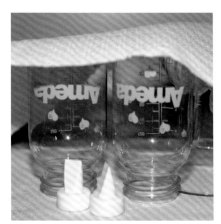

Fig. 311   Air dry and cover pump parts in the hospital

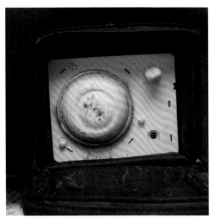

Fig. 312   Black mold growing on internal pump parts

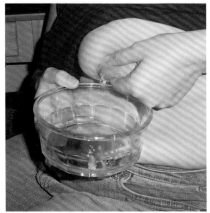

Fig. 313   Hand expression is an important skill

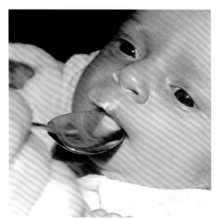

Fig. 314   0.6 ml of colostrum delivered with a spoon

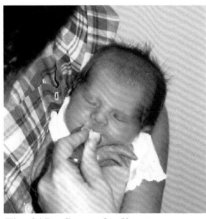

Fig. 315   Spoon feeding to rouse sleepy baby

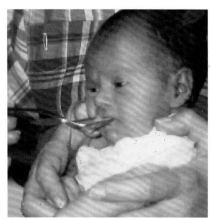

Fig. 316   Spoon feeding has roused baby

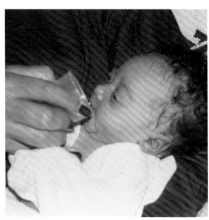

Fig. 317   Cup feeding

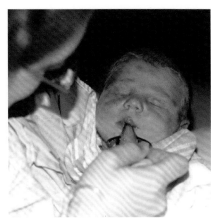

Fig. 318   Feeding with a paladai

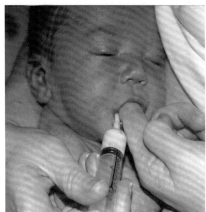

Fig. 319   Finger feeding with 12 cc Monoject™ curved-tip syringe

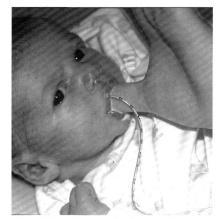

Fig. 320   Finger feeding with a feeding tube along the thumb

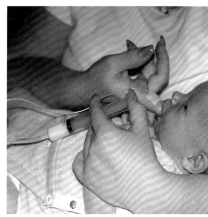

Fig. 321   Finger feeding with feeding tube on 12 cc syringe

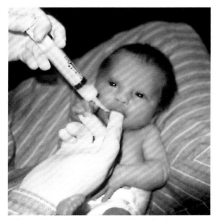

Fig. 322   Finger feeding infant is failing to thrive

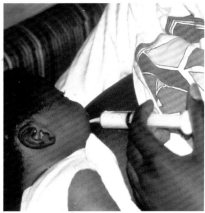

Fig. 323   Syringe feeding at breast

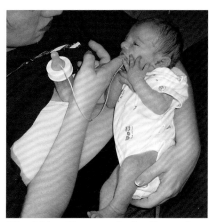

Fig. 324   Homemade feeding tube device

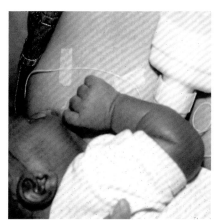

Fig. 325   Adopted infant at breast with SNS ™ supplementer

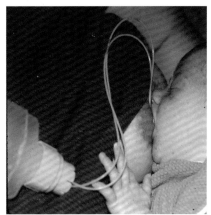

Fig. 326   Using 2 tubes on the same breast to increase flow rate

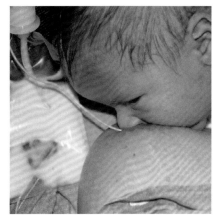

Fig. 327   Lact-Aid™ supplementer

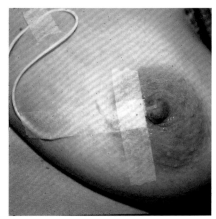

Fig. 328   Reverse positioning of feeding tube

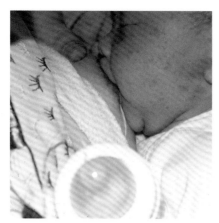

Fig. 329 Reverse positioning of tube with lower lip & tongue contact

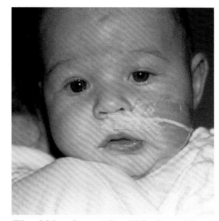

Fig. 330 3 month-old baby with nasogastric tube

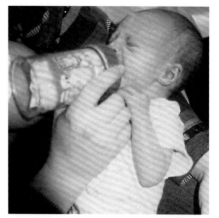

Fig. 331 Stress cue while bottle feeding

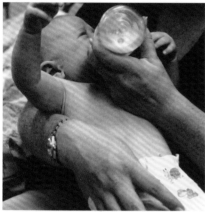

Fig. 332 Stress cue while bottle feeding

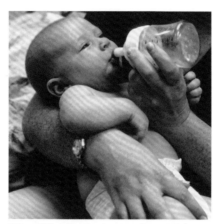

Fig. 333 Less stress when pacing techniques are used

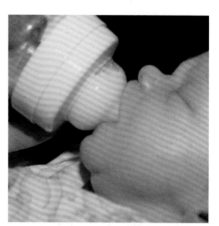

Fig. 334 Stress cue while bottle feeding preterm twin

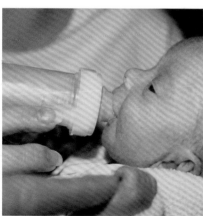

Fig. 335 Holding the bottle horizontally to slow the flow rate

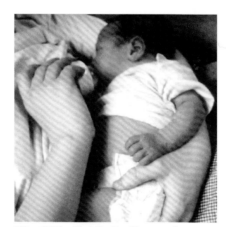

Fig. 336 Bottle feeding at the breast

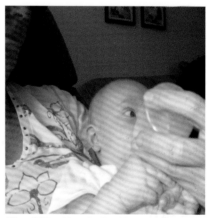

Fig. 337 Bottle feeding facing away from feeder's body

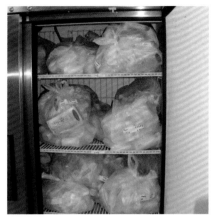

Fig. 338   Raw milk in the freezer

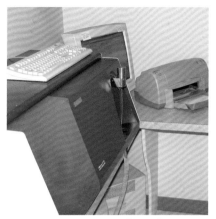

Fig. 339   Foss MilkoScan for nutritional analysis

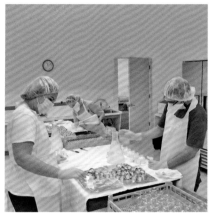

Fig. 340   Pasteurizing human milk

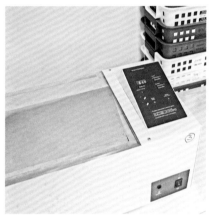

Fig. 341   Holder pasteurizer

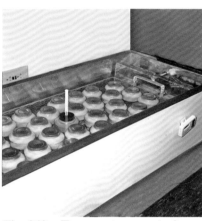

Fig. 342   Temperature control during Holder process

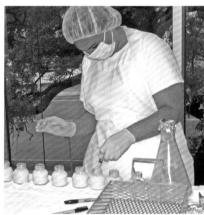

Fig. 343   Bacteriologic sampling after pasteurization

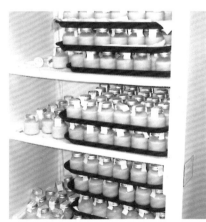

Fig. 344   Frozen pasteurized milk awaiting bacteriological results

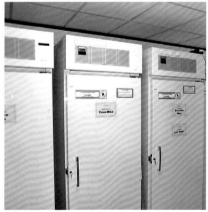

Fig. 345   Bank of freezers at a milk bank - milk is ready to dispense

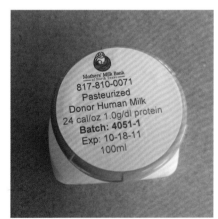

Fig. 346   High Calorie Donor Milk

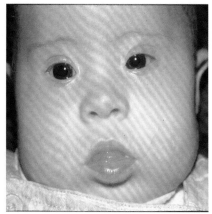

Fig. 347   Infant with Down Syndrome -- 4 mo old

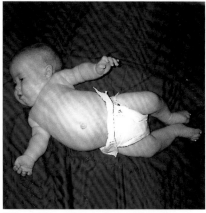

Fig. 348   "Pear-shaped" body

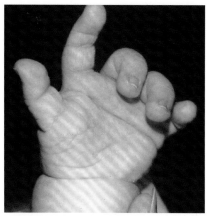

Fig. 349   Palmar crease

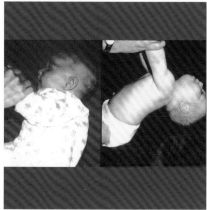

Fig. 350   Normal tone/ head lag in infant with Down Syndrome

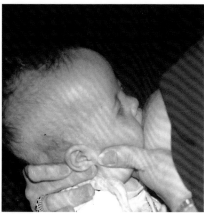

Fig. 351   Dancer hand position stabilizes feeding

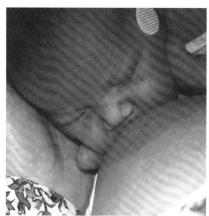

Fig. 352   Cheek counter-pressure reduces intra-oral space

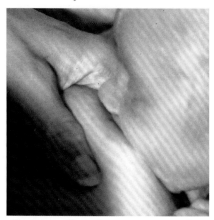

Fig. 353   Deep breast compression

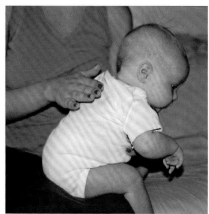

Fig. 354   Avoid increasing abdominal pressure in infants with reflux

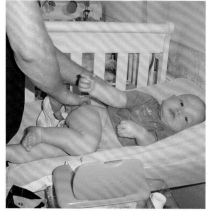

Fig. 355   Diaper on the side to decrease abdominal pressure

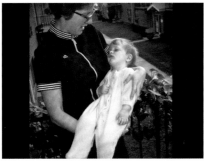

Fig. 356   Hypotonia as a marker for illness

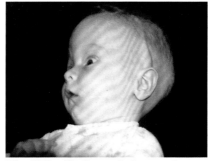

Fig. 357   Hydrocephalus -- shunt to drain cerebrospinal fluid

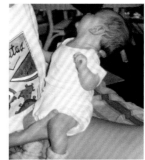

Fig. 358   Hypertonia -- arching causes hyperextension

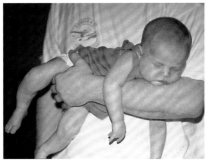

Fig. 359   "Colic hold" helps draw baby into flexion

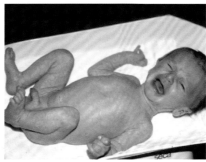

Fig. 360   FTT -- 35 day-old only 142 g above birthweight

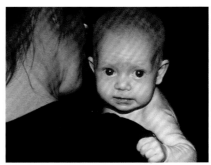

Fig. 361   FTT- 75 days old 60 g below birth weight

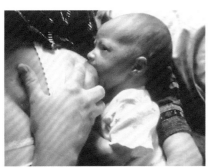

Fig. 362   FTT -- note retracted lips, worried expression

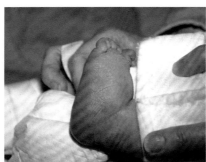

Fig. 363   Infant with Turner's Syndrome -- unusually shaped foot

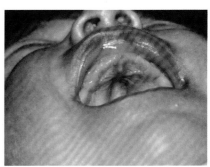

Fig. 364   Naturally occurring grooved (channel) palate

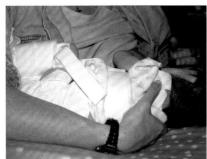

Fig. 365   Cross-cradle positioning with hip cast for hip dysplasia

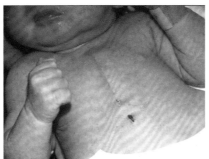

Fig. 366   Heart surgery scar 14 day-old infant

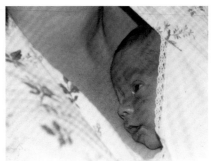

Fig. 367   Skin-to-Skin (Kangaroo) Care benefits preterm infants

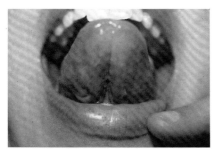

Fig. 368 Normal range of motion -- tongue lift

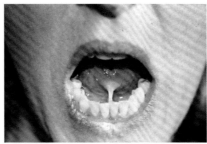

Fig. 369 Tongue-tied adult attempting to lift tongue

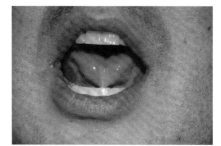

Fig. 370 Tongue-tied father of tongue-tied infant

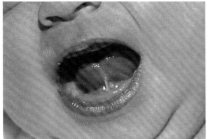

Fig. 371 Heart-shaped tongue tip

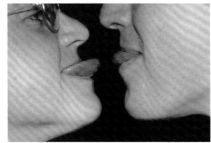

Fig. 372 Variability of tongue length -- short tongue on the right

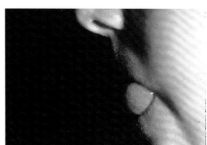

Fig. 373 Tongue-tied 12 year-old -- limited extension

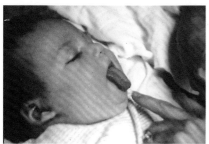

Fig. 374 Tongue extension -- long tongue

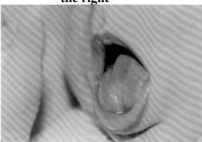

Fig. 375 Tongue-tie -- distortion during extension

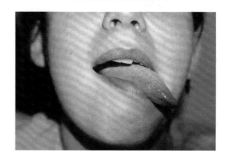

Fig. 376 Normal lateralization

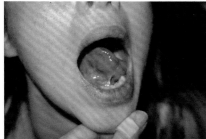

Fig. 377 Limited ability to lateralize

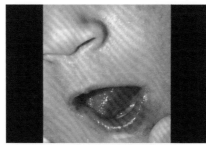

Fig. 378 Observe lateralization in infants

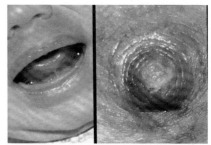

Fig. 379 Tongue-tie and damage to mother's nipple

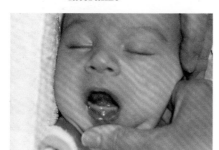

Fig. 380 The infant's tongue lifts to the upper gum ridge

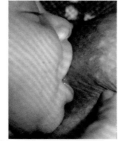

Fig. 381 Normal tongue cups and extends beyond gum ridge

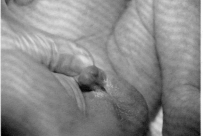

Fig. 382 Hypospadius -- another mid-line defect

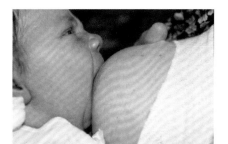

Fig. 383   Case study of FTT infant
with tongue-tie -- no latch

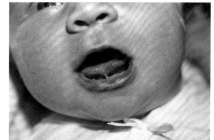

Fig. 384   Her tight lingual
frenulum

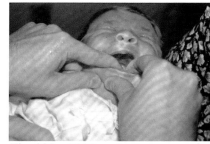

Fig. 385   ENT evaluates range of
motion of her tongue

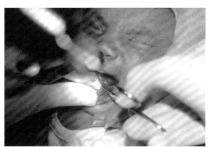

Fig. 386   Clipping the frenulum

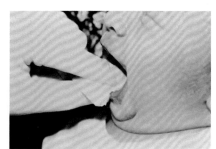

Fig. 387   Brief pressure with gauze
pad after frenotomy

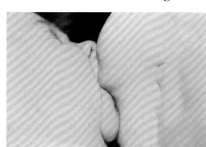

Fig. 388   Breastfeeding 10 minutes
after frenotomy

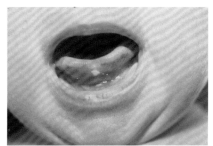

Fig. 389   Frenotomy site 1 week
later

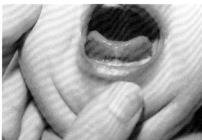

Fig. 390   Tongue healed at 2 weeks

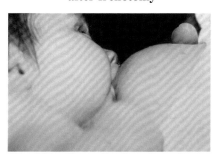

Fig. 391   Breastfeeding 3 weeks
after frenotomy

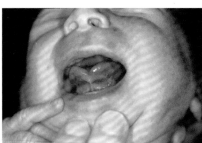

Fig. 392   Evaluate function not
appearance -- baby fed
well

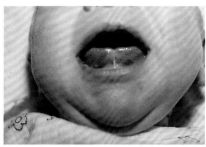

Fig. 393   Case study -- infant with
tongue-tie

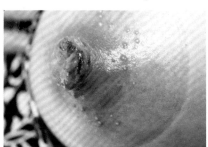

Fig. 394   Her mother's damaged,
infected nipple

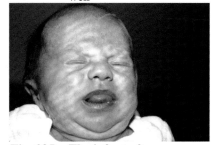

Fig. 395   The infant after
frenotomy

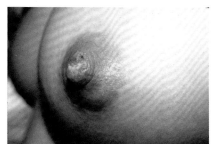

Fig. 396   Her mother's healing
nipple

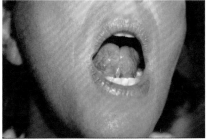

Fig. 397   Tongue-tied adult shown
in Fig. 369 after frenotomy

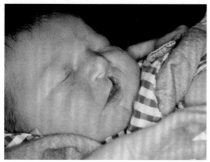

Fig. 398   Cleft lip

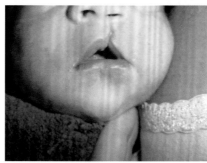

Fig. 399   Cleft lip

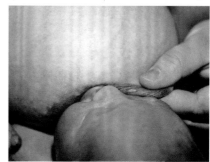

Fig. 400   "Teacup hold" to plug the gap and help form a seal

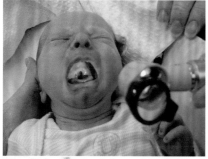

Fig. 401   Cleft of the soft palate

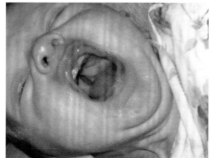

Fig. 402   Cleft of the soft palate

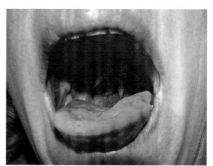

Fig. 403   Bifid uvula in adult female

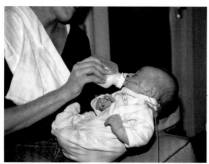

Fig. 404   Flexed at the hips to prevent hyperextension

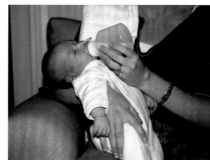

Fig. 405   Aversive feeding behavior

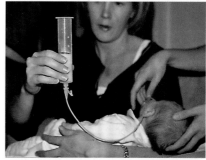

Fig. 406   Nasogastric tube-feeding to protect growth

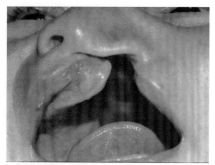

Fig. 407   Complete cleft of the lip and palate

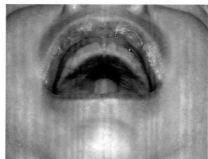

Fig. 408   Grooved (channel) palate

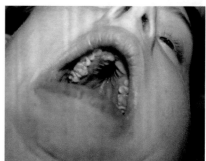

Fig. 409   Grooved palate in 12 year-old with Down Syndrome

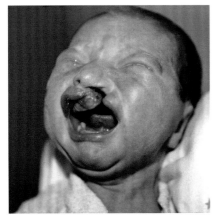

Fig. 410   Complete cleft of the lip
            and palate -- A case study

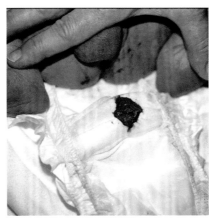

Fig. 411   Scant, dark stools on
            Day 4

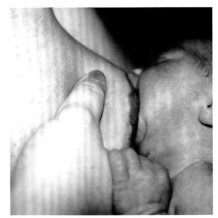

Fig. 412   Upright feeding position
            and breast compression

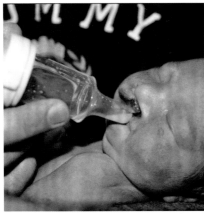

Fig. 413   Feeding colostrum with
            a Special Needs® Feeder

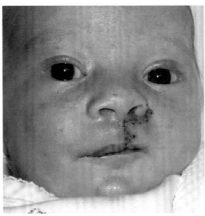

Fig. 414   After early repair of the
            cleft lip (courtesy K. Bird)

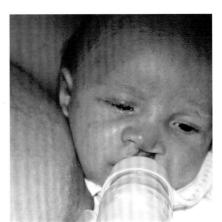

Fig. 415   Bottle-feeding at breast
            with the Pigeon® Feeder

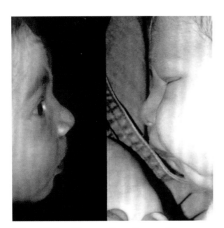

Fig. 416   Normal and receding
            chins

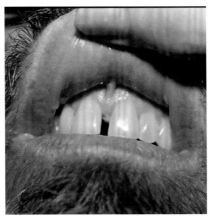

Fig. 417   Tight labial frenum --
            affects tooth spacing

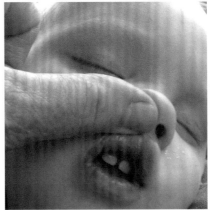

Fig. 418   Tight labial frenum --
            affects tooth spacing

Index

209